Surgical Diagnosis and Management

A GUIDE TO

GENERAL SURGICAL CARE

David C. Dunn MB, MChir, FRCS
Consultant Surgeon, Addenbrooke's Hospital;
Associate Lecturer and Director of Surgical Studies,
University of Cambridge School of Clinical Medicine;
Penrose May Teacher, Royal College of Surgeons, England;
Formerly Director of Medical Studies,
St John's College, Cambridge

Nigel Rawlinson MB, BChir, FRCS
Registrar, Department of Neurosurgery,
Frenchay Hospital, Bristol;
Formerly Anatomy Demonstrator,
Department of Anatomy,
University of Cambridge

SECOND EDITION

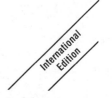

b

Blackwell
Science

International Edition

To Anne and Pat plus six

© 1985, 1991 by
Blackwell Science Ltd
Editorial Offices:
Osney Mead, Oxford OX2 0EL
25 John Street, London WC1N 2BL
23 Ainslie Place, Edinburgh EH3 6AJ
238 Main Street, Cambridge
  Massachusetts 02142, USA
54 University Street, Carlton
  Victoria 3053, Australia

Other Editorial Offices:
Arnette Blackwell SA
224, Boulevard Saint Germain
75007 Paris, France

Blackwell Wissenschafts-Verlag GmbH
Kurfürstendamm 57
10707 Berlin, Germany

Zehetnergasse 6
A-1140 Wien
Austria

First published 1985
Reprinted 1989
Second edition 1991
Reprinted 1992, 1993, 1994, 1995, 1996
Four Dragons edition 1991
Reprinted 1992, 1994, 1996

Set by Setrite Typesetters, Hong Kong
Printed and bound in Great Britain
at the University Press, Cambridge

DISTRIBUTORS

Marston Book Services Ltd
PO Box 269
Abingdon
Oxon OX14 4YN
(*Orders*: Tel: 01235 465500
    Fax: 01235 465555)

USA
Blackwell Science, Inc.
238 Main Street
Cambridge, MA 02142
(*Orders*: Tel: 800 215-1000
    617 876-7000
    Fax: 617 492-5263)
Canada
Copp Clark, Ltd
2775 Matheson Blvd East
Mississauga, Ontario
Canada, L4W 4P7
(*Orders*: Tel: 800 263-4374
    905 238-6074)
Australia
Blackwell Science Pty Ltd
54 University Street
Carlton, Victoria 3053
(*Orders*: Tel: 03 9347 0300
    Fax: 03 9349 3016)

British Library
Cataloguing in Publication Data
Dunn, David C.
  Surgical diagnosis and management.
  2nd ed.
  1. Medicine. Surgery. Diagnosis
  I. Title   II. Rawlinson, Nigel
  617.075

  ISBN 0–632–02782–7 (BSL)
       0–632–03081–X
  (International Edition)

Contents

Preface to the Second Edition, v

Preface to the First Edition, vi

Acknowledgements, viii

The Layout of this Book, ix

1 The Daily Management of Patients in Surgical Wards, 1
  1.1 Admitting the surgical patient, 3
  1.2 Preparing for the operation, 11
  1.3 The management of patients with pre-existing medical diseases, 16
  1.4 The operation and afterwards, 33
  1.5 Postoperative complications: presenting symptoms, 36
  1.6 Gastrointestinal and respiratory complications, 45
  1.7 Cardiovascular complications, 51
  1.8 Urinary complications, 63
  1.9 Infections, abscesses and fistulae, 68
  1.10 The intensive care unit, 80

2 Prescriptions and Other Tasks, 83
  2.1 Management of intravenous fluids, 85
  2.2 Prescribing drugs for surgical patients, 98
  2.3 Sutures and drains, 112
  2.4 Relatives, discharges, deaths and documents, 122

3 The Head and Neck, 133
  3.1 Lumps in the head and neck, 135
  3.2 Cervical lymphadenopathy, 151
  3.3 Lumps in the thyroid gland and goitres, 157
  3.4 Parathyroids, 173
  3.5 Conditions of the mouth, 178
  3.6 Conditions of the tongue, 189

4 The Breast, 197
  4.1 Assessment of breast lumps and benign disease, 199
  4.2 Carcinoma of the breast, 212
  4.3 Other breast presentations, 222
  4.4 Conditions of the male breast, 226

5 The Chest, 229
  5.1 Chest drainage and thoracotomy, 231
  5.2 Dysphagia, 238

6 Abdominal Pain and Related Symptoms, 259
6.1 Stomach and duodenum, 261
6.2 Liver, pancreas and spleen, 288
6.3 Adrenal glands, 328
6.4 Central abdominal pain, 334
6.5 Colorectal presentations and skeletal pain, 346

7 Perineum and Groins, 373
7.1 Perianal pain, 375
7.2 Lumps in the groin and other hernias, 388

8 Urinary Tract, 405
8.1 Disorders of the kidney, 407
8.2 Conditions of the bladder and urethra, 421
8.3 Male genitalia, 446

9 Vascular Disease, 469
9.1 Chronic ischaemia of the leg, 471
9.2 Management of the ischaemic limb, 478
9.3 Aneurysms, emboli and arterio-venous fistulae, 489
9.4 Other arterial conditions, 498
9.5 Venous disorders, 503
9.6 Lymphoedema, 510

10 The Skin, 513
10.1 Benign lesions of the skin, 515
10.2 Pigmented naevi and malignant skin conditions, 525
10.3 Skin infections and hyperhidrosis, 533

11 Conditions of Children, 543
11.1 Surgical conditions of children, 545
11.2 Congenital obstruction of the gut, 555

12 Trauma, 567
12.1 Dealing with a major accident, 569
12.2 Head injuries, 573
12.3 Chest and abdominal injury, 585
12.4 Spinal and pelvic injuries, 600
12.5 Trauma to the skin and limbs, 606

List of Surgical Procedures, 620

Index, 623

Preface to the Second Edition

The format and layout used in the First Edition have proved popular and have been maintained. The text has been revised and updated throughout and new sections have been included on acquired immune deficiency syndrome, liver surgery, liver and kidney transplantation, lymphoedema, mesenteric adenitis and the management of patients on anticoagulants. The sections on carcinoma of the breast, splenectomy, urology, diabetes and head injuries have been extensively revised. The section on intravenous fluid management has been modified to take account of the modern practice of using litre bags rather than half-litre bags of fluid. The section on postoperative complications has been compressed and unified. Other modifications reflect the modern increasing desire to avoid blood transfusion where possible. The rest of the text has stood the passage of time remarkably well, although it has all been subjected to careful scrutiny in the light of modern practice.

David C. Dunn
Nigel Rawlinson

Preface to the First Edition

The stimulus to the production of this book has been the repeated demands of our medical students and housemen for a concise practical text which lists the methods of diagnosis and management of the main general surgical conditions they will have to deal with. It has been derived from a popular series of seminars in surgery given in Cambridge.

The combination of authors is unusual. One (D.C.D.) has been a consultant since 1974 and the other (N.R.) was his houseman when the work started. We hope that this combination has helped us to concentrate on a layout which answers the needs of the houseman and medical student, needs which have often become obscure to senior doctors. Most surgical texts, for instance, fail to deal with questions which regularly confront the houseman, such as how much blood should be cross-matched for an operation, and how long patients will be in hospital and off work.

The book is designed to be easy to use for rapid reference and a similar layout is used for each subject, with headings suggested by the questions our students ask, such as:
What is that condition?
What makes you think that the diagnosis is likely?
How will you prove whether you are right or not?
What is the management, before, during, and after the operation?
What do I tell the patient when I'm obtaining his consent?

The headings are explained on pp. ix and x, as are the 'Codes' given for each operative procedure.

We have tried hard to make sure that the facts in the book are as accurate as possible and are grateful to our many colleagues who have checked the text. Inevitably, however, some errors may have crept in and we hope that our readers will write to us about these so that they may be corrected later.

The housesurgeon and patient have generally been described as 'he' in this book, a choice which is merely convenient and one which we hope will not upset our many excellent female junior staff.

Both authors have found the exercise of cooperating on this book to be interesting and illuminating. We hope our readers will also benefit from what we have produced.

David C. Dunn
Nigel Rawlinson

Acknowledgements

We are again grateful to many students, housemen and housewomen at Addenbrooke's and Bristol who have helped us review the text. We are also particularly indebted to several sub-editors who have reviewed and revised sections of the book. These include Mr T. Chen (Urology), Mr Peter Friend (Hepatic Surgery), Mr. Laitung (Burns), Dr M. Lindop (Anaesthesia, Postoperative Management, Intensive Care), Dr Robert Marcus (Haematology), Mr S. Tsui (Trauma), Dr R. Warren (Infections and Antibiotics), Mr F. Wells (Chest Surgery and Oesophagus), Dr T.K. Wheeler (Cancer of the Breast), Dr F.M. Rawlinson, Dr J.A. Emmerson and Dr L.D. Wijesinghe. Once again we owe a great debt to our wives and families, who have put up with all the extra work which has been needed to produce this new edition. Finally Mrs Ros Britton has cheerfully incorporated innumerable edits, corrections and recorrections in the text and brought the whole project to fruition. Without her cheerful skill and help, this edition would never have been completed.

D.C.D
N.R

The Layout of this Book

The first two chapters deal with the routine of patient management before and after any operation. In the subsequent chapters individual surgical conditions and their management are described. Each is presented under the following headings.

The condition

This section gives a brief descriptive outline of the disorder being dealt with.

Recognizing the pattern

When an experienced clinician is faced with a patient complaining of a symptom, he makes a diagnosis by taking an accurate history and by a careful examination. As he does this, however, he is constantly comparing the findings in the patient with a 'typical' picture he associates with various disease states. When he recognizes one of several familiar patterns of symptoms, he will ask subsidiary questions to strengthen or weaken his developing hypothesis as to the cause of the symptom. This process depends on a background knowledge of the typical pattern of each disease. In this section such typical patterns are presented.

Proving the diagnosis

The usual investigations necessary to prove the diagnosis are given.

Management

The general management of each condition is discussed and, because this is a surgical textbook, this will usually involve an operative procedure. A brief description of the preoperative preparation is given, followed by a short account of the operation itself. In most cases the latter is general, rather than very detailed. In a few cases, however, where it is considered that a junior doctor might be called upon to do the procedure himself, more details are included.

Codes

The 'Codes' given at the end of each operative procedure are an attempt to provide the houseman with some guidelines for answering those questions which frequently arise at the time of any operation. Notes on their use are given below and should be read before drawing any conclusions.

We are sensitive to the fact that these figures may prove controversial and there is considerable variation between the practices of individual consultants. Where the junior doctor finds that the figures for his unit are markedly different, we suggest that he alters them in the text for his own future reference.

The figures do not represent the *personal* experience of the senior author (DCD) but are the sort of statistics he would give to a patient asking for them, regardless of which surgeon was operating. We hope that other surgeons will be tolerant if they feel they are an inaccurate representation of their own experience.

Notes on the use of 'codes'

Please read this carefully before drawing any conclusions from the figures given for each operation.

Blood. Refers to the amount of blood it is advisable to have available for the operation. It does not represent the amount usually lost.

GA/LA. GA, general anaesthetic; LA, spinal or local infiltration anaesthetic.

Opn time. Refers to the amount of time that might be allowed for this operation during an operating list. The actual time taken varies very widely according to the pathology encountered and the individual surgeon's operative technique.

Stay. Refers to the approximate time a patient can be told to expect to be in hospital. The length of stay will be prolonged if there are complications. It also varies with individual surgeons and hospitals and with the pressure on available beds.

Drains out and sutures out. Different surgeons vary widely in their practices but the figures given are thought to be reasonable to the authors and may help when no other information is available. Further general information is given in Section 2.3.

Off work. The figure for this is necessarily very approximate. Nevertheless, such information is usually difficult to find so an attempt has been made to provide it. It must be emphasized that the figure given is only an estimate suitable to give the patient as a prediction. It should not be used in any legal arguments about whether or not a particular patient should be back at work.

1 The Daily Management of Patients in Surgical Wards

1.1 **Admitting the surgical patient**
Introduction
Managing people who need operations
Admitting the patient
Some common pitfalls in surgical management

1.2 **Preparing for the operation**
Preoperative management
Organizing the operating list

1.3 **The management of patients with pre-existing medical diseases**
Respiratory disease
Asthma
Cardiovascular disease
Diabetes
Patients on steroid drugs
Patients on anti-coagulants
Haemophilia
Other bleeding disorders and prothrombotic states
AIDS
Hepatitis B

1.4 **The operation and afterwards**
The housesurgeon in theatre
The immediate postoperative period
The daily postoperative ward round

1.5 **Postoperative complications: presenting symptoms**
Postoperative pyrexia
Postoperative pain
Discharging wound
Nausea and vomiting
Constipation
Breathlessness
Confusion
Collapse
Oliguria/anuria

1.6   Gastrointestinal and respiratory complications
Paralytic ileus
Acute dilatation of the stomach
Pulmonary collapse and bronchopneumonia
Inhalation of vomit
Pneumothorax

1.7   Cardiovascular complications
Haemorrhage
Blood transfusion reactions
Myocardial infarction
Left ventricular failure
Stroke
Deep venous thrombosis
Pulmonary embolus

1.8   Urinary complications
Urinary tract infection
Postoperative retention of urine
Postoperative renal failure
Urinary fistula

1.9   Infections, abscesses and fistulae
Wound infection
Wound dehiscence
Infected intravenous drip site
Subphrenic abscess
Hepatic abscess
Pelvic abscess
External intestinal fistula
Bed sores
Septicaemia

1.10 The intensive care unit
The houseman's role in the intensive care unit (ICU)
The ICU chart
Daily management of patients on ICU

1.1 Admitting the Surgical Patient

Introduction

The first two chapters of this book deal with the daily tasks a surgical houseman has to perform. They should be useful to those who are starting a surgical housejob. They will also help medical students to understand what is going on in a surgical ward and to prepare themselves for the task of being a surgical houseman after qualification. In the subsequent chapters the diagnosis and management of individual general surgical conditions are dealt with, the layout being as described in the preface.

Managing people who need operations

Both medical teachers and laymen tend to assume that every young doctor regards the human body as a collection of mechanical tubes and pipes and overlooks the importance of the 'individual'. It has been our experience, however, that most doctors find their work fascinating simply because they are dealing with a human body enclosing a mind and a spirit as well as a complex, delicate, biological system.

The management of patients in surgery is dominated by this difference between the mechanical and the human, the difference between a technician and a surgeon. To obtain good results in surgery the mechanics must, of course, be correct. The anastomosis must not leak, the electrolytes must be kept in the correct range. Over and above this, however, the patient has to believe in his management and obtain confidence from his medical helper. Efforts spent on developing a trusting, friendly and honest relationship can pay huge dividends during the patient's illness. Every practising doctor knows this and has experience of patients surviving by their own will or dying because they have given up. Maintaining the patient's morale can be just as important as maintaining his blood pressure.

During this book we have not dwelt too much on this important and overriding principle in medicine, mainly because the relationship of one human being with another cannot be satisfactorily dealt with in a book of this type. It is, however, of supreme importance, and the ability to develop good relationships with patients will transform the knowledgeable bad doctor into the excellent and successful practitioner whom most medical students aspire to be.

The houseman plays a central role in the organization of a surgical firm. While the more senior members of the firm have to split their time between the ward, the outpatient department and theatre, the houseman's main priority is the ward. He or she is the link between the patient, the surgical staff, the nurses and the paramedical staff and must co-ordinate all aspects of patient care.

The daily ward work

The routine ward work can be split into five parts.
1 Admitting the patient.
2 Preoperative management.
3 Organizing the operating list.
4 The housesurgeon in theatre.
5 The daily postoperative ward round.

Admitting the patient

Make sure that you have seen the outpatient notes and the consultant's letter before you start the routine clerking. Check that any X-rays, scans or investigations taken previously are available on the ward. Note which diagnosis the patient has been labelled with, but make your assessment critically and avoid blindly following a predetermined diagnostic pathway. By keeping an open mind you will be able to spot things which have been missed in the often hurried outpatient assessment.

A full routine clerking is then carried out on all patients. Some points require special attention when an operation is being planned and these are listed below.

Detecting future problems

History
You are looking for any indication that the patient may not be fit for surgery or may be liable to develop problems postoperatively. Particular points are listed below.

Systems

1 Chest
Look for the following.
● Pre-existing chest disease.
● Shortness of breath on minor exertion or at rest.
● Cough, and is it productive?
● A history of asthma.
● Smoking habit.

2 Cardiovascular system

Is there a history of the following?

- Chest pain or angina.
- Symptoms of cardiac failure (such as oedema, nocturnal dyspnoea, orthopnoea or palpitations).

3 Alimentary system

Ask about the following.

- Anorexia and weight loss. This may indicate poor nutrition resulting in slow healing. In such patients check the serum proteins. The operation may need to be delayed until a protein deficit has been restored (see p. 96).
- Bowel habit. Any patient prone to constipation who will be restricted to bed may well require suppositories to keep the bowels moving.
- Heartburn and reflux. A patient with reflux may aspirate under anaesthesia and the anaesthetist should be warned.

4 Micturition

Check whether there is a history of difficulty of micturition or dysuria. These may give a clue to potential postoperative urinary retention or infection. After the operation the detection of a distended bladder may be difficult if there is a lower abdominal incision.

5 Periods

Heavy periods are a common cause of anaemia in women.

6 Locomotor system

Does the patient suffer from arthritis? Are there any particularly stiff joints? Intubation may be difficult in the presence of cervical joint disease. It may be difficult or impossible to put patients in the lithotomy position on the table when they have stiff hips, knees or back.

Past history

Find out about the following.

- Previous operations, and whether they were followed by any complications such as deep venous thrombosis or infection.
- Previous anaesthetics. Were there any problems such as drug reaction, excessive vomiting, scoline sensitivity or malignant hyperpyrexia?
- Previous history of rheumatic or scarlet fever which may have damaged the heart valves. With such a history you must examine the heart carefully. Prophylactic antibiotics may be needed for a significant valvular lesion.

● Previous history of jaundice. You might have to test the scrum for Australia antigen.

Medical conditions
Does the patient suffer from any other diseases which will influence your management? These are dealt with in Section 1.3 and include diabetes, heart disease and chest disease.

Drug history
Many drugs interfere with the action of routine anaesthetic agents and others such as diuretics may lead to preoperative electrolyte disturbances.

Check whether the patient is on the contraceptive pill. There is a theoretical danger of postoperative venous thrombosis in patients on oestrogen therapy and many surgeons will not do routine operations unless the patient has been taken off the 'pill' for 4−6 weeks before admission. This is usually arranged when the patient is seen in clinic. Others will give prophylactic anti-coagulation therapy in these circumstances.

Allergies
Ask about allergies to:
anaesthetics,
antibiotics,
applications (e.g. iodine or elastoplast).
Check whether the allergy is genuine by determining what sort of reaction the patient had when he was exposed to the agent. Many patients say they are allergic to antibiotics because they felt ill at the time, due to the infection which was being treated. Where there is any possibility of allergy, however, the patient's record should be marked and that drug avoided.

Family history
Is there any family history of reaction to anaesthetic? Some problems such as scoline apnoea can be inherited. Any patient who has a relative who developed problems under anaesthesia is going to be anxious. Discovering this and reassuring him may make management easier.

Also ask about any history of malignant hyperpyrexia, bleeding disorders or porphyria in the family.

Social history
Important points are as follows.
● The patient's job. What exactly does this involve? This will determine when the patient can go back to work.

Patients can return to light office work earlier than they can to heavy manual work.

- Home facilities. Find out about the layout of the toilet and bathroom in the patient's house. This will give you an idea of how difficult it will be for him to manage once he leaves hospital.
- Support. What sort of support is available from the family or friends postoperatively?
- Habits. Check how much the patient drinks and smokes. A heavy drinker will be resistant to the normal doses of anaesthetic agents. A heavy smoker will be very liable to develop a chest infection postoperatively, and preoperative physiotherapy may be indicated to minimize this risk.

The examination

Always try to improve on the findings made during the rapid outpatient assessment. Finding a supraclavicular lymph node, for instance, may save a patient with cancer from an unnecessary abdominal operation.

Details in the general examination which may be important are as follows.

General condition

Look for signs of dehydration, anaemia or cachexia. These may require correction before the operation is undertaken.

Mental state

Any patient will be anxious about the operation and in some this anxiety is extreme. Careful explanation and reassurance is required. A mild hypnotic or tranquillizer given on the night before the operation is often helpful.

Cardiovascular system

Look for cardiac irregularities, hypertension and cardiac failure. If the blood pressure is high on the first examination come back and measure it again. If it is still high, put the patient on a 4-hourly blood pressure chart. High blood pressures often settle once the patient gets used to his new environment. If it remains high the anaesthetist must be informed.

Chest

Assess the shape of the chest looking for signs of emphysema. Check that there are no signs of pleural fluid, lung consolidation or bronchospasm.

Abdomen

The presence of abdominal scars provides a useful check on the patient's history. They may also indicate that a routine operation will be more difficult than usual and require more operative time because of adhesions.

All patients should have a rectal examination before abdominal surgery. Make a note of the amount and hardness of the faeces. Constipation should be relieved before the operation is undertaken. In males note the size of the lobes of the prostate. This information will be of value if the patient develops urinary problems postoperatively. Once in retention, the size of the prostate is much more difficult to assess.

Joints and teeth

Examine the teeth. Note if they are false and identify any crowned or loose teeth that will require care during intubation.

Is there any limitation in the movement of the mandible or in the neck? Both of these may affect the ease and speed of intubation.

A more detailed consideration of medical diseases present before surgery is given in Section 1.3.

Investigations

Five investigations should always be considered before an operation, though not necessarily undertaken. These are as follows.

1 Haemoglobin

This is especially important in women who are menstruating and in elderly patients. Look for both polycythaemia and anaemia.

2 Urea and electrolytes

These should be estimated:
(a) if the history suggests fluid or electrolyte disturbance;
(b) if the patient is on diuretics;
(c) in the presence of cardiac arrhythmia;
(d) if there will be prolonged postoperative intravenous infusion;
(e) if he is to be treated with drugs excreted by the kidney which are potentially toxic (e.g. gentamicin).

3 Liver function tests

The serum albumin gives a good indication of the state of nutrition of the patient and should be undertaken where this is in doubt. Other liver function tests may form part of the work-up for general liver disease such as hepatic metastases or cirrhosis.

4 Chest X-ray
A chest X-ray should be performed in patients:
(a) with acute respiratory symptoms;
(b) with suspected or established cardio-respiratory disease who have not had a chest X-ray in the previous 12 months;
(c) with suspected or established malignancy and possible metastases;
(d) who are recent immigrants from countries where tuberculosis (TB) is endemic and who have not had a chest X-ray in the previous 12 months;
(e) in whom tracheal obstruction may be present.

5 Electrocardiogram (ECG)
The indications for this investigation are:
(a) evidence of cardiac failure;
(b) hypertension treated or untreated;
(c) an irregular pulse;
(d) history of angina, myocardial infarction or congenital heart disease;
(e) diabetes mellitus;
(f) men over 50, or women over 60 undergoing major surgery.

The extent of other investigations required depends on what is found during the history and examination and on which operation is intended.

Some common pitfalls in surgical management

Diagnosis
Avoid accepting the diagnosis with which the patient has been labelled. This is a common source of error. The mind tends to follow patterns of behaviour and once set off on the wrong track is very resistant to change. Never accept the general practitioner's (GP's) diagnosis or the outpatient diagnosis as proven, but try to work it out again for yourself.

In taking a history do not accept non-specific terms such as 'a cold', 'pneumonia' or 'cystitis'. Find out precisely what the patient means by these terms. Often you will find that they mean something quite different to the patient from what they mean to you. If you accept the patient's statement without question you may be led on the wrong diagnostic path. An example would be the patient who has had 'pneumonia'. You may accept this as an episode of inflammation and infection in the lungs but, by enquiring further, you may discern that the patient has an obstructed bronchus causing recurrent chest infections and the diagnosis is in fact carcinoma of the bronchus. Patients may say they have had an episode of 'pleurisy'. In fact they have had a pulmonary embolus and this must be taken into account in your future management.

Management

In postoperative management avoid prescribing antibiotics for a fever before you know what it is due to. When a patient is ill with a fever it is tempting to give antibiotics as soon as possible. However, if the fever is due to pus formation, the antibiotics will dampen it down and improve the symptoms but the abscess remains, and the symptoms will recur as soon as the antibiotics are stopped. By giving antibiotics you are simply prolonging the recovery period. Similarly, antibiotics given for a chest infection may produce symptomatic relief for a while, but unless the obstructing plug of mucus is removed from a bronchus the patient will not recover and permanent lung damage may result.

Beware of the patient's previous drugs. In particular, diuretics are widely used in the elderly and these patients may frequently have pre-existing electrolyte imbalances, which can lead to a fatality unless corrected before an anaesthetic.

1.2 Preparing for the Operation

Preoperative management

The following is a useful checklist to run through for each patient on the next day's operating schedule.

1 Identification

Check that the correct patient is having the correct operation on the correct side. Mark such things as hernias, lumps in the breast, varicose veins and small lumps and bumps, using a permanent skin marker.

2 The A's, B's and C's

A

Anaesthetist

The anaesthetist needs to be told a number of facts on the afternoon of the day before surgery.

1 A brief summary of the patient's general health, outlining any relevant problems, past medical history, drugs and examination findings.

2 The proposed surgery.

3 The position of the patient on the list.

4 When the patient last ate or drank (in emergency cases).

The anaesthetist also needs to be asked a number of questions.

1 If he will be writing up the premedication.

2 If he requires any further preparation.

3 If any extra monitoring needs to be arranged for theatre.

Antibiotics

Is cover required? See p. 107.

Anti-coagulation

Does the surgeon require the patient to have prophylactic anti-coagulation? Generally speaking this may be required in patients who have a previous history of thrombotic disease. For indications, see p. 56.

B

Blood

Is the haemoglobin available?

Biochemistry

Are the electrolytes available and within the normal range? A blood sugar series should be available in diabetics.

Bacteriology

Make sure the result of a culture swab is available on any patients who have preoperative sepsis.

Cross-match

Check that this has been arranged and that the blood will be ready on time (see individual operations).

Chest X-ray

If required.

Cardiogram

If required.

Consent

This is not simply a signature. Time must be spent explaining simply and concisely what the operation will involve. Use the opportunity to tell the patient something about what to expect in the postoperative period. Mention such things as drains and nasogastric tubes, explaining why they are needed. Tell him how long he will be in bed and unable to eat or drink, and how long he is likely to stay in hospital. This information is given in the relevant section later in the book.

3 Investigations

Make sure that the results of all the investigations that have been asked for preoperatively are available before the operation starts. These often contain some surprises that affect what should be done.

Organizing the operating list

Having admitted each individual patient, it is the house-surgeon's job to organize the operating list and to co-ordinate the various personnel in the departments involved.

The following headings summarize the main steps and may be used as a checklist. This should be done on the day before the operations are scheduled.

1 Surgeon

Be sure you know the following from him:
(a) all the patients on the list;
(b) what operations he intends to perform. Check you know the precise description and the most complicated

alternative procedure likely to be performed. Find out whether he will want any special instruments or preoperative investigations;

(c) the order of the list;

(d) what time he wants to start;

(e) in cases where you are uncertain, check with him whether or not blood is required.

2 Anaesthetist

Is he fully informed as on p. 11?

3 Assistant

One assistant of adequate experience should be available (some procedures will require more).

4 Theatre

All the information collected needs to be passed on to the theatre staff. This is done by providing an operating list (see Fig. 1). They need to know:

(a) the surgeon's name;

(b) the anaesthetist's name;

(c) the place and time at which the list will take place;

(d) the name and age of the patients (children require special instruments);

(e) the order of the list;

LIST OF OPERATIONS

DATE 24.12.91

SURGEON: Mr Cutfaster   ANAESTHETIST: Dr Snooze

TIME 8.30 a.m.

THEATRE 8

Number	Patient's Name	Number	Age	Ward	Operation
1	Andrew SMITH	54321	6 months	D2	LEFT inguinal hernia (baby)
2	Jane BLOGGS	68624	55	C8	Cholecystectomy and exploration of common bile duct. Operative cholangiogram.
3	Susan McARTHUR	72643	60	D8	Laparotomy for abdominal mass. ?RIGHT hemicolectomy ? oophorectomy.
4	Henry SMITH	629953	39	D8	RIGHT nephrectomy for hypernephroma ? Exploration of inferior vena cava.

Fig. 1. Specimen operating list.

N.B. When making up the list write clearly with no abbreviations. Always indicate the side of the operation in capital letters.

(f) the operation intended, and any alternatives thought likely;

(g) any special equipment needed, e.g. nerve stimulator in parotid surgery, staple gun for bowel anastomosis, monitoring equipment, etc.

5 Wards

A copy of this list is sent to all the wards involved.

6 Peroperative investigation

The relevant departments need to be informed of any special investigations that will be undertaken during an operation, e.g. histopathology for frozen section, radiology for operative cholangiogram.

7 Blood

Certain operations cannot be started unless compatible blood is available. Cross-matching is therefore one of the first things to organize once the list is known. For a routine transfusion during the week, 24 hours' notice should be given. The blood sample should arrive in the laboratory by late morning the day before the operation. Most haematology departments are unable to cross-match blood at weekends so blood required for Monday morning lists needs to be cross-matched on, or before, Friday. If necessary this may mean bringing the patient up specially. Blood may be cross-matched in special cases on the same day as the operation. This is done by arrangement with the laboratory and at least 2 hours must be allowed between the time the laboratory receives the sample and the time when the blood is required.

The whole policy of cross-matching blood for operations is at present under review. Patients who have previously had blood grouping and antibody screening performed can, in theory, have safe compatible blood provided rapidly without the need for traditional cross-match, provided that no 'atypical' antibodies have been found. This may reduce the need for blood to be held in theatre in case patients bleed, especially in low risk cases. If this system is introduced in your hospital it will be essential to make sure the patient is screened before he goes to theatre and that the laboratory is informed of the possible need for blood.

Blood is cross-matched in case haemorrhage occurs, rather than because it is expected to occur. Individual surgeons' preferences vary but, in general, blood should be cross-matched in the cases listed below.

1 Extensive procedures.

2 Operations in well-vascularized areas.

3 Operations on or adjacent to major blood vessels where rapid haemorrhage may be encountered.

A rough guide to the amount of blood many surgeons would wish to have available is set out in Table 1. Further details are given under each individual procedure.

Table 1. Quantities of blood that should be available for operations

Cholecystectomy Amputation — lower leg Thyroidectomy Parathyroid exploration Vagotomy	Group and save serum
Mastectomy Staging laparotomy Transurethral prostatectomy Nephrectomy	2 units
Gastrectomy Whipple's procedure Colectomy Anterior resection Vascular surgery distal to common iliac vessels	4 units
Abdomino-perineal resection Aortic surgery	6 units

1.3 The Management of Patients with Pre-existing Medical Diseases

It is important to identify any patients with an illness that could influence the postoperative course, and to do so in time to allow adequate treatment before the operation. The procedure may have to be delayed until the patient is made as fit as possible. The following medical conditions will be considered in this chapter.

1 Respiratory disease: acute and chronic.
2 Cardiovascular disease.
3 Diabetes.
4 Patients on steroids.
5 Haemophilia.
6 Patients with acquired immune deficiency syndrome (AIDS).

Respiratory disease

Acute

Coughs, colds, sore throats and acute infections are all contraindications to elective surgery. Recovery usually takes place very quickly, especially in children, and unless the operation is urgent it should be delayed until the patient is fit. This usually means a delay of 2−4 weeks. The final decision as to whether a patient is fit for anaesthetic is left to the anaesthetist.

Chronic

[margin note: made worse by immobility abdominal distension cough]

Any patient with chronic respiratory disease has an increased risk of developing problems after an operation. Factors adversely affecting the chest include immobility, abdominal distension, an inability to cough due to pain and suppression of the cough reflex by analgesics.

The risks are increased by certain factors.

[margin note: Divide — severity operation < site anaesthetic]

1 *The nature and extent of the disease.* Chronic airways obstruction is more of a problem than restrictive chest disease.
2 *The severity of the operation.* A prolonged anaesthetic or postoperative recovery enhances the risk of chest infection.
3 *The site of the operation.* Chest problems are more common after thoracic or abdominal operations, where coughing is very painful.
4 *Type of anaesthetic.* General anaesthetics cause more problems than local anaesthetics. The inhalation agent depresses

16

the function of the cilia in the bronchi and leads to the retention of secretions. Secretions are also more viscid following the use of atropine.

5 *Continued smoking.* The risks of surgery will be considerably increased if the patient continues to smoke until the operation.

The risk of chest infection can be decreased by good preoperative chest physiotherapy incorporating breathing and coughing exercises.

Assessment   Patients at risk should be recognized and the severity of their condition assessed.

Investigations

1 *Full blood count.* The haemoglobin may be elevated reflecting secondary polycythaemia due to chronic hypoxia. This indicates severe respiratory impairment. The white cell count is raised in an acute infective exacerbation.

2 *Microbiology.* It can be helpful to know the organisms in the patient's sputum and their antibiotic sensitivity.

3 *Blood gases.* Both hypoxia and hypercarbia in a blood gas sample reflect severe respiratory impairment.

4 *Chest X-ray.* Emphysema can be seen on a chest X-ray as a hyper-expanded chest with radiolucent lung fields and a depressed diaphragm. Any focus of infection will show up as an area of radio-opacity in the lung fields. The chest X-ray is also an important preoperative base-line investigation for comparison with later postoperative X-rays.

5 *Respiratory function tests.*

Vitalography

The vitalograph measures the rate at which a patient can exhale. The patient is instructed to take a full inspiration and then blow as hard and for as long as possible into the mouthpiece. The instrument plots the volume exhaled against time. From the best plot obtained one can determine the volume of air exhaled in the first second (FEV 1 = forced expiratory volume in 1 second) and the total volume exhaled (FVC = forced vital capacity). The peak expiratory flow rate (PEFR) is another simpler measurement and is related to the FEV 1. Normal values depend on age, weight, sex, etc., and nomograms are available.

Airways obstruction or volume restriction affects the shape of the graph in a characteristic way (see Fig. 2). A useful measure from the graph is the ratio of FEV 1 to FVC. (Normal value > 75%.)

Airways obstruction reduces the rate at which air can be

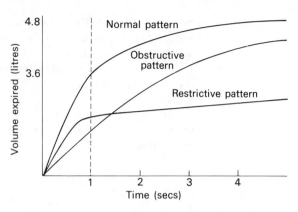

Fig. 2. The vitalograph plots the volume exhaled against time.

expelled more than the total volume. Thus the ratio of FEV 1 to FVC is less than 75%. If it is less than 50% significant obstruction is present and an attempt should be made to improve the situation before an anaesthetic. Previous vitalographs may also be useful for comparison.

Restrictive airways disease (e.g. fibrosing alveolitis). The vital capacity is decreased more than the FEV 1 and the ratio may therefore be above 75%.

Management

Preoperative management

1 Non-urgent surgery should be planned in the summer months when the patient's chest is at its best.

2 The patient should stop smoking. Ideally the patient should stop at least 1 month before surgery. The attempt to stop must, therefore, be made from the outpatient appointment. This is best achieved by putting the responsibility for the patient's postoperative health in his own hands. Explain that he is very likely to develop pneumonia after his anaesthetic if he continues smoking. Most patients understand this and try to do something about it.

3 Try to admit the patient 3 or 4 days before the operation for assessment and preoperative treatment. This consists of the following:

(a) *Physiotherapy.* This may be both active (breathing exercises and loosening of secretions) and passive (postural drainage).

(b) *Bronchodilators.* There is usually an element of reversible airways obstruction and bronchodilators are therefore used. Nebulized salbutamol (2 ml 0.5% solution 4-hourly by inspiration) is effective and simple to use. Aminophylline suppositories at night help nocturnal dyspnoea and bronchospasm.

(c) *Mucolytic agents*. These are of doubtful value, although steam inhalations can help.

(d) *Antibiotics*. Generally speaking these should be avoided preoperatively as they will result in the emergence of resistant strains of bacteria. Where an operation has to be carried out urgently in spite of an active chest infection, antibiotics will obviously be needed.

4 If the operation can be performed under a local an aesthetic, rather than a general, this may have advantages.

5 The operative time should be kept to a minimum.

Postoperative care

1 Encourage *early mobilization* as this will improve chest expansion and decrease ileus.

2 Continue *active physiotherapy*.

3 Good *analgesia* is important as it helps coughing. Sufficient should be given to make the coughing pain-free. Intercostal nerve blocks are very effective in patients with upper abdominal incisions. They improve chest expansion and aid coughing without depressing the cough reflex. With high-dependency nursing available, various epidural or intravenous infusion techniques may be used.

4 *Bronchodilators*.

5 Prompt *treatment of infection*. Watch for any signs of infection, i.e. postoperative increase in respiratory rate, pyrexia, purulent sputum or shortness of breath. Antibiotics may be given but they are no substitutes for good physiotherapy. Ampicillin or co-trimoxazole are suitable to start with and others can be used once the results of sensitivity tests are known.

6 *Respiratory stimulants* (e.g. doxapram given by continuous intravenous infusion) may be used in severe cases. Such therapy is usually given in conjunction with the anaesthetist.

Asthma

Asthma is intermittent reversible airways obstruction which may be precipitated by inhalation of an allergen (in the young, atopic individual) or may be intrinsic (in the older patient with no history of allergy and no specific external precipitating factors).

Assessment

Find out about the following points.

1 Any known precipitating factors.

2 The frequency and severity of attacks and the treatment needed to reverse them.

3 What normal maintenance treatment is required to prevent attacks?

Management

1 A mild well-controlled asthmatic is rarely a problem.
2 Severe asthmatics should be admitted early to allow time for assessment and for the patient to settle on the ward.
3 Reassurance and good premedication are important. Anxiety may well precipitate an attack.
4 Discuss the case with the anaesthetist and ask him if he wants any particular preoperative medication. Tell him about the patient's present therapy.
5 Listen for bronchospasm postoperatively and treat it early. Similarly, treat any developing chest infection quickly.

Cardiovascular disease

The following problems will be considered.
1 Myocardial ischaemia:
   (a) history of infarction;
   (b) angina.
2 Hypertension.
3 Left ventricular failure.
4 Cardiac arrhythmias, e.g. atrial fibrillation.
5 Heart murmurs.
These pre-existing conditions should be spotted in the general assessment of the patient during the history and examination. If present, a full cardiovascular assessment is required.

Assessment

All patients with a cardiovascular abnormality should have the following investigations.
1 Haemoglobin: to exclude anaemia.
2 Chest X-ray:
   (a) assess heart size and shape;
   (b) look for pulmonary congestion;
   (c) look for unfolding of the thoracic aorta (seen in long-standing hypertension);
   (d) look for calcification in the cardiac valves or aorta.
3 ECG:
   (a) look for evidence of arrhythmia;
   (b) look for changes of ischaemia;
   (c) look for conduction defects.

Management

1 Myocardial ischaemia

Infarction
An elective operation should not be undertaken in the first 3 months after a myocardial infarct, as there is a significantly increased risk of reinfarction during that time. The risk is increased if the patient is hypertensive, if the operation is

likely to be prolonged, or if the operation involves thoracic or abdominal surgery. Patients who have had a myocardial infarction more than 6 months previously have a small risk of reinfarction but should nevertheless be managed as below.

Angina

If the patient has a history of angina, assess its severity using the following parameters.

(a) The frequency of attacks.

(b) The duration of attacks.

(c) The rate of improvement with rest or glyceryl trinitrate.

(d) How severe the circumstances were which brought on the attack.

Management of patients with myocardial ischaemia

(a) Before the operation, inform the anaesthetist. Use adequate premedication to reduce anxiety.

(b) During the operation, excessive blood loss or overtransfusion should be avoided.

(c) Postoperatively, give adequate sedation and avoid fluid overload.

2 Hypertension

Drugs

Patients receiving treatment for hypertension usually stay on this treatment while in hospital. It is important that the anaesthetist knows which drug is being used as it will influence his management (e.g. beta-blockers may mask any sympathetic response to hypotension). He will also have to decide whether any alternative therapy should be given when the patient is taken off oral drugs just before operation.

Control

Check the blood pressure is well controlled. It should be taken on at least two occasions by the houseman preoperatively.

Electrolytes

If the patient is on long-term diuretics check the electrolytes. Such patients are often potassium-depleted and this must be corrected before any anaesthetic is given.

Secondary effects

Look for left ventricular hypertrophy, myocardial ischaemia, ECG changes and impaired renal function.

3 Left ventricular failure

If this is acute it should be brought under control before the patient has an anaesthetic, using diuretics, oxygen and, in severe cases, diamorphine. Only emergency surgery would be carried out in such a patient.

If it is chronic, the following must be done:
(a) assess the present degree of failure;
(b) note the treatment the patient is receiving;
(c) check the urea and electrolytes, especially the potassium;
These facts must be related to the anaesthetist.
(d) be especially careful to avoid fluid overload post-operatively. It may be an advantage to run the patient rather more dehydrated than usual.

4 Arrhythmia (e.g. atrial fibrillation)

If the patient has an acute arrhythmia the operation should be delayed until this has been successfully treated. Long-standing arrhythmias may not be reversed, but at least a stable cardiac state should be established. If the patient is stable, note the treatment he is on and pass the information on to the anaesthetist.

5 Heart murmurs

Assess the origin of the murmur and the lesion likely to be producing it (by clinical assessment and evaluation of the ECG and chest X-ray). If you are in doubt about the interpretation of the murmur seek expert advice.

In addition, assess the physiological significance of the murmur by looking for secondary effects such as dilatation of the chambers of the heart, or left or right ventricular failure. Check the patient's notes for evidence of previous problems from a cardiac lesion.

Management of patients with valvular disease and septal defects
1 Treat any cardiac failure or arrhythmia.
2 Antibiotics. Any diseased valve may act as a site for subacute bacterial endocarditis. Thrombus on its surface may be colonized by organisms during a transient bacter-aemia or septicaemia.

Prophylactic antibiotics are given to those patients with a murmur who are having any procedure likely to cause such a bacteraemia, e.g.
(a) oral or dental surgery (*Streptococcus viridans*),
(b) large bowel surgery,
(c) cystoscopy, prostatectomy, genito-urinary surgery (*Streptococcus faecalis*),
(d) biliary surgery,
(e) abortion (*Streptococcus faecalis*)
The drugs used are those indicated by the possible infecting organism. They should be given intravenously with

the premedication. Amoxycillin and gentamicin, erythromycin or vancomycin are possible drugs to use.

3 As in all cardiac disease, avoid any undue strain on the heart (e.g. hypovolaemia or fluid overload) as this may precipitate heart failure.

Diabetes

Diabetic treatment is normally planned and adjusted for the individual patient to follow his usual lifestyle, while maintaining a normal blood sugar. Admission for a surgical operation disturbs this balance of 'treatment versus lifestyle', due to the catabolic response to surgery. Diabetics also have an increased risk of developing problems at the time of surgery due to the following factors.

1 Infection.

2 Cardiovascular disease.

3 Renal disease: diabetic nephropathy may affect the elimination of drugs by the kidney.

4 Autonomic neuropathy: this causes postural hypotension, affects the bladder causing retention, and has been implicated in sudden cardio-respiratory arrest in diabetics undergoing surgery.

Assessment

Determine how severe and how unstable the particular patient's diabetes has been.

In addition look for evidence of diabetic complications. Assess the following:

(a) cardiac function (by history, examination, chest X-ray and ECG);

(b) renal function (by measurement of the blood pressure, looking for the presence of oedema, testing the urine for protein and checking the serum urea and electrolytes);

(c) the neurological system (look for autonomic neuropathy by taking blood pressure supine and upright).

Ideally, diabetic patients needing major surgery should be admitted at least 24 hours before operation for assessment, including a blood sugar series and regular urinalysis to check their stability. More time will be needed if their method of diabetic treatment is to be changed (see later).

Monitoring sugar levels

1 Urinalysis

This method is unreliable as it is retrospective. The urine reflects the blood sugar content some hours previously. A catheter specimen which is fresh is slightly more reliable but still inferior to blood sugar estimations.

The value of regular urinalysis is that it will safeguard against incorrect blood sugar measurements. Remember that it will only reflect hyperglycaemia and not hypoglycaemia.

2 Blood sugar estimation
All patients should have a blood sugar specimen analysed to provide a base-line. However, repeated laboratory tests are expensive and may take time. For serial monitoring, the sugar level in the blood can be tested either by the visual 'sticks' (Dextrostix or BMstix) or a reflectance meter (glucometer). The latter is reliable provided that there are sufficient staff trained and experienced in its use.

Management

The aim of management is to maintain good control and prevent hypoglycaemia and ketoacidosis. Ketoacidosis is prevented by supplying adequate calories and insulin, and hypoglycaemia is prevented by ensuring that the insulin given is covered by sufficient glucose input.

Patients can be divided into three main groups.
1 Diabetics controlled by diet.
2 Diabetics controlled by oral hypoglycaemics.
3 Insulin-dependent diabetics.

Procedures can be divided into:
(a) small operations, where the patient may eat as soon as he wakes up;
(b) large operations, where the patient may have no oral intake for a variable length of time postoperatively.

The precise management will depend on which combination of these factors is present.

Regimes

1 Diabetics controlled by diet

General
The diet should be adjusted to one containing 250−500 less calories to compensate for bed rest.

Small operations
No specific measures.

Large operations
(a) Measure the blood sugar just before anaesthetic.
(b) Regular 3−4 hourly blood sugar measurements postoperatively for 24 hours.
(c) Usually there is no problem, but the combination of stress and bed rest may cause a rise in blood sugar and make the patient temporarily insulin-dependent (see Section 3, p. 25).

For patients withdrawn from oral feeding, a standard intravenous regime (e.g. 1 litre of normal saline, 2 litres of 5% dextrose, each with 20 mmol potassium) will give the patient 100 g of carbohydrate. Insulin may or may not be added to this.

2 Diabetics controlled on oral hypoglycaemics

Small operations
(a) Stop long-acting oral hypoglycaemics (e.g. chlorpro pamide) 2 days preoperatively.
(b) Stabilize on tolbutamide.
(c) No hypoglycaemic on the day of operation.
(d) Measure blood sugar just before anaesthetic, postoperatively and 4 hours later.
(e) Restart oral hypoglycaemics as soon as oral intake is established.

Large operations
Patients must be stabilized and managed on short-acting insulin. Ideally they should be admitted 48 hours before the operation for conversion to a short-acting soluble insulin (e.g. 10−12 units of Actrapid 8-hourly). Further management is then as for patients on insulin.
N.B. The effect of chlorpropamide lasts at least 24 hours. These patients therefore start with a small dose of insulin and increase to the required dose gradually.

3 Insulin-dependent diabetics
Discuss the preoperative management with the anaesthetist. There are different ways of managing such diabetics and the anaesthetist may well have a preference.

Small operations
If possible plan the operation early in the list.
(a) Omit any long-acting insulin the night before the operation.
(b) Low insulin requirement: omit the morning dose of insulin. Set up an intravenous infusion for the pre- and perioperative period of 1 litre 5% dextrose with 16 units Actrapid and 20 mmol KCl, infused at 100 ml/hour.
   Patients having small operations later in the day can have a light breakfast covered by half the normal dose of insulin in the morning. They are then starved and an infusion is set up as above.
(c) Check the blood sugar before operation, immediately after operation and 4-hourly until eating normally.

(d) As soon as oral intake is re-established after the operation, restart the insulin.

Large operations
The following is a suggested regime using a continuous insulin infusion and blood sugar monitoring, but other methods are possible.
Plan the operation early in the list.
(a) The day before the operation give the patient his normal dose of insulin in short-acting form.
(b) On the morning of the operation start an intravenous infusion of 5% dextrose with 16 units Actrapid and 20 mmol KCl, infused at 100 ml/hour.
(c) Postoperatively, the insulin is given by continuous infusion from an insulin pump 'piggy backed' into the side of the drip (strength: soluble insulin 1 unit/ml in saline). The infusion is governed as in Table 2.

This system needs good nursing care as the glucose and insulin are given independently and there is a risk that they may get out of phase (in particular, there is a danger of hypoglycaemia).

An insulin infusion is ideal, especially for a long period of care when the patient is going to have no fluid or restricted fluid by mouth. Once the patient begins to drink and becomes re-established on a diet, a twice- or thrice-daily soluble insulin regime can be restarted and adjusted according to blood sugar levels. The initial total daily insulin should roughly equal the patient's preoperative dose. It should be increased by about 20% in the presence of infection or when the patient is taking high-dose steroids. Fifty units Actrapid plus 50 ml 0.9% saline via intravenous infusion pump are administered according to the scale shown in Table 2. One litre 5% dextrose i.v. is infused concurrently

Table 2. Sliding scale for insulin infusion rate according to blood sugar measurement

Ward glucometer test (mmol/litre)	Insulin i.v. (units/hour)
<2	Give 50 ml 50% glucose i.v.
2– 5.9	None
6– 8.9	0.5
9–10.9	1.0
11–16.9	2.0
17–28	4.0

N.B. The dose may need doubling or quadrupling if the patient is severely ill, shocked or taking steroids or sympathomimetic drugs.

over 8–10 hours. The saline requirement is given through a second line. Potassium requirements can be added as usual.

Measure the blood sugar 2-hourly postoperatively until stable, adjusting the infusion rate according to the above chart. Once stable, measure it 6-hourly. Monitor the potassium levels.

Alternative regime: insulin given intramuscularly (blood sugar monitoring)
The insulin requirement is given intramuscularly according to the sliding scale shown in Table 3.

Table 3. Sliding scale for insulin given by subcutaneous injection according to blood sugar measurement

Blood sugar (mmol/litre)	Soluble insulin units i.m.
Less than 5	No insulin
5–15	8
15–20	16
More than 20	Review

N.B. The blood sugar levels are measured 4-hourly and the dose of insulin given on the basis of the results of these tests.

Emergency surgery in diabetics
The management is really the same as above, although there is no time to make preparation. Patients on oral hypoglycaemics may have to manage with short-acting insulin and must be covered over their operation by a 5% dextrose and insulin infusion as described above. Regular blood sugar levels must be taken. Do not forget that chlorpropamide has a prolonged action.

If a patient is admitted as a surgical emergency in ketoacidosis, the operation must be delayed until this is corrected, if necessary by hourly subcutaneous injection of insulin. Not only does this improve the patient's chances, but it may change the clinical picture and the possible diagnosis. Ketoacidosis can itself produce abdominal pain mimicking an acute abdomen.

Patients on steroid drugs
If the patient has been on regular steroids in the 6 weeks preceding the operation he may have adrenal suppression and be unable to respond to stress and trauma in the usual way. Additional steroid cover is then required.

The dose given is influenced by the severity of the operation and the length of the previous steroid treatment. A commonly used regime for a major operation is listed below.

Hydrocortisone 100 mg i.m. with premedication.
Hydrocortisone 100 mg 8-hourly over the day of the operation.
Hydrocortisone 50 mg 8-hourly on the second postoperative day.
Hydrocortisone 50 mg 12-hourly on the third postoperative day.
Then 25 mg 12-hourly gradually decreasing to the patient's normal dose over a further week. (It is useful to remember that 5 mg of prednisolone is equivalent to 20 mg of hydrocortisone.)

If the patient's blood pressure falls postoperatively and other causes have been excluded, suspect adrenal insufficiency and give extra hydrocortisone (e.g. 100 mg hydrocortisone i.v.) until the blood pressure is restored. A short synacthen test can be done to check adrenal response to adrenocorticotrophic hormone (ACTH).

Patients on anti-coagulants

The precise management depends on the policy of the local surgical unit, anaesthetists and haematologists. Patients are usually on anti-coagulants as prophylaxis against venous or arterial thrombosis. This is discussed fully on pages 107–110. In each case a fine balance needs to be kept between effective anti-coagulation and minimal risk of haemorrhage during surgery.

The anti-coagulant effect of both heparin and warfarin can be reversed. The action of heparin is reversed with protamine sulphate. The action of warfarin is reversed with fresh frozen plasma.

In patients taking warfarin for the prevention of arterial thrombosis three courses of management are possible.

1 If emergency surgery is planned, 0.5 litres of fresh frozen plasma should be available during the operation. The anaesthetist, theatre and laboratories should be informed.

2 If routine surgery is planned, the patient is admitted earlier and the dose of warfarin reduced to make the international normalized ratio (INR) between 2 and 2.5. Fresh frozen plasma should be available if difficulties arise.

3 Warfarin therapy can be stopped 2 days before surgery and anti-coagulation continued with heparin. The reversal of heparin does not involve the addition of a large volume of plasma to the intravascular compartment, so this regime is recommended in those patients whose cardiac function is compromised. The precise dose of heparin required is variable (about 100 units/kg) and is usually titrated against the Factor Xa assay or the protamine sulphate neutralization

test. The kaolin partial thromboplastin time (KPTT) is not accurate in the presence of recent warfarin therapy.

In patients taking warfarin for the prevention of venous thrombosis it is usual to either reduce the dose, as above, or discontinue the drug. Anti-coagulation can then be continued with heparin (5000 units subcutaneously three times daily). Postoperatively, once the patient's condition is stabilized, oral anti-coagulation can be restarted using the regime on p. 109.

Haemophilia

Classical haemophilia is due to a deficiency of Factor VIII. Christmas disease is due to a deficiency of Factor IX. The severity of the condition varies between different patients, but all need special management when surgery has to be undertaken. Capillary bleeding initially ceases due to platelet aggregation (primary haemostasis). Due to the plasma clotting factor deficiency, the clotting cascade is inadequately activated and insufficient fibrin is produced to stabilize the clot. Continued bleeding therefore occurs in the post-operative period unless replacement therapy is given.

Management　　Any patient with a history suggestive of a bleeding diathesis, or a family history of haemophilia, should have a full clotting screen undertaken before an operation is contemplated. Patients with proven haemophilia are managed in close co-operation with the haematology department, which must be given as much advance warning as possible. They will usually arrange for the defective factor to be replaced. This may be done using concentrates of Factor VIII or Factor IX. Some patients develop antibodies to the missing factors, making management much more difficult. The patient is screened for such antibodies before operation, and if present elective surgery is usually contraindicated.

Patients with mild haemophilia can have their own Factor VIII levels stimulated by giving a non-vasoactive vasopressin analogue deamino-D-arginine vasopressin (DDAVP).

If the clotting factor deficiency is corrected, the care of haemophiliacs is similar to that of other patients. However, after major surgery, Factor VIII levels may need to be measured and Factor VIII given twice daily. Factor IX may need to be given once a day. The morning dose should be given first thing before the patient is bathed and the wound dressed. Intramuscular injections should be avoided. Sutures should be left in longer than usual (10 days) as there is a tendency to bleed around the eighth or tenth day and this may be precipitated by removal of the sutures. Similarly, bleeding may occur after the removal of drains. If effective anti-haemophilic therapy is assured, drains should only be used where they would otherwise be indicated and not inserted specially because of the haemophilia.

Other bleeding disorders and prothrombotic states

A number of other bleeding disorders may require careful preoperative management. They are rare and include:

(a) disorders of the clotting cascade (e.g. Factor X or XI deficiency);

(b) disturbances of platelet vessel wall interreaction (e.g. von Willebrand's disease);

(c) abnormalities of platelet function (e.g. thrombasthenia).

A careful personal and family history of excess bleeding, especially after tooth extraction or tonsillectomy, will often raise suspicion of the presence of one of these disorders. A basic clotting screen (bleeding time, prothrombin time, partial thromboplastin time (PTT) and fibrinogen) will frequently produce initial confirmation of clinical suspicions.

It is increasingly recognized that congenital and acquired disorders of coagulation are common causes of postoperative thrombosis. Such conditions, frequently due to a reduction of the level of naturally occurring anti-coagulants (such as protein C, S, and anti-thrombin III) will require careful pre- and postoperative management. Once again a personal or family history of deep venous thrombosis or pulmonary embolism, especially before the age of 40 years, will give a clue as to whether further detailed investigations are required.

AIDS

Acquired immune deficiency syndrome (AIDS), caused by the human immunodeficiency virus (HIV), is a major new disease which has profound implications for both patients and staff. Infection can be acquired by drug abuse, through homosexual or heterosexual intercourse or due to treatment with blood products contaminated with HIV. Quite apart from the effects of the disease, the consequences of diagnosis on an individual's mortgage, insurance, compensation and family can be devastating.

Transmission of the disease occurs with difficulty and requires intimate contact with infected human blood, serum or semen. Once infection has occurred, the virus may remain dormant for many years. Eventually, most, if not all, carriers develop the full-blown immune deficiency syndrome in which there is a deficiency of T cell helper activity.

This syndrome can present in a wide variety of ways due to lowered resistance to other infections. These may involve any of the surgical specialties. Among the common presentations are atypical pneumonia (pneumocystis), orogenital candidiasis, progressive lymphadenopathy and Kaposi's sarcoma. Although at the time of writing there is no cure for this infection, active treatment can improve the patient's length and quality of life. Patients have a right to confidentiality particularly as there is still intolerance by society to this diagnosis.

Diagnosis

The diagnosis should be suspected in any patient presenting with an unusual condition who might be in a high-risk group for infection. The main high-risk groups are listed below.

1 Homosexual males.
2 Bisexual males.
3 Intravenous drug abusers.
4 Haemophiliacs.
5 Recipients of blood products before HIV testing started.
6 Residents of African countries south of the Sahara.
7 Sexual partners of any of the above.
8 Children of infected mothers.
9 Prison inmates, past or present.

Proving the diagnosis

The patient's informed consent must be obtained prior to HIV testing. Occasionally the virus can be isolated from the host tissues, but this is unreliable.

HIV antibodies appear in serum up to 3 months after infection. The patient can transmit infection during this seronegative phase. HIV antigen can also be detected in serum, but this test is less widely available than that based on the antibody.

Management

It is unethical for a doctor to refuse treatment to a patient infected with HIV on the grounds that there is a risk of the doctor becoming infected (General Medical Council, 1988). Therefore adequate precautions must be taken to prevent cross infection from any patient who might be at risk of having HIV infection.

Precautions

1 Plastic aprons.
2 Disposable gowns.
3 Visors or glasses.
4 Double gloves.
5 Overshoes or impermeable footwear.
6 Modified operating technique.

Modifications to operative techniques

1 Use less unprotected sharp instruments, e.g. staples instead of sutures, scissors instead of knives.

2 Unsheathed needles should be avoided.

3 Scalpels and sharps should never be handed from one person to another, but always replaced in a 'receiver' before transfer.

4 Disposable sharps and knives with integral handles (without removable blades) should be used. Particular care should be taken if the wound contains bone fragments, wires or other sharp objects.

5 Sharps bins should be taken to the patient and not sharps to the bin.

6 Health workers should be warned of the possibility of HIV infection.

7 Open cuts or scabs should be covered with dressings or the worker excluded from contact with the patient.

In the event of accidental injury the wound should be thoroughly washed with soap or disinfectant and water, and made to bleed using a tourniquet. Blood should be taken from the injured individual and from the patient and stored for future testing. The situation should be explained to the patient, as a negative test will be reassuring to the injured health worker.

Areas contaminated with infected blood should be cleaned with a 1 in 10 solution of sodium hypochlorite (household bleach).

Patients with HIV infection *do not* need to be individually isolated.

Hepatitis B

Similar precautions should be taken with patients who are seropositive for hepatitis B infection. Health workers at risk should be immunized against hepatitis B. Reimmunization may be needed when the antibody titre falls after 5 years. (Some 5% of individuals never make antibody, so a confirmatory check after immunization is advisable.) Suitable disinfectants for hepatitis B are glutaraldehyde or hypochlorite.

The Operation and Afterwards

The housesurgeon in theatre

The housesurgeon should ensure that the operating list runs as smoothly as possible. A bleep can be very distracting to the surgeon and should not be worn in theatre.

Before scrubbing up:
1 check whether the patient requires a bladder catheter;
2 check that any necessary preoperative antibiotics have been given;
3 fill in a histology form for frozen section if this is required.

If the operating list is running late, inform any other department that might be affected, e.g. those providing peroperative radiology or frozen section histology.

Assisting at operation

The principle of assisting is to make the operation as easy as possible for the surgeon. If you are the first assistant try and follow the operation, imagining you were having to do it yourself, and thus anticipating what is required.

When sutures are being tied have a pair of scissors ready to cut the ends when asked to do so. Always use the tips of the scissors. If you use the blade higher up there is a danger of inadvertently cutting neighbouring structures. Skin sutures should be cut so that the ends are as long as the distance between each suture. In this way they can be seen easily for removal, but are not in the way of the next knot.

Catgut sutures should generally be cut so as to leave 5 mm ends. They tend to unravel as they swell postoperatively and will come undone if they are cut too short. Nylon sutures, on the other hand, if properly tied with a double 'surgeon's knot', can be cut off close to the knot. Silk sutures should be cut with 2 mm only to spare, as long ends enhance the danger of knot sepsis.

Ensure that the area the surgeon is operating on is as well exposed as possible, using suitable retractors or forceps to display the structures. Keep the field clear of blood using swabs or suction.

Never try and 'dictate' what the surgeon should do next; simply make it as easy as possible for him to achieve what he has decided to do.

There is usually less to do as a second assistant and you may find yourself holding on to a retractor for hours. This is an important role, as a good demonstration of the operative field may make all the difference between a successful or unsuccessful operation for your patient. Do it willingly and cheerfully.

The immediate postoperative period

Checklist
The houseman should check the following things after each operation.

1 *Laboratory specimens.* Have they been labelled and the forms signed? Make sure any microbiology specimens have gone to the laboratory.

2 *Operation note.* Has it been written?

3 *Prescription chart.* Check this in order to be certain of the following:
  (a) adequate analgesia and night sedation are written up;
  (b) an intravenous fluid regime is written up if the patient requires it.

4 *Intravenous lines, arterial lines, drains and catheters.* After a large operation make a mental note of the position of these. Are they all necessary in the postoperative period and how long will the surgeon require them to be left in?

5 *Nursing observations.* Note which observations are required postoperatively and inform the nurses of any particular problems such as the presence of a chest drain or drains requiring measurement of output.

The daily postoperative ward round
The houseman should see every patient under his care at least once a day. This enables him to keep in touch with the patient's progress, and to pick up any postoperative problems as they arise.

The following is a basic plan for such a round, designed to check quickly on every aspect of patient care. If you find something positive the methods of management can be followed up in Sections 1.5–1.10.

1 History
Ask about pain and vital functions.

(a) Pain: if the patient has any new or unexpected pain, diagnose the cause. Ask particularly about pain in the legs or chest (thrombo-embolism), or increasing pain in the wound (wound infection). Has adequate analgesia been prescribed?

(b) Breathing: shortness of breath, cough, haemoptysis.

(c) Eating: appetite, nausea, vomiting.

(d) Bowels: passage of flatus, motions.

(e) Urine: has the patient passed urine? Has the patient had any dysuria or difficulty?

2 Examination

Check the following:

(a) temperature charts for pyrexia, change in pulse rate, blood pressure and respiratory rate;

(b) chest: examine for signs of infection, collapse or oedema;

(c) wound: check for developing localized tenderness;

(d) bowel sounds (after abdominal surgery);

(e) legs: check for localized tenderness over the soleal muscles;

(f) mental state.

3 Fluid balance

Examine the fluid chart and check the input (oral, i.v.) against the output (urine, nasogastric tube, drains and insensible loss). Is the patient in positive or negative fluid balance?

4 Drains and tubes

Check the position of intravenous lines, drains and any urinary catheter. Are they all draining? Can any be removed? Have any become infected?

5 Drugs

Check the prescription sheet for any unnecessary drugs which can be deleted.

6 Investigations

Order any tests which may be necessary (e.g. haemoglobin, urea and electrolytes, serum proteins).

Postoperative Complications: Presenting Symptoms

Some of the common problems you will be called upon to deal with in the postoperative period are dealt with in this section. They are listed in Table 4. Further notes on subsequent management are given in Sections 1.6–1.9.

Postoperative pyrexia

The temperature chart is a very good indicator of developing postoperative problems and should be inspected every day. The time of onset of the fever will help you to decide the cause.

Early postoperative fever, days 0–2
A mild pyrexia in the first 24 hours after operation is commonly due to tissue damage and necrosis, or haematoma formation at the operative site. A higher and more persistent pyrexia may be due to pulmonary collapse, or specific infections related to the surgery, e.g. urinary infection after bladder surgery or biliary infection after a cholecystectomy. A fever due to blood transfusion may also appear in this early period.

Fever, days 3–5
A pyrexia developing in this period is likely to be due to either developing sepsis (e.g. wound infection or pelvic or subphrenic abscess formation) or bronchopneumonia.

Fever, days 5–7
Problems presenting at this time include those associated with failure of a bowel anastomosis, e.g. leakage and fistula formation, and a fever due to venous thrombosis either in the limbs or in the pelvic veins.

Fever after the first week
This is less likely to be due to a problem directly related to the operation, although the development of wound or deep sepsis can be delayed if the patient has received prophylactic antibiotics. Other causes include the development of distant sepsis such as a hepatic abscess or cerebral abscess. Thrombotic disease may also be delayed in onset and appear at this time.

Table 4. Common postoperative problems

Common presentations	Causes	Page reference
Pyrexia	Pulmonary collapse or bronchopneumonia	47
	Wound infection	68
	Intra-abdominal abscess (pelvic or subphrenic)	72, 75
	Urinary tract infection	63
	Inflamed drip site	71
	Thrombo-embolism	55
	Blood transfusion reaction	52
	Septicaemia	77
Postoperative pain	Wound haematoma or infection	68
	Chest	38
	Heart	38, 53
	Abdomen	39
	Legs	39
	Deep venous thrombosis (DVT)	55
Discharging wound	Abscess	68
	Fistula	66, 75
	Dehiscence	69
Nausea and vomiting	Drugs	39
	Intestinal obstruction	337
	Acute dilatation of the stomach	46
Constipation	Paralytic ileus	45
	Drugs	40
Breathlessness	Pulmonary collapse	47
	Bronchopneumonia	47
	Pulmonary embolism	58
	Left ventricular failure	54
	Inhalation of vomit	49
Confusion	Anoxia	41
	Toxaemia	
	Drugs, alcohol withdrawal	
	Electrolyte disturbances	
Collapse	Inhalation of vomit	49
	Haemorrhage	51
	Septicaemia	77
	Pulmonary embolus	58
	Myocardial infarction	53
	Stroke	55
Oliguria/anuria	Postrenal, renal and prerenal failure	65
	Retention of urine	63

Making the diagnosis	Carry out the following routine.

Making the diagnosis

Carry out the following routine.

1 Ask about symptoms of cough, sputum, dysuria, urinary frequency or calf pain.

2 Examine:

(a) the respiratory and pulse rates;

(b) the chest;

(c) the wound;

(d) the drip site and drain sites;

(e) the calves for tenderness localized over the soleus muscle;

(f) the abdomen and rectum if an abdominal operation has been performed.

3 Consider performing these investigations: specimens of sputum, urine, blood (if temperature above 38°C) and a wound swab for microscopy, culture and sensitivity.

The condition

Some common causes of postoperative pyrexia are shown in Table 4. Further details of these conditions are given in subsequent chapters.

Postoperative pain

Pain relief is almost always required in the postoperative period and analgesic therapy is discussed on p. 101.

The cause of any pain must be determined in the same way as in other circumstances but there are important causes in a postoperative patient.

1 Wound pain

worse on most
72h than settles
it continues, infection

Pain in the wound is worse on movement and is usually maximal in the first 72 hours. Thereafter it usually settles. If the pain is getting worse after this, check for signs of wound infection. Occasionally, patients suffer quite severe 'spasms' of pain in an abdominal wound. This is more common in those who are excessively tense and is probably due to involuntary muscle guarding in response to the pull of the sutures. The pull of the muscles then increases the pain.

Treatment

Analgesia for wound pain; small doses of tranquillizers (e.g. diazepam 2−5 mg 8-hourly) are helpful for muscle spasms.

2 Chest pain
wound pleuritic
cardiac

Excluding any pain due to a thoracic wound, two other types of chest pain occur postoperatively.

(a) *Pleuritic.* Sharp, localized and severe pain increased by inspiration. This is either due to infection involving the pleura or pulmonary infarction after an embolus. (see pp. 47 and 58).

(b) *Cardiac pain* (due to myocardial ischaemia). The patient may complain of a retrosternal tight pain with or without radiation into the arm (see p. 53).

3 Abdominal pain

Possible causes of increasing abdominal pain include:
(a) intra-abdominal sepsis (see pp. 68–75);
(b) anastomotic leakage (p. 75);
(c) retention of urine (p. 63);
(d) constipation (p. 10);
(e) new intra-abdominal pathology, e.g. ischaemic bowel (p. 340), intussusception (p. 342), intestinal obstruction (p. 337).

4 Legs

(a) Deep or superficial venous thrombosis (p. 55).
(b) Sciatica
(c) Postoperative arterial thrombosis or embolism.

Discharging wound

A copious discharge from the wound may be due to the release of a wound abscess. You should also consider the possibility of the development of an intestinal fistula (see p. 75), a urinary fistula (p. 66) or a deep wound dehiscence (p. 69).

Nausea and vomiting

The condition

The common causes of postoperative vomiting are as follows:
1 Drugs:
    (a) analgesics (opiates),
    (b) anaesthetic agents,
    (c) other drug therapy, e.g. digoxin toxicity.
2 Intestinal obstruction:
    (a) paralytic ileus,
    (b) mechanical.

Making the
diagnosis

1 Note which drugs the patient has received.
2 Check possible drug interactions. For example, an elderly patient may be on digoxin and develop hypokalaemia with intravenous fluid and diuretics. This may precipitate digoxin toxicity.
3 Assess the oral input and listen for bowel sounds. Nausea and vomiting when the patient has just started drinking after abdominal surgery may be due to a persistent paralytic ileus. In that case the abdomen will be distended and bowel sounds absent.

4 If nausea and vomiting occur after the patient has been tolerating oral fluids, consider the possibility of a mechanical obstruction due to fibrinous adhesions, intussusception or volvulus. Here there is usually colicky pain with active bowel sounds, and localized tenderness. On abdominal X-ray there is a localized area of distended loops and fluid levels on the erect film.

Treatment

1 Pass a nasogastric tube to drain the stomach.
2 Paralytic ileus (see p. 45)
3 Mechanical obstruction (see p. 337)
4 Drug-induced vomiting. Treat with an anti-emetic (e.g. prochlorperazine 12.5 mg i.m. 4−6 hourly, or metoclopramide 10 mg i.m. 4−6 hourly). The latter should be limited to 3−4 doses, as an excess causes extrapyramidal side effects.

Constipation

Constipation occurs frequently after an operation and can cause great discomfort to the patient. A rectal examination is essential. Faecal impaction causes considerable distress and the cause is not always apparent to the patient. The early use of suppositories while the patient is still immobile often avoids the need for enemas or manual evacuation later on.

Opiate analgesics are a major cause of such constipation.

Treatment

Daily bulking agents, such as Normacol, should be given to those at risk (i.e. the elderly, those with a tendency to constipation, and those confined to bed for a long period). Once the patient has become constipated the following agents may be tried (in order).
1 Glycerine suppositories.
2 Dulcolax suppositories.
3 Phosphate enemas.
4 Manual evacuation.

The management of postoperative ileus is dealt with on p. 45. Drugs used in bowel preparation before surgery are reviewed on p. 110.

Breathlessness

Breathlessness in a postoperative patient is usually due to one of the following factors.
1 Pulmonary collapse (p. 47).
2 Bronchopneumonia (p. 47).
3 Pulmonary embolism (p. 58).
4 Left ventricular failure either due to fluid overload or myocardial infarction (p. 54).

5 Pneumothorax (p. 49). This occasionally complicates the insertion of a central venous pressure line or intercostal anaesthetic blocks, or may even occur spontaneously.

Confusion

The condition
It is quite common for a surgical patient, often elderly, to become confused after an operation. This is distressing both for the patient and the relatives, though fortunately it is usually short-lived. The distress is increased by the fact that medical and nursing staff do not always appreciate that there is usually a cause which may well be amenable to treatment.

Causes
1 Anoxia (bronchopneumonia, pulmonary embolus).
2 Toxaemia (sepsis, urinary tract infection, chest infection).
3 Drugs (analgesics, sedatives, steroids).
4 Alcohol withdrawal.
5 Electrolyte imbalance.
6 Uraemia.
7 Pain (wound, retention of urine).

Making a diagnosis
The symptoms of confusion are disorientation, agitation and rambling conversation. Review with the above causes in mind. Always examine the chest. Bronchopneumonia is a frequent cause of confusion in the elderly. Check for a past history of alcohol abuse and see what drugs have been given. Remember that more than one of the causative factors may be operating.

Proving the diagnosis
The investigations may include:
(a) haemoglobin and haematocrit;
(b) urea and electrolytes;
(c) liver function tests;
(d) blood sugar;
(e) blood gases;
(f) microbiology where appropriate, e.g. blood cultures, samples of sputum and urine;
(g) appropriate X-rays.

Management
1 Talk to the patient. Gentle reassurance is required. A confused, elderly patient is usually aware of his own strange behaviour and terrified he is going to be permanently insane. Explain to him that such confusion is not uncommon and not his fault. Reassure him that he will recover from it in a few days. Even in his confusion he will usually understand this and be grateful for it later.
  Also, do not forget to reassure the relatives.

41 SECTION 1.5

2 Check the drug chart for anything which may be causing the confusion and, if possible, stop the drug concerned.

3 Treat any organic cause found.

4 If the patient is still agitated or potentially hostile despite the above measures, then sedation is needed. Suitable drugs include chlorpromazine (200 mg i.m.) and diazepam (10 mg i.m.). Chlormethiazole is an alternative and the drug of choice for delirium tremens.

Collapse

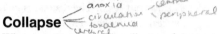

The condition

When a patient suddenly collapses after an operation there is often a degree of panic and it is important to take charge and make a careful assessment.

The collapse is usually associated with cerebral impairment, either due to cerebral depression by anoxia, toxaemia or drugs, or due to a fall in the cerebral blood supply. Whatever the initial cause, the final picture tends to be similar as one system failure results in failure of another. (See Fig. 3.)

Common primary causes to think of include the following conditions.

1 Anoxia:
   (a) inhalation of vomit (p. 49);
   (b) bronchopneumonia (p. 47).

2 Central circulatory failure:
   (a) myocardial infarction (p. 53);
   (b) pulmonary embolism (p. 58).

3 Peripheral circulatory failure:
   (a) haemorrhage (reactionary or secondary) (p. 51);
   (b) oligaemia (e.g. pancreatitis, mesenteric infarction).

4 Toxaemia:
   (a) septicaemia (p. 77);
   (b) drug overdose (e.g. opiates, digoxin).

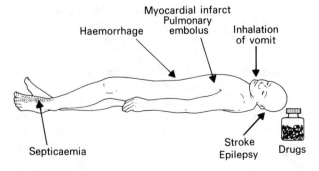

Fig. 3. Postoperative collapse.

5 Cerebral causes:
(a) stroke (p. 55);
(b) epilepsy.

Making the diagnosis

Make a quick appraisal of the following.
1 *Circulation.* Blood pressure (BP), pulse rate and character. Listen to the heart. Jugular venous pulse (JVP).
2 *Peripheral resistance.* Are the extremities warm (vasodilated) or cold (vasoconstricted)?
3 *Respiration.* Rate and character. Quiet or dyspnoeic? Laboured? Tracheal tug? Are there any physical signs in the chest?
4 *Oxygenation.* Pink or cyanosed?
5 *Cerebral function.* Level of consciousness.

If the blood pressure and pulse are adequate then the cause is anoxia, toxaemia or a cerebral problem such as a stroke.

If there is circulatory collapse (low BP and tachycardia), then you have to decide whether this is due to central (cardiac) failure or peripheral failure (oligaemia or vasodilation).

In central failure there is venous hypertension (raised JVP, peripheral oedema, pulmonary oedema).

Peripheral failure may be due to inadequate blood volume (in which case the patient is cold and sweating and the peripheries are vasoconstricted), or due to toxic vasodilation (in which case the blood pressure is low but the peripheries are warm and well perfused).

The following investigations may help in making further progress:
(a) ECG,
(b) chest X-ray,
(c) electrolytes,
(d) haemoglobin and white cell count.
While arranging these remember to cross-match blood if this is likely to be needed.

Management

Initial management involves attention to the airway and setting up an intravenous infusion as necessary. The further management depends on the cause of the collapse. Various possibilities are dealt with in subsequent sections as listed on pp. 42–43.

Oliguria/anuria

It is not uncommon for a patient to have a diminished urine output after a major operation, due to the effects of fluid and blood loss and the physiological response of the adrenal cortex to stress (see i.v. fluid therapy, p. 91). This temporary oliguria should recover after 12−24 hours. An output of less than 500 cm^3 in 24 hours is not satisfactory and should be investigated.

There are three possible causes to consider for poor postoperative urine output.

1 Retention of urine.

2 Prerenal failure.

3 Acute renal failure.

These are dealt with in Section 1.8. Retention of urine is diagnosed by finding a full bladder on examination and confirming this by catheterization. If no evidence of retention is found then renal failure must be suspected and appropriate steps taken.

1.6 Gastrointestinal and Respiratory Complications

Paralytic ileus

The condition

Paralytic ileus ('ileus') is atony of the intestine causing intestinal obstruction. It has a complex aetiology and is common after any operation when the stomach or bowel have been handled, or where there has been peritonitis. The condition is exacerbated by chemical derangement (hypokalaemia, uraemia, diabetes), by reflex sympathetic inhibition (e.g. after retroperitoneal haematoma or injury) or by anticholinergic drugs.

There may be an ileus for a variable period after abdominal surgery. Oral feeding can only be restarted once bowel function has returned and you will be called upon to make a decision about this.

Management

Surgeons differ widely in their attitudes towards reintroducing fluids after abdominal operations. Immediately after the operation, unless a nasogastric tube is present, the patient is either kept 'nil by mouth', or only allowed small volumes of water to drink (e.g. 15 cm^3/hour) or ice to suck, occasionally. The fluid requirements are given intravenously. If a nasogastric tube is in place, the patient may drink more and this keeps the mouth and pharynx comfortable. The tube should be aspirated before each drink is given. You should check that it is draining freely and not blocked. If in doubt, test by giving fluid to drink and then re-aspirating it up the tube.

Recovery from ileus

The end of the ileus is demonstrated by:
(a) the return of bowel sounds;
(b) passage of flatus;
(c) the patient beginning to feel hungry;
(d) a decrease in the nasogastric aspirate (if a tube is present);
(e) an increase in the urinary output as fluid is absorbed from the bowel.

Listen to the abdomen daily. When bowel sounds return, oral fluids may be increased slowly. The nasogastric tube can be removed once the oral intake exceeds the nasogastric drainage over a few hours. Large volumes of aspirate may persist if the tip of the tube has passed into the duodenum, or if a pyloric bypass operation such as a pyloroplasty or gastroenterostomy has been performed.

As the ileus recovers the patient frequently has some abdominal distension and 'wind' pains, and will require reassurance about these. They are relieved when flatus is passed. Peppermint water can be helpful at this stage.

Prolonged ileus

If the ileus persists for more than 4 days, there may be some other cause operating such as continuing peritonitis, intra-abdominal abscess formation, anastomotic leakage, or mechanical intestinal obstruction. A prolonged ileus is also common where a truncal vagotomy has been performed or large amounts of narcotic agents have been given.

Providing none of the above causes are apparent, encourage the patient to mobilize, pushing his drip stand before him. Rectal suppositories may help. Metoclopramide (10 mg i.m.) is a good anti-emetic, as it not only has central action but also helps gastric emptying. A prolonged ileus may eventually necessitate the introduction of intravenous feeding.

Simple constipation

This is dealt with on p. 40.

Acute dilatation of the stomach

The condition This is a rare complication of any laparotomy. There is over-distension of the stomach affected by ileus. It contains several litres of fluid, mucus and air. The contents resemble extracellular fluid and contain little acid. As distension progresses the duodenum becomes kinked causing mechanical obstruction to outflow. The stomach wall becomes thinned out and congested, with occasional mucosal erosions. Eventually there is circulatory collapse and a risk of aspiration pneumonitis.

Acute dilatation is seen occasionally after splenectomy, vagotomy or operations on the biliary tree, but can occur after any abdominal procedure. It may rarely also occur after trauma, childbirth, the application of plaster of Paris, during acute infection or in diabetic coma.

Recognizing the pattern The most important factor is to think of the possibility. The condition can occur any time in the first week after an operation and can be rapid in onset. Do not be misled by the presence of a nasogastric tube as this may not have been aspirated efficiently. The patient complains of progressive distension, hiccups and vomiting. The vomiting becomes effortless, and is of dark brown fluid.

On examination
The upper abdomen is distended. The patient may be dehydrated with a tachycardia and hypotension. There may be dullness and poor air entry to the lower lobe of the left lung due to elevation of the left hemi-diaphragm.

Proving the diagnosis

The diagnosis is proved by passing a nasogastric tube and aspirating large volumes of dark-coloured fluid.

An abdominal X-ray shows a very large gastric air bubble. A chest X-ray may show a raised left hemi-diaphragm and some basal collapse.

The following investigations are important.
1 Urea and electrolytes to check the potassium.
2 Haematocrit to assess the degree of hypovolaemia.

Management

1 The nasogastric tube is left in place and aspirated regularly to keep the stomach empty. The patient immediately feels better. No fluids should be given orally for 24 hours. Clear fluids can then be gradually reintroduced. The gastric ileus recovers rapidly once the stomach is decompressed.
2 Intravenous fluid is given to provide both the body require-ment and to replace that lost by vomiting and aspiration. This should correct the hypovolaemia. Watch the potassium level.
3 The treatment of inhalation of vomit is given on p. 49.

Pulmonary collapse and bronchopneumonia

The condition

Pulmonary collapse (Fig. 4) is due to the blockage of bronchi with retained secretions and absorption of air from the distal

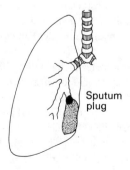

Sputum plug

Fig. 4. Pulmonary collapse.

47 SECTION 1.6

segment. It usually happens within 48 hours of operation. If the sputum plug persists then secondary bronchopneumonia ensues.

Recognizing the pattern

The most constant feature is an early postoperative pyrexia which may be quite high (e.g. 39°C). If initial treatment fails to dislodge the blockage, the pyrexia remains high and eventually purulent sputum is produced.

The patient may complain of shortness of breath and a dry cough. He may feel there is something he wants to cough up but is unable to.

On examination
The patient has a raised respiratory rate and a tachycardia. Examination of the chest usually fails to show anything very significant in the early stages, though later on deviation of the trachea to the affected side, clinical signs of collapse and coarse crepitations may be present.

Proving the diagnosis

The collapsed segment may be visible on chest X-ray after a few days. As soon as a sample of sputum is produced it should be sent off to the microbiologists for culture in case antibiotics are required later.

Management

The condition can be prevented by adequate analgesia and encouraging coughing in the first few hours after operation. If this fails however, the impacted secretions must be removed. Physiotherapy is used to help the patient cough. This is both active (chest percussion and breathing exercises) and passive (postural drainage). Adequate analgesia is essential if this is to be successful. For an upper abdominal incision the best pain relief is achieved with intercostal nerve blocks. Strong narcotic drugs should be given as needed. Steam inhalation is useful to make the mucus less tenacious.

In severe cases a catheter can be passed into the bronchi, either through the nose or down an endotracheal tube, and the secretions aspirated directly. Failing this, bronchoscopy is indicated.

If the pyrexia persists for more than 48 hours then antibiotic therapy should be instituted to treat secondary infection. In those with no previous chest disease, *Pneumococcus* is the most likely organism and penicillin is a suitable drug (benzyl penicillin 600 mg i.v. or i.m. 6-hourly). In those with chronic chest disease there could be a number of bacteria responsible and ampicillin or co-trimoxazole are suitable.

Inhalation of vomit

This usually occurs in the early postoperative period and may be associated with acute gastric dilatation or a pre-existing hiatus hernia with reflux. Inhalation of vomit causes an aspiration pneumonitis (Mendelson's syndrome). The chemical inflammation causes bronchospasm, pulmonary oedema, and respiratory and circulatory collapse, the extent of which depends on the volume and the acidity of the aspirate.

Recognizing the pattern

There is often a history of unconsciousness, vomiting or difficult intubation. There is progressive deterioration in respiratory function with cyanosis, tachycardia and dyspnoea. There are generalized bronchospasm, poor air entry and diffuse crepitations in the chest. The blood pressure is low and the peripheral vessels are vasoconstricted.

Proving the diagnosis

A chest X-ray shows generalized shadowing in the lungs, particularly at the bases.

Management

1 Oxygen.
2 Bronchodilators (aminophylline 250 mg i.v. given over 5 minutes).
3 Hydrocortisone (100–200 mg i.v.).
4 Intravenous colloid infusions to maintain blood pressure.
5 Antibiotics (ampicillin and flucloxacillin i.v.).
6 Artificial ventilation may be needed if respiratory failure ensues.

Pneumothorax

The condition

Pneumothorax can occur during or after an operation. It can arise:
(a) spontaneously;
(b) due to rupture of the lung occurring during positive pressure ventilation;
(c) following insertion of a central venous pressure line;
(d) if the pleura has been opened accidentally (e.g. in nephrectomy or cervical sympathectomy).
    Spontaneous pneumothorax and tension pneumothorax are described on p. 587.

Recognizing the pattern

The chest on the affected side is immobile and hyperresonant with decreased breath sounds.

Proving the diagnosis

The air in the pleural space is visible on a chest X-ray.

Management
A pneumothorax large enough to impair breathing is treated by chest drainage. The insertion and management of a chest drain is discussed in Section 5.1. Where the pneumothorax is not complicated by the presence of blood or fluid in the chest, a small tube placed anteriorly in the second intercostal space provides a satisfactory method of management. The tube is connected to an underwater seal drain.

1.7   Cardiovascular Complications

Haemorrhage

The condition of postoperative haemorrhage may be:

(a) primary — bleeding at the time of operation from uncontrolled vessels;

(b) reactionary — occurs within 24 hours of operation. This is from uncontrolled vessels after vasospasm relaxes. Such haemorrhage also occurs as the blood pressure rises after recovery from anaesthesia, and with increases in venous pressure on moving and coughing;

(c) secondary — occurs 7–14 days after operation and is due to re-opening of a vessel by separation of the thrombus or to erosion due to infection. Such haemorrhage is often preceded by a 'warning' minor bleed.

Making the diagnosis

The pattern of presentation depends on the rate of bleeding.

Minor bleed

With a slow haemorrhage there will be a tachycardia with mild hypotension made worse by an upright posture. The patient often notices blood in the bed or a blood-soaked dressing.

Major bleed

Acute severe haemorrhage presents as collapse. The patient becomes semiconscious, appearing restless, pale, cold and sweaty. The pulse is weak and there is tachycardia with a low blood pressure and low JVP/CVP (central venous pressure). The patient may become breathless.

Look for external bleeding (e.g. from the wound) or increasing abdominal distension suggesting intra-abdominal haemorrhage. Check whether there is blood issuing from any drains.

Early detection of haemorrhage is important as it significantly reduces morbidity and mortality. Regular reliable observations should be carried out on any patient at risk, half- to one-hourly, for at least 12 hours after an operation.

Management

1 Stop the bleeding. Pressure dressings may help. If the loss is rapid the patient may need to go back to theatre for laparotomy or exploration of the wound. Wound dressings

must be changed regularly as blood-soaked dressings are a good medium for infection.

2 Replace the lost blood volume. Set up as many infusion lines as are required. Normally at least one large one (14- or 16-gauge) is needed. Cross-match some blood urgently. Initial fluid replacement should be with plasma expanders or blood as discussed on pp. 87–9. Give oxygen and ideally catheterize the patient to monitor the urine output.

3 A chronic slower bleed may require blood transfusion over the next 24 hours.

Blood transfusion reactions

The condition

A reaction to blood transfusion is quite common and occurs for a number of reasons. The most serious, though rarest, reaction is that following transfusion of incompatible blood due to an error of identification. This causes intravascular haemolysis with haemoglobinaemia and haemoglobinuria and later circulatory collapse, acute renal failure and jaundice. Disseminated intravascular coagulation and a bleeding tendency can develop.

More commonly, milder reactions occur due to the presence of pyrogens in the donor blood, or recipient antibodies to donor white cells. This results in a mild febrile reaction. Atopic individuals may have antibodies to exogenous antigen, e.g. milk or egg protein present in the donor plasma, which may cause an urticarial reaction. This very occasionally causes acute anaphylactic shock.

Making the diagnosis

A mild pyrexia (37.5–38.0°C) commonly occurs during or within 2 hours of blood transfusion. It is usually harmless, lasting a few hours, and the patient is otherwise well. Sometimes, an itchy urticarial rash may develop. There may be a past history of allergy.

The symptoms and signs of a haemolytic reaction include pain in the transfused limb, constricting pain in the chest, and pain in the loins. On examination there is flushing, pyrexia, rigors, hypotension and bronchospasm. There may be persistent bleeding, and this can be the first indication of incompatible blood transfusion during operation.

Management

The following guidelines may be helpful.

1 Mild pyrexia with no other symptom or signs:
    (a) leave the blood transfusion running;
    (b) watch for any deterioration in the routine observations;
    (c) reassure the patient.

2 Pyrexia with an itchy urticarial rash, no other abnormalities:

(a) slow the transfusion down;

(b) the itching and rash may be relieved by anti-histamine drugs. In an acute situation chlorpheniramine (10 mg i.m.) can be used. If the patient has a past history of repeated urticarial reactions to blood he may be started before transfusion on chlorpheniramine (4 mg orally 8-hourly);

(c) if the rash persists, remove the unit of blood.

3 Patients with more serious symptoms which suggest either a haemolytic reaction or anaphylactic shock:

(a) take the blood and the giving set down. Send it with a fresh sample of the patient's blood and urine to the laboratory for analysis;

(b) give hydrocortisone (200 mg i.v.), adrenalin (1:1000 0.5−1.0 ml s.c./i.v.), aminophylline (250 mg i.v. slowly if bronchospasm is present), and oxygen;

(c) watch the pulse, blood pressure, clotting time and urine output very carefully and treat accordingly.

Overall, if you are in doubt, change the unit being transfused.

Myocardial infarction

The condition
Myocardial infarction may occur after operation. People who have a past history of infarction or angina are particularly at risk.

Recognizing the pattern
The history
The history is of continuous constricting chest pain which may radiate down the arms or into the neck.

On examination
The patient may be pale, cold, sweating and apprehensive. There is a tachycardia and the blood pressure may fall. Listen for a pericardial rub and exclude an arrhythmia or left ventricular failure. The severity of the clinical picture varies widely, however, and there may be very little cardiovascular instability.

Proving the diagnosis
The ECG shows:
(a) ST elevation,
(b) T wave inversion,
(c) Q waves.

Cardiac enzymes are elevated over the next 2 or 3 days as follows:

(a) creatine phosphokinase, Marsh−Bender factor (CPK.MB): up 2−4 hours, maximum 36 hours;
(b) lactate dehydrogenase (LD_1): up 10 hours, maximum 92 hours.

Management

Initial management is analgesia with diamorphine, oxygen and bed rest. Further management is beyond the scope of this book and a textbook of medicine or cardiology should be consulted.

Left ventricular failure

The condition

Left ventricular failure occurs in surgical patients who have been overloaded with fluid, e.g. following intravenous re-hydration or blood transfusion, particularly where there is a past history of heart failure or myocardial ischaemia. When the left ventricle fails the lungs become oedematous and the patient dyspnoeic.

Recognizing the pattern

The history
The patient, who is often elderly, complains of severe shortness of breath. This may come on acutely or slowly, and is worse on lying flat.

On examination
The patient is dyspnoeic, often very distressed, and cyanosed. There is a tachycardia with a triple rhythm, and bilateral fine basal crepitations with or without bronchospasm in the lungs. In the absence of chronic obstructive airways disease, acute bronchospasm in the elderly is often due to pulmonary oedema.

There may also be associated signs of right heart failure, such as a raised JVP, hepatomegaly and peripheral oedema.

Proving the diagnosis

A chest X-ray shows hilar congestion. An ECG must be performed. In severe cases blood-gas measurements are helpful.

Management

Sit the patient up and give oxygen. Intravenous diuretics (e.g. frusemide 80−120 mg) and diamorphine (5−10 mg i.v.) are effective in the acute attack. Aminophylline (250 mg i.v. over 5 minutes) is useful in resistant cases.

Preventative measures are important. The elderly need less fluid and this must be remembered during the adminis-tration of intravenous fluid therapy (see Section 2.1). Blood transfusion should be undertaken with caution and it may be better to use packed cells rather than whole blood. At night the patient should be propped up in bed and aminophylline suppositories may be useful.

Stroke

The condition A stroke is due to intracerebral haemorrhage, thrombosis or embolism with subsequent ischaemia or infarction of cerebral tissue. Preoperative predisposing factors include hypertension and vascular disease. During or after operation severe hypovolaemia may result in intracerebral thrombosis. Emboli may arise from the myocardium, heart valves, great vessels, or carotid and basilar arteries.

Recognizing the pattern The patient usually suffers a sudden collapse and becomes unconscious.

On examination
There may be neurological signs of hemiplegia (e.g. paralysis on one side, up-going plantar responses, difficulties with speech). There may also be evidence of raised intracranial pressure such as a progressively slowing pulse, rising blood pressure and the appearance of papilloedema and pupil dilation.

Proving the diagnosis This is usually made obvious by the neurological deficit. A skull X-ray may also show shift of the pineal gland (if this is calcified).

If there is doubt the diagnosis can be confirmed by a computerized axial tomography (CAT) scan.

Management 1 The initial management is conservative, comprising nursing care particularly of the skin and mouth, catheterization, attention to fluid balance and regular observations to pick up any serious elevation of intracranial pressure.
2 Treat any excessive hypertension.
3 The patient may be referred to the neurologists for further management. They may decide to treat raised intracranial pressure with dexamethasone.
4 Physiotherapy. Most patients who have had a stroke have long-term problems and are going to be dependent on others for some time. Active physiotherapy is important in assisting them to cope with their disabilities.

Deep venous thrombosis

The condition Virchow's triad states that intravascular thrombosis is more likely to occur if the following three conditions are in evidence.

1 Increased coagulability of the blood.

2 Decreased flow in the vessel.

3 Local injury to the intima.

Once a localized thrombus has formed in a vein it may extend proximally and there is a danger that fragments of the clot will break off as emboli.

Thrombo-embolism is particularly common after any surgical procedure since the criteria of the triad are all likely to be fulfilled. There is an increase in blood viscosity after an operation, associated with dehydration and alteration in the serum proteins. The patient is immobile and there may be local injury to vessels while lying on the operating table or during abdominal and pelvic surgery. In addition, there is an increase in blood coagulability following the physiological response to trauma.

The risks are particularly increased by long operations in the pelvic or hip regions. Other risk factors include a past history of deep venous thrombosis or pulmonary embolus, obesity, smoking, carcinomatosis and taking the contraceptive pill.

Common sites of postoperative phlebothrombosis are in the pelvis and in the venous plexus in the soleal muscles of the calf.

Recognizing the pattern

A characteristic sign of venous thrombosis is a persistent tachycardia and a mild 'rumbling' fever. Other signs depend on the site of the thrombus formation.

Pelvic phlebothrombosis is difficult to diagnose. Apart from the systemic signs, there is little to find. There may be some tenderness rectally.

Acute thrombosis of the iliac veins or femoral veins leads to a grossly swollen painful leg. There is localized tenderness over the involved vein. Axillary vein thrombosis similarly presents with marked swelling of the arm.

When thrombosis occurs in the soleal plexus there is tenderness in the soleal muscle, which is swollen and turgid compared with the other side. The enlargement can be measured accurately with a tape measure.

Proving the diagnosis

The diagnosis may be difficult to prove. A number of investigations can be used.

1 Ultrasound examination of the femoral veins may show decreased flow on one side. When the femoral vein is thrombosed, however, the distal leg is almost always grossly swollen and the diagnosis is not difficult to make.

2 ^{131}I-fibrinogen is of value in early deep venous thrombosis

but does not detect thrombi which have formed before the ^{131}I is given.

3 A venogram can demonstrate the presence of thrombus in the deep veins of the leg. This investigation can also cause deep venous thrombosis and it does not demonstrate thrombus in veins that are completely blocked.

Management

1 Anti-coagulation

Any suspicion of venous thrombosis should be treated with anti coagulants unless there is a contraindication. Initial treatment is with heparin. After 5 days anti-coagulation is maintained with warfarin. Suitable regimes are described on p. 107.

When the leg is acutely painful and swollen, the patient should be kept in bed with the leg elevated until the swelling and temperature have settled. Thereafter mobilization should be encouraged as soon as pain allows it. When ambulant, the leg is firmly supported with heavy-duty 'Blue line' elastic stockings.

2 Analgesia

Deep venous thrombosis is frequently very painful and analgesics will be required.

3 Prevention

This is very important. Identify any patient who is at risk (see above). During the operation avoid prolonged calf compression (rest the heels on a pad to elevate the calves; do not lean on the calves). It is also possible to aid venous return by intermittent calf compression with inflatable stockings. Subcutaneous heparin should be given to 'at-risk' patients (5000 units subcutaneously 8-hourly). This is started with the premedication and continued at least until the patient is fully mobile. Passive leg exercises should be encouraged whilst the patient is in bed, and the foot of the bed should be elevated to increase the venous return. Early mobilization should be the rule for all surgical patients.

In certain procedures the surgeon may not wish to give subcutaneous heparin because of the risk of bleeding and you should always check with him before starting therapy.

Dextran 70 may also be used for prophylaxis as it inhibits platelet adherence; 500 cm^3 can be given intravenously during the operation, followed by 500–1000 cm^3 in the next 24 hours.

Pulmonary embolus

The condition Pulmonary embolism occurs when a thrombus from the peripheral venous system becomes detached, passes through the right side of the heart, and impacts in the pulmonary arterial circulation. The consequences depend on the size of the embolus and the site at which it lodges.

A small embolus causes a localized pulmonary infarction and pleurisy if the periphery of the lung is involved. Small emboli may herald larger ones; subsequently repeated small emboli can cause pulmonary hypertension (Fig. 5a).

A large embolus blocks the main pulmonary arteries and thus causes a major block to the whole circulation. The effects are shown in Fig. 5b. There is decreased output from the left ventricle and a rise in venous pressure.

Emboli occur as an implication of deep venous thrombosis

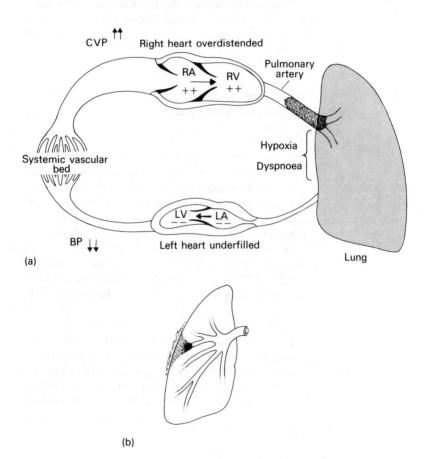

Fig. 5. (a) A minor embolus produces a pulmonary infarct. (b) A major pulmonary embolus affects the whole circulation.

but in 50% of cases the site of the primary problem is not obvious. Indeed, when the site is evident with signs of localized tenderness and swelling, the thrombus is usually adherent to the vein wall and the risk of embolism is smaller.

Minor pulmonary embolus

Recognizing the pattern

A small pulmonary embolus causes pleuritic pain, haemoptysis and breathlessness (the latter because the patient cannot take a deep breath due to the pain).

On examination
There is tachycardia and there may be a pleural rub. Beneath the rub there may be an area of dullness to percussion.

Proving the diagnosis

The symptoms, together with haemoptysis, prove the diagnosis, although the latter may not be apparent in the first day or two.
1 *ECG.* There is no major effect on the circulation and the ECG is usually normal.
2 *Chest X-ray.* In an early case the chest X-ray is normal. However, as the infarct develops a wedge-shaped shadow may appear, extending out to the edge of the lung.
3 *Pulmonary perfusion scan*, see p. 60.

Management

The patient is anti-coagulated with heparin and then warfarin (p. 107). The heparin usually helps to relieve the pain.

Major pulmonary embolus

Recognizing the pattern

The history
A large embolus may cause collapse or sudden death. The patient experiences tight retrosternal chest pain (angina) and becomes acutely dyspnoeic. He or she is often terrified and feels as though death is imminent.

On examination
The acute block in the pulmonary arterial tree causes right ventricular distension and a gallop rhythm is heard over the praecordium. The decreased pulmonary blood flow results in cyanosis, dyspnoea and a low blood pressure. The back pressure behind the right side of the heart is visible as a markedly raised JVP. There is a tachycardia.

Proving the diagnosis

The diagnosis of a large pulmonary embolus rests mainly on the clinical findings. Frequently there is no time to carry out any other investigations apart from an ECG.

1 An *ECG* shows evidence of right ventricular strain with an S wave in lead I, Q wave and inverted T wave in lead III ('S1, Q3, T3').

2 *Blood gases.* The arterial PO_2 is low. The PCO_2 is also lowered due to hyperventilation.

3 *Ventilation perfusion scan.* Ventilation can be investigated by giving the patient radiolabelled xenon to breathe. Perfusion can be investigated using technetium-labelled albumin aggregates. An embolus shows up as an area which is ventilated but not perfused. Areas of consolidation are neither ventilated nor perfused.

4 A *chest X-ray*, like the ventilation scan, shows no abnormality in the presence of an early embolus.

5 *Emergency angiography.* A pulmonary angiogram can be performed by threading a catheter up any peripheral vein. This may show the presence of the clots in the major pulmonary arteries. This confirms the diagnosis and the catheter can be used to infuse thrombolytic agents (see below). Whenever possible this investigation should be done if pulmonary embolectomy is to be carried out.

Management

1 Resuscitation
A large embolus can cause acute circulatory collapse and cardiac arrest. The patient may require intubating and ventilating with oxygen. An intravenous cannula should be inserted to provide a route for drugs. If the patient has a cardiac arrest, efficient heart massage may break up the clot and push it further into the pulmonary tree, thus allowing some circulation to be restored. Immediate embolectomy may be appropriate. This is discussed further below.

2 Analgesia
Heparin is an effective analgesic in pulmonary embolism. It may be dangerous to give any other analgesia because of the risk of exacerbating the hypotension.

3 Anti-coagulation
The patient is heparinized and anti-coagulated as on p. 107.
   If the patient does not improve and cardiac failure persists, further measures to remove the clot are indicated. This may be attempted using thrombolytic agents or by open pulmonary artery embolectomy.

4 Thrombolytic agents
Many emboli can be dissolved by agents such as streptokinase or tissue plasmin activator. Streptokinase may be given by direct infusion into the pulmonary artery or into the systemic

circulation through a peripheral vein. It breaks up the embolus by activating plasminogen. The usual dose is 250 000 units in the first hour, followed by 100 000 units each subsequent hour. It is given either intravenously or into a pulmonary artery catheter. Hydrocortisone is also given (e.g. 100 mg i.v. 4–6 hourly) to prevent any sensitivity reactions. When streptokinase therapy is stopped, heparin must be given to allow plasminogen levels time to return to normal.

Streptokinase therapy is dangerous in patients who are:
(a) within 5 days of a major operation;
(b) within 10 days of a hip replacement;
(c) within 4 weeks of a diagnostic cannulation of a major artery;
(d) hypertensive;
(e) pregnant, within 10 days of delivery, or lactating;
(f) in hepatic or renal failure;
(g) actively bleeding from the bowel or urinary tract.

These patients may be treated by pulmonary embolectomy, but the relative risks will have to be weighed up on an individual basis.

Epsilon aminocaproic acid (EACA) can be used as an antidote for excessive thrombolysis (dose = 6 g i.v. plus 3 g 4–6 hourly).

Tissue plasminogen activator (TPA) has been used successfully in arterial thrombosis and myocardial infarction and may be used for extensive venous thrombosis. It is less allergenic than streptokinase and carries less risk of bleeding since it only binds and dissolves cross-linked fibrin.

5 Pulmonary artery embolectomy

Massive pulmonary emboli can be removed surgically as an emergency. This is only indicated when the patient fails to respond to anti-coagulation or streptokinase therapy, when there is insufficient time to allow streptokinase to work because of the patient's desperate condition, or when streptokinase therapy is considered to be too dangerous.

The operation may be done in one of two ways.

Operation: inflow stasis pulmonary embolectomy

This operation is performed if there are no facilities for cardiopulmonary bypass. The superior and inferior venae cavae are exposed through a midline sternotomy and controlled with tapes. The pulmonary artery is opened and the clot sucked out. The venous inflow can be restored and interrupted several times in order to remove all the emboli.

Codes

Blood	10 units as soon as possible . . . .
GA/LA	GA . . . .
Opn time	1−2 hours . . . .
Stay	Variable . . . .
Drains out	Chest drain 48 hours, pericardial 4−5 days . . . .
Sutures out	7−10 days . . . .
Off work	Variable, 2−3 months . . . .

Operation: cardiopulmonary bypass

This is the safest way to remove major emboli surgically. The sternum is split and the right atrium and aorta cannulated. After cardiopulmonary bypass has been established the pulmonary artery is opened and all clot removed.

Codes

Blood	10 units . . . .
GA/LA	GA . . . .
Opn time	2−4 hours . . . .
Stay	Variable . . . .
Drains out	Chest drain 48 hours, pericardial 4−5 days . . . .
Sutures out	7−10 days . . . .
Off work	Variable, 2−3 months . . . .

1.8   Urinary Complications

Urinary tract infection

The condition   Urinary tract infection is a common complication in the postoperative period. Urinary catheterization is an important predisposing factor, although it can occur following any episode of hypovolaemia, with decreased renal perfusion, low urinary output and urinary stasis. The organism is commonly a Gram-negative bacillus such as *Escherichia coli*.

Recognizing the pattern   Women are more frequently affected than men. The patient complains of frequency and urgency of micturition, and burning dysuria. She is usually pyrexial and this may be the first sign if a catheter is in place. Other symptoms include suprapubic pain and pain in the renal angle due to ascending infection. Advanced infection can result in septicaemia and rigors. The urine looks cloudy and may smell offensive. There may be haematuria.

Proving the diagnosis   The white cell count is elevated with a neutrophil leucocytosis. Microscopic examination of a specimen of urine shows white cells and protein casts. The causative organism may be cultured.

Management   The patient is encouraged to drink as much as possible (e.g. 4–5 litres a day). Antibiotics are commenced once the bacteriological specimen has been taken. The choice of drug is discussed on p. 106. Any indwelling catheter should be removed if this is feasible.

Further investigations, such as an intravenous urogram (IVU) and cystoscopy, are indicated if the infection does not settle or recurs.

Postoperative retention of urine

The condition   This is a common postoperative problem and the most frequent cause of oliguria following surgery. The patient finds it difficult to initiate micturition while under the influence of drugs, in strange surroundings, when movements are painful, and when he is immobilized in bed. Benign prostatic hypertrophy is an important predisposing cause, although postoperative urinary retention also occurs in women. Patients at risk should be recognized during the

63

initial clerking. Other causes of acute retention are mentioned on p. 430.

Making the diagnosis

The patient in classical acute retention is anuric and in great discomfort with an intense desire to micturate. The bladder is palpable as a tender mass arising out of the pelvis.

This classic picture is not, however, always present and the condition can be difficult to diagnose. The patient may not be anuric. In acute retention with overflow the patient produces urine but the amounts are small (50–100 cm^3) and passed very frequently. This pattern, recorded on the fluid chart, should alert you to the possible diagnosis. An abdominal incision covered with dressings may make it impossible to palpate the enlarged bladder and thus obscure the cause of pain. Suprapubic dullness to percussion can be a useful sign in these circumstances. Finally patients with chronic retention may not be in any discomfort, but have a distended bladder and frequency.

Proving the diagnosis

The diagnosis is proved by passing a urethral catheter and releasing a large volume of urine (more than 500 cm^3 in an adult). Very occasionally an ultrasound examination can be helpful to define the enlarged bladder.

Patients at risk should not be subjected to continual questions about whether they have passed urine or not. Privacy, reassurance and adequate analgesia are helpful. If retention is developing, a tranquillizer (such as diazepam 5–10 mg i.m.) can be useful and conservative measures, such as sitting in a hot bath, and allowing the patient to sit out on the toilet, should be tried.

There are two indications for catheterization.

1 The patient is in pain from the distended bladder and demands relief.

2 There is doubt about the diagnosis and renal failure must be excluded.

In other circumstances it is always worth waiting for the patient to pass urine naturally.

The method of passing a urethral or suprapubic catheter is described on pp. 431–432. If there is very little urine in the bladder and adequate amounts are not produced after catheterization, the patient may be in renal failure and should be managed accordingly (see below).

Patients who have been in retention should have the catheter removed after 24–48 hours. In elderly males, if two trials of catheter removal are unsuccessful, the patient should be considered for a prostatectomy (pp. 435–439).

Postoperative renal failure

Failure to produce urine after an operation, once obstruction has been excluded, may be due to prerenal failure (see Fig. 6).

Prerenal failure

The condition

The blood supply to the kidneys may become inadequate postoperatively due to dehydration, blood loss or systemic hypotension. These causes are reversible, but if they are not dealt with early the condition may progress to acute renal failure.

Making the diagnosis

Having established that the urine output is inadequate, the diagnosis of prerenal failure is made by finding concentrated urine and signs of a cause.

Examine the patient looking for hypotension, dehydration (dry tongue, skin turgor) or cardiac failure (JVP, CVP). Assess the peripheral perfusion (warm or cold hands?).

Inspect the charts, looking for a negative fluid balance, and check whether there has been any excess blood loss or a period of hypotension.

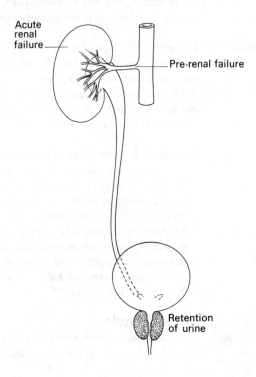

Acute renal failure

Pre-renal failure

Retention of urine

Fig. 6. Causes of oliguria/anuria.

Test the urine. If renal function is normal it will be very concentrated (specific gravity over 1020).

Management

Insert a CVP line (p. 94). Replace fluid with saline, blood or plasma until the CVP is at the upper range of normal. This may restore urine production. If not, and the patient is no longer hypovolaemic, a large bolus of frusemide (250–500 mg i.v.) may be effective. If there is still no urine, treat as acute renal failure.

Acute renal failure

In a surgical patient this usually follows a period of renal hypoperfusion (prerenal failure) as above. It can also be a complication of incompatible blood transfusion, extensive trauma or drug therapy. The condition is associated with acute necrosis of the renal tubules.

Making the diagnosis

The diagnosis is made after catheterization has excluded retention, and careful fluid status assessment and correction have excluded renal hypoperfusion. If there is still less than 500 cm^3 of urine output in the day, acute tubular necrosis has occurred. This may be confirmed by measuring urine and plasma osmolarities and finding a ratio of less than 1:1.

Management

1 Provided any hypovolaemia has been corrected, a large bolus of frusemide (e.g. 250–500 mg i.v.) should be given and may restart urine production.
2 The management of established renal failure is complex and best described in medical textbooks. It includes:
(a) restricted fluid intake: 500 cm^3 a day plus any fluid losses;
(b) restricted protein intake (less than 20 g/day);
(c) adequate carbohydrate intake (3000 kcal/day);
(d) daily assessment of blood and urinary electrolytes and adjustment of electrolyte intake accordingly. Sodium losses are replaced but potassium is not given;
(e) peritoneal dialysis or haemodialysis if necessary. Peritoneal dialysis can be used in a patient who has had laparotomy from about 4 or 5 days after the wound has been closed. Continuous haemofiltration is preferred in the intensively ill patient.

Urinary fistula

The condition

This either follows breakdown of a urinary tract anastomosis or accidental damage to the ureters during operation.

Making the diagnosis	The condition presents with an increased discharge through the wound or drain site. This has the characteristic appearance and smell of urine. There is less constitutional upset than with an intestinal fistula.
Proving the diagnosis	The urea content of the fluid is high (like urine) and above the level of the patient's serum urea. If further proof is necessary it can be obtained by giving an intravenous injection of indigo carmine, which is excreted by the kidney and will appear through the fistula.
Management	Urinary fistulae will close spontaneously (like bowel fistulae, p. 75) providing there is no distal obstruction. Such closure may take several weeks. The presence or absence of distal obstruction can be ascertained by performing a 'fistulogram'.

If the fistula fails to heal, operation is needed and the precise nature of this depends on the site of the fistula. Free distal urinary drainage must always, however, be established.

1.9 Infections, Abscesses and Fistulae (Fig. 7)

Wound infection

The condition

Infection still complicates about 2% of surgical incisions, depending on the type of procedures being performed. A wide variety of organisms (*Staphylococcus*, coliforms, streptococci, including *Streptococcus milleri*, *Bacteroides* and anaerobes) are involved.

Predisposing factors

1 Preoperative:
  (a) malnutrition;
  (b) diabetes;
  (c) carcinomatosis;
  (d) infection near the site of incision;
  (e) steroid therapy.
2 Operative:
  (a) contamination of the wound with faeces, pus, etc.;
  (b) infection from staff instruments or airborne agents;
  (c) poor surgical technique, e.g. haematoma formation, or too tight suturing causing tissue necrosis.
3 Postoperative: infection on the ward (either from the patient himself, other patients or the staff).

Making the diagnosis

There is a history of increasing pain and tenderness in the wound.

On examination the patient has a climbing, swinging pyrexia with localized tenderness in the wound, which is also swollen, hot and red. There may be fluctuation on palpation or pus may discharge.

Proving the diagnosis

1 White cell count. This will be elevated in active infection.
2 A specimen of pus must be sent to microbiology for culture.

Management

1 The collection should be drained. Remove some of the stitches and probe the wound to let out all the pus.
2 The wound is dressed daily, or more frequently if dressings become saturated. The wound is not resutured but left to heal by secondary intention.
3 Analgesia.
4 If the patient has systemic illness or spreading cellulitis, then antibiotics should be given.

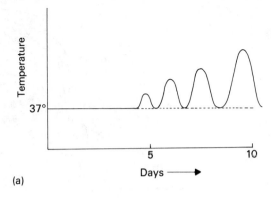

(a)

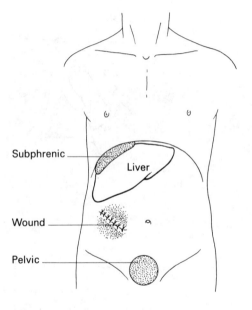

Subphrenic

Liver

Wound

Pelvic

(b)

Fig. 7. (a) Postoperative sepsis. (b) Sites of postoperative abdominal sepsis.

Wound dehiscence

The condition
Breakdown of the wound may be either partial or complete (see Fig. 8). In partial breakdown the skin closure holds, but breakdown of the muscle layers gives rise to an incisional hernia later. In complete dehiscence the abdominal incision bursts open to reveal bowel. The aetiology is similar to that for wound infection. Exacerbating factors include obesity,

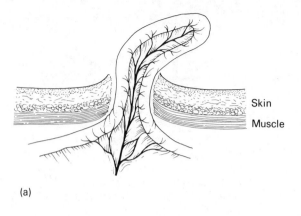

(a)

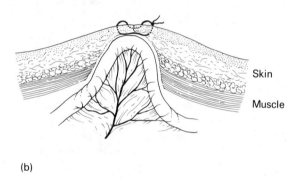

(b)

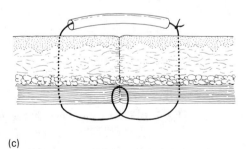

(c)

Fig. 8. (a) Complete wound dehiscence. (b) Incomplete wound
dehiscence. (c) Figure-of-eight suture.

raised intra-abdominal pressure (from coughing, difficulty
in passing urine or constipation), ascites draining through
the wound, wound infection and haematoma. However,
most wound dehiscences are due to faulty technique. Factors
include pulling the sutures too tight, inserting sutures too

close to the edge of the muscle, and insecure knots. Wound dehiscence is much less common since deep-tension, one-layer, monofilament-suture techniques have been used.

Making the diagnosis	This occurs typically 4−10 days after operation. The patient may feel something 'give' in the wound. There is a sudden increase in pain and a pink fluid discharge from the wound. In complete dehiscence there is protrusion of loops of bowel. The patient becomes shocked and distressed.
Management	1 Lie the patient down and give reassurance. 2 Strong opiate analgesia is required. 3 Cover the wound with a sterile pack soaked in warm saline. 4 The wound requires urgent resuture in theatre with deep-tension sutures.

Operation: resuture of abdominal wound
The dressings and sutures are removed and the whole wound is re-opened. All the muscle layer sutures are taken out. A laparotomy is performed and any intraperitoneal pus is removed. Bacteriological specimens are collected for aerobic and anaerobic culture. The abdomen is then closed in one layer with deep-tension figure-of-eight sutures tied over either gauze or rubber to prevent them cutting into the skin (see Fig. 8c). The subcutaneous layer is usually drained.

Codes

Blood	0 ....
GA/LA	GA ....
Opn time	1 hour.........................
Stay	2 weeks or more.................
Drains out	3−5 days ....
Sutures out	14−21 days ....
Off work........	6 weeks........................

Postoperative care
The sutures are left in place for at least 14 days. The wound tends to discharge and may require regular dressing. Antibiotics should be started at the operation and continued until the wound is healed. They can be modified according to the results of the culture.

Infected intravenous drip site
A drip site may become infected and is one of the causes of postoperative pyrexia. The organism is often a *Staphylococcus* or *Streptococcus*.

Recognizing the pattern	*The patient* The patient complains of pain in the limb that is being infused. The intravenous infusion usually slows or stops completely. *On examination* The patient is pyrexial and the involved skin is red, swollen and tender. There may be spreading cellulitis over the vein proximally, and even pus around the entry of the cannula. Regional lymph nodes may become enlarged tender and inflamed.
Management	The cannula must be removed and the tip cultured. If the infusion is still required, re-site the drip in the other arm. Flucloxacillin is given. Systemic analgesia is often needed and a poultice applied to the inflamed vein is comforting.

Subphrenic abscess

The condition	A subphrenic abscess commonly follows generalized peritonitis, particularly after acute appendicitis or a perforated peptic ulcer. It may also occur through infection of a haematoma after an operation such as splenectomy. Such abscesses are commonly just underneath the hemi-diaphragm but may also occur beneath the liver in the lesser sac or in the hepato-renal pouch.
Recognizing the pattern	*The patient* The patient initially recovers from the operation and then 7–21 days later develops a swinging fever and general malaise, nausea and loss of weight. He may complain of pain in the upper abdomen which can radiate to the shoulder tip. He may also become breathless due to a pleural effusion above the abscess or collapse of the lower lobe of one lung. *On examination* There is a swinging pyrexia for which no obvious cause is found. Occasionally, there may be tenderness or even oedema in the abdominal wall in the subcostal region. The liver may be displaced downwards and there may be physical signs of a pleural effusion or collapse of the lung.
Proving the diagnosis	The old aphorism 'pus somewhere, pus nowhere else, pus under the diaphragm' is a useful reminder of the possibility of a subphrenic abscess. The presenting symptoms and signs do not always suggest this possibility. Investigations which can be helpful are as follows. 1 Ultrasound is effective in localizing the collection of pus.

2 White cell count. There is typically polymorphonuclear leucocytosis of around 20 000.

3 Chest X-ray and screening of the diaphragm. A chest X-ray shows a high diaphragm on the affected side. There may be a gas space and fluid level beneath it. There may also be pleural effusion. Movements of the diaphragm can also be screened in the X-ray department using an image intensifier. There is diminished movement of the diaphragm over the abscess.

Management

1 The best management is to drain the abscess. This may be done percutaneously under ultrasound control or by open operation. The former can be very effective, but if adequate drainage is not established operation is indicated. Before this is done the abscess should be localized as accurately as possible, as this will affect the incision which should be used.

2 An early subphrenic abscess with no air or fluid level may be treated with broad-spectrum antibiotics (e.g. gentamicin, benzylpenicillin and metronidazole). Such treatment not infrequently leads to gradual resolution of the abscess. If the patient remains toxic and ill, however, for more than 5 days, conservative management should be abandoned and the abscess drained. Gentamicin levels should be measured twice weekly. Reduce the dose in renal impairment.

Operation: drainage of subphrenic abscess
The abscess may be approached by a posterior or anterior route.

1 Posterior approach
The patient is positioned lying on his side with the abscess uppermost. The twelfth rib is removed and the subhepatic space or subphrenic space approached retroperitoneally. When the abscess is encountered it is opened and drained in the most dependent direction.

2 Anterior approach
The abdomen is opened through a subcostal incision and the abscess approached extraperitoneally and drained.

Once the abscess has been opened, covering antibiotics can be given, although they are not essential. Large abscess cavities are usually drained using a large red rubber tube drain to encourage track formation.

Codes
Blood . . . .   0 . . . .
GA/LA . . . .   GA . . . .

Opn time	1 hour...........................
Stay	1–2 weeks ....
Drains out	10–14 days ....
Sutures out	7 days ....
Off work........	4 weeks........................

Postoperative care

If the abscess is large, sinograms may be performed down the drain after 10 days and the progress of the cavity followed. The drain can then be gradually withdrawn as the abscess heals up behind it.

Hepatic abscess

The condition

This often occurs as metastatic infection from intraperitoneal sepsis, usually in a debilitated patient. The incidence is low since antibiotic treatment was introduced. The more common causes of hepatic abscesses include appendicitis, diverticular disease, ulcerative colitis and ascending cholangitis.

Recognizing the pattern

The patient is usually very ill with a high swinging fever and rigors. He may complain of right upper quadrant pain and develop mild jaundice. The liver may be enlarged and tender.

Proving the diagnosis

1 The white cell count is raised.
2 Liver function tests are abnormal. In particular the alanine transaminase (ALT) is raised.
3 The abscess cavity may be demonstrated on ultrasound.
4 A liver scan will show an hepatic abscess if this is over 2 cm in diameter.
5 An erect chest X-ray shows a high right diaphragm and fluid in the pleura above it.
6 Blood cultures may occasionally be positive.

Management

The patient should be given broad-spectrum antibiotics and the abscess drained as soon as it is localized. This may be done percutaneously under ultrasound or CAT scan control, or by open operation.

Operation: drainage of hepatic abscess

The abscess is usually approached through an extrahepatic route over the right lobe of the liver. As the abscess is approached, oedema and fibrosis are encountered and this may be broken into, opening up the cavity in the liver. A red rubber drain is inserted.

Codes

Blood	2–4 units	
GA/LA	GA	
Opn time	1 hour	
Stay	14–21 days	
Drains out	10–21 days	
Sutures out	7 days	
Off work	6–12 weeks	

Postoperative care

The postoperative care is similar to that described above for a subphrenic abscess.

Pelvic abscess

The condition

This is an abscess in the rectovesical pouch commonly following peritonitis, e.g. after a pelvic appendicitis or colonic perforation. Infection of a pelvic haematoma following poor haemostasis is another common cause.

Making the diagnosis

A patient who has had generalized peritonitis becomes unwell with pyrexia and malaise 4–10 days postoperatively. There may be a history of mucus discharged per rectum. The abscess may rupture through the rectum or vagina.

On examination the patient has a swinging pyrexia, and rectal or vaginal examination may reveal a palpable mass which may be pointing and may indeed burst on examination.

Management

Daily rectal examinations should be performed to monitor the progress of the developing abscess. The abscess may point up into the wound or down into the rectum. When a fluctuant area is felt in the rectum it can be broken into with a finger under a short general anaesthetic. If the patient has systemic symptoms antibiotics may be given but these delay the ripening and discharge of the abscess. Premature attempts to drain the abscess through the rectum may damage adjacent loops of bowel, leading to fistula formation. An alternative route for drainage in women is through the posterior fornix of the vagina.

External intestinal fistula

The condition

This is a communication between the bowel lumen and the body surface. It develops postoperatively due to the following factors.

1 Disruption of a bowel anastomosis (due to tension, ischaemia, infection or distal obstruction).

2 Inclusion of the bowel when suturing the abdominal wall.

3 Erosion of the bowel by an abdominal drain.

4 Perforation of ischaemic bowel (e.g. due to damage to the mesentery at operation or after strangulation in a hernia).

Making the diagnosis

Five to ten days after operation there is an increased discharge through the wound or down a drain which becomes faecal and offensive. Persistent discharge causes general malaise, dehydration, hypoproteinaemia and weight loss. If the track is not completely walled off generalized peritonitis may occur.

Proving the diagnosis

The presence of a fistula can be demonstrated by ingestion of methylene blue dye, Ribena or blackcurrant juice, which will be revealed in the discharge from the fistula a few hours later. Barium studies are also helpful.

Management

Fistulae tend to heal spontaneously providing there is no distal obstruction and providing the patient can be kept in positive nitrogen balance. Healing usually takes 3−6 weeks. A fistula will not heal under the conditions listed below.
1 The tract becomes epithelialized.
2 There is obstruction beyond the fistula site.
3 In the presence of persistent infection (e.g. TB, a foreign body, Crohn's disease, actinomycosis).
4 In the presence of malignant disease along the tract.

In the absence of these problems, conservative management should be followed.
1 Protect the skin from auto-digestion (especially with a high intestinal or pancreatic fistula). This can be achieved by covering the surrounding skin with karaya gum ('stom-adhesive') and attaching an ileostomy bag to the fistulous opening.
2 Parenteral nutrition. This has transformed the management of intestinal fistulae. When a fistula is diagnosed a central venous line should be set up in almost all instances. Oral feeding can then be restricted and the patient's nutritional state maintained until the fistula heals (see p. 96).
3 Adequate fluid and electrolyte replacement of the volume lost down the fistulous track must be given. Daily electrolyte estimations should be performed.
4 Surgical closure may be required if the fistula fails to close off with the above conservative treatment. In that case it will be necessary to excise the fistulous track and deal with any obstruction or other cause of failure to heal.

Operation: excision of fistula

The skin is incised around the external opening and the track dissected out and removed. Any obstructive lesion must be dealt with. The defect in the bowel is oversewn and the abdominal wall closed. A drain is put down to the fistula site. In the presence of persistent peritonitis it may be safer to bring out the bowel opening as an ileostomy (to be closed later). A repair of a large bowel fistula may need covering with a proximal colostomy.

Codes

Blood	2 units ....
GA/LA	GA ....
Opn time	1−2 hours ....
Stay	10−14 days ....
Drains out	Wound drain and intra-abdominal drain 7−10 days ....
Sutures out	7−10 days ....
Off work........	4−6 weeks ....

Bed sores

Bed sores occur over pressure areas in patients who are immobilized in bed for a long period. Five factors play a part: pressure, moisture, anaemia, malnutrition and injury.

Making the diagnosis

The area initially becomes erythematous and does not blanch on pressure. The skin then ulcerates and may become secondarily infected.

Management

Bed sores are avoided by good nursing care with regular attention to pressure areas and regular turning in bed. The patient should not be allowed to lie on damp sheets. Sheepskin pads under the heels and sacrum help. Patients who are going to be immobilized for a long period of time should be nursed on a water bed or ripple mattress.

For established bed sores, avoid pressure on the area. Regular gentle massage to the surrounding skin is necessary. Infra-red therapy may help. Keep the area dry either with dressings or by leaving the wound open to the air. Antibiotics are required if there is spreading cellulitis or systemic illness and the patient must be mobilized as soon as possible.

Extensive chronic bed sores may require excision and rotational skin grafting.

Septicaemia

The condition

This is an overwhelming infection spreading from the primary source into the bloodstream due to Gram-negative organisms, staphylococci or streptococci. Gram-negative septicaemia is common after biliary or urological surgery.

Recognizing the pattern

The patient is collapsed with a pyrexia (39–40 °C), a tachycardia and a normal or low blood pressure. The extremities are initially warm due to vasodilation, but may later become cold due to hypoperfusion. The patient may have rigors. Look for a cause. Inspect the urine; is it cloudy and thick? Examine the chest and abdomen; is there a CVP line that may be infected?

Proving the diagnosis

1 Blood cultures. Take two specimens of blood each of 10–20 ml minimum, from different sites. Inoculate the culture set provided (which may contain identifiable aerobic and anaerobic bottles). The blood should be taken using a strict aseptic technique. The forearm vein should first be identified and the skin then cleansed. The site of the venepuncture should not be contaminated again after this. The tops of the bottles should be cleaned unless they are already sterile. If the vein is not clearly visible, a heat-sensitive strip which changes colour over the vein may be useful. Otherwise use sterile gloves if further palpation is needed.

The blood collected is injected into the anaerobic bottle first. As the injection is made, avoid introducing any bubbles into the syringe. At this point you can also check that there is a good vacuum. The needles should not be changed unless a re-sheathing protector is available (because of the risk of needle stick injury). The aerobic bottle is injected. Specimens should be sent to the laboratory as soon as possible for incubation.

2 Other microbiology samples should be sent depending on the suspected site of infection.

3 If there is a CVP line in use and it is suspected that this is the source of the infection, it should be removed and the tip cultured. Re-site it if required.

4 Perform a white cell count.

Management

1 Intravenous antibiotics. These must be started immediately after the blood cultures have been taken. The choice depends on the sort of surgery which has been undertaken. For gut-related septicaemia penicillin, gentamicin and metronidazole or a cephalosporin and metronidazole provide broad cover. For urological surgery the metronidazole is unnecessary. If staphyloccocal sepsis is likely, flucloxacillin should be substituted for penicillin (or vancomycin if methicillin-resistant *Staphylococcus aureus* (MRSA) is locally common). Cephalosporins cover ordinary staphylococci but not MRSA. The initial antibiotics are modified when the sensitivities of the organism are known.

2 Intravenous support of the circulation. In severe cases a CVP line is used to monitor this.

3 Watch the urine output. The patient should be catheterized.

4 It is well worth while discussing the case with the microbiologists, particularly if the origin of the organism found is not known.

5 Treat the cause of the septicaemia as required.

1.10　The Intensive Care Unit

The houseman's role in the intensive care unit (ICU)

Intensive care units (ICU) are designed to look after the very ill. The department is often organized by the anaesthetic department, and run by senior specialized nursing staff.

The care of the patient is undertaken jointly by the surgeon and the intensive care staff, but the ultimate responsibility for a surgical patient normally resides with the consultant surgeon. In the intensive care unit the house-surgeon's role is to act as a co-ordinator and to monitor all aspects of patient care, making sure that nothing is left out. Although most of the management decisions are made by others, it is important to keep everybody in touch with events and to keep up to date with the patient's progress yourself.

The intensive care unit often seems very impersonal, with a large part of the management based on observation charts, results and machinery. In the midst of all this do not forget to examine the patient. Also remember that even if patients cannot speak (because they are intubated) they may well be able to see and hear all that is going on. Make sure you keep them fully informed about how they are progressing and avoid discussion or teaching within earshot.

The ICU chart

The information and observations about each patient are usually recorded on a large chart (see Fig. 9) and you should rapidly make yourself familiar with the layout of the one used in your hospital. It is usually divided up into sections covering circulation and respiration, neurological observations, and fluid balance.

Daily management of patients on ICU

1　The chart

Inspect the chart, thinking in terms of systems.

(a) *Circulation*. Are the pulse, blood pressure and CVP stable and, if not, why not? Has there been any response to therapy given in the last 24 hours?

(b) *Respiration*. If the patient is on a ventilator, the tidal volume, minute volume, respiratory rate and ventilator pressure are recorded. Check the blood gases. These will

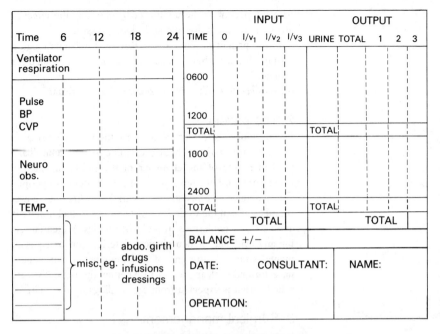

Time	6	12	18	24	TIME	0	l/v_1	l/v_2	l/v_3	URINE	TOTAL	1	2	3
							INPUT				OUTPUT			
Ventilator respiration					0600									
Pulse BP CVP					1200									
					TOTAL					TOTAL				
Neuro obs.					1800									
					2400									
TEMP.					TOTAL					TOTAL				
					TOTAL						TOTAL			
	misc. eg.	abdo. girth drugs infusions dressings			BALANCE +/−									
					DATE: CONSULTANT: NAME:									
					OPERATION:									

Fig. 9. The type of chart used in the intensive care unit.

give an indication of whether or not the ventilation is satisfactory. The anaesthetist usually makes decisions about this but you should keep yourself in the picture. The blood gases are usually recorded separately on the result sheet.

(c) *Fluid balance.* Check the total input versus the total output in the last 24 hours. If there has been excessive loss, is this being replaced? Is the urine output adequate? A patient in intensive care should produce at least $0.5 \text{ cm}^3/\text{kg}$ body weight/hour ($35 \text{ cm}^3/\text{hour}$ for a 70 kg patient) and preferably $2-3$ times this volume.

(d) *Intravenous regimen.* Has it been written up for the next 24 hours and does it need adjusting according to the fluid balance?

(e) *Investigations.* Check the day's result, particularly the urea and electrolytes, the haemoglobin and the most recent chest X-ray. The intravenous chart may well need further adjustment after looking at the electrolytes. Check the serum albumin; low values cause fall in oncotic pressure and predispose to pulmonary oedema.

Check whether the patient's blood clotting studies and platelet numbers are satisfactory.

(f) *Drug treatment.* Review the analgesia given and ascertain whether it has been satisfactory either by communicating with the patient or the nurses, or by checking the effect of analgesia on the pulse rate and blood pressure.

Is the patient on antibiotics? Review any bacteriological results. Should they be started, stopped, continued or changed?

(g) *Temperature.* What is the source of any pyrexia?

2 The patient

Having looked at the chart to assess the patient's progress over the previous 24 hours, examine the patient. Take particular note of the character of the pulse, the jugular venous pressure, the lung bases, and any evidence of peripheral oedema. Note his state of hydration. Check for bowel sounds and that the wound is satisfactory, and feel if there is any localized tenderness in the calf muscles. Watch closely for any evidence of neurological deterioration or signs of mental strain. At the end of this examination you should have formed a clear idea as to whether the patient's state reflects what is expected from the readings on the chart.

3 Surgical management

Keep a close eye on the following:

(a) wound dressings;

(b) abdominal or wound drains;

(c) stitches; when should they be removed (these tend to be forgotten in intensive care)?

(d) state of postoperative ileus.

As the patient recovers he should generally be moved off the intensive care unit as soon as it is practicable. Patients get little rest while being intensively cared for and the mental strain is considerable. Make sure a bed is being kept somewhere for the patient to return to in the general ward.

If there is one overriding rule, it is to keep in constant liaison with the intensive care registrar and, through him, to keep the rest of your team informed.

2 Prescriptions and Other Tasks

2.1 Management of intravenous fluids
Normal daily requirements
Common crystalloid preparations
Other types of intravenous fluid
Prescribing the daily requirement
Modified requirements
Monitoring the effect of therapy
Central venous pressure (CVP)
Intravenous feeding

2.2 Prescribing drugs for surgical patients
How to write a prescription
Drug management
Analgesics
Hypnotics and sedatives
Antibiotics
Anti-coagulants
Bowel preparation

2.3 Sutures and drains
Sutures
Needles
Drains

2.4 Relatives, discharges, deaths and documents
Dealing with relatives
Patient discharge
Dealing with death
Confirming death
Death certificates, the coroner and cremation forms
Other medical certificates and legal statements
Surgical audit

2.1 Management of Intravenous Fluids

The indications for setting up an intravenous infusion in a surgical patient are as follows.

1 To give the normal fluid and electrolyte requirement in a postoperative patient who is unable to drink.
2 To replace abnormal losses, e.g. haemorrhage or vomiting.
3 As a route for intravenous drugs.
4 To give parenteral feeding.

Normal daily requirements (Fig. 10)
The normal fluid requirement for an adult has to replace:
(a) the 'insensible' loss of water in faeces and from the lungs — about 500 cm^3;
(b) urinary output — about 1000 cm^3;
(c) insensible loss from the skin plus perspiration — 500–3000 cm^3 depending on the patient's temperature and environmental conditions.

A suitable basic intravenous regime for a fit 70 kg adult is:
water   3 litres
sodium   100 mmol
potassium   60 mmol

A useful approximation which can be remembered and used to check the fluid intake against body weight is:
40 ml fluid/kg adult body weight (babies need more, old people less)
2 mmol sodium/kg
1 mmol potassium/kg

The diagrams in this section will illustrate the contents of a litre unit.

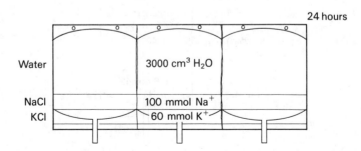

Fig. 10. Daily requirements for water, sodium and potassium ions.

The daily intake can be presented in a variety of ways using the commonly available crystalloid preparations.

Common crystalloid preparations

These are solutions of electrolytes in water. They disperse throughout the extracellular fluid space and are not confined to the circulation. They are dispensed in 500 or 1000 cm^3 units.

Normal saline (0.9% = isotonic)

The contents are shown in Fig. 11.

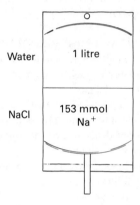

Fig. 11. 1 litre of normal saline.

Dextrose saline (4% dextrose + 0.18% saline)

The contents are shown in Fig. 12.

N.B. Some bags of 'dextrose saline' are in fact 0.9% saline with 5% dextrose (Fig. 13), which is hyperosmolar. Be

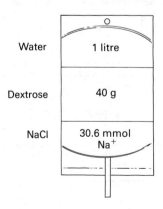

Fig. 12. 1 litre of 4% dextrose, 0.18% saline.

aware of this and prescribe the percentage clearly on the fluid chart.

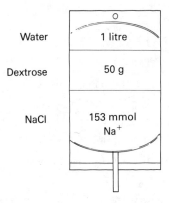

Fig. 13. 1 litre of 5% dextrose, 9% saline.

5% dextrose

The contents of 1 litre are shown in Fig. 14.
N.B. This is effectively water, i.e. volume replacement only. Any of these fluids may have potassium added, either in 10 mmol batches of KCl or 1 g batches of KCl (1 g = 13.4 mmol).

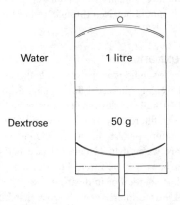

Fig. 14. 1 litre of 5% dextrose.

Hartmann's solution (Fig. 15)

This is more 'Physiological' and contains potassium, calcium and bicarbonate as well as sodium chloride.

Other types of intravenous fluid

Colloid solutions stay in the blood circulation and increase blood volume by both the added volume of fluid and the

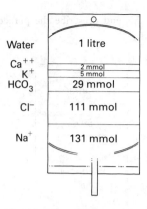

Water	1 litre
Ca^{++}	2 mmol
K^+	5 mmol
HCO_3	29 mmol
Cl^-	111 mmol
Na^+	131 mmol

Fig. 15. 1 litre of Hartmann's solution.

increase in colloid osmotic pressure drawing fluid into the circulation from the tissues. They are, therefore, useful for the maintenance of blood volume, though obviously, apart from blood, they have no oxygen-carrying capacity.

Plasma protein fraction

This is a 5% solution of protein containing 88% albumin. One litre contains 145 mmol Na^+ and 0.25 mmol K^+.

It should be given through a filter but carries no hepatitis risk.

Dextran

These solutions are polymers of glucose of different molecular weights, the usual fluids being dextran 40 (average mol. wt 40 000) and dextran 70 (average mol. wt 70 000). Dextran 40 is filtered by the kidney but dextran 70 is not and therefore persists in the circulation longer. Dextran binds more water than Haemaccel (see below) and anaphylactic reactions may be rarer. The dextran is presented either in saline solution or in dextrose.

Dextran interferes with cross-matching of blood once in the circulation, and therefore any serum for cross-matching should be taken before the infusion is started.

Haemaccel

Haemaccel is a solution of partially degraded gelatin (Fig. 16).

This has a half-life in the circulation of 3−4 hours and a lower water binding capacity than dextran 70. It may also be more likely to cause an anaphylactic reaction.

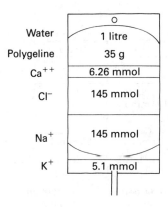

	O
Water	1 litre
Polygeline	35 g
Ca^{++}	6.26 mmol
Cl^-	145 mmol
Na^+	145 mmol
K^+	5.1 mmol

Fig. 16. 1 litre haemaccel.

Blood

This is used to replace blood lost. Whole blood may be used or the volume may be reduced by infusing packed red cells. The latter are useful for treating elderly anaemic patients.

Blood contains sodium and potassium. If large amounts of blood are transfused quickly it is important to watch the serum potassium, which may become elevated causing acidosis. The serum calcium also becomes depressed due to the infusion of excess citrate in the stored blood. Finally, the clotting factors are diluted by large transfusions of stored blood and should be assessed after such therapy.

Prescribing the daily requirement

This is usually given in one of two regimes, A or B.

Regime A (Fig. 17)

This gives the patient some energy in the form of dextrose: two litres of 5% dextrose solution = 100 g of dextrose, which yields 400 kcal. Although this is insufficient for energy requirements postoperatively, it is all right in the short term as the body utilizes endogenous stores. However, should the patient be off oral fluids for more than 4−5 days, intravenous nutrition must be considered (see below).

Regime B (Fig. 18)

An alternative regime gives the patient 3 litres a day, 90 mmol of sodium and 60 mmol of potassium and 120 g of dextrose. As can be seen, this is not quite enough to meet the sodium requirements although in the short term this may not matter as the kidney has good powers of conservation.

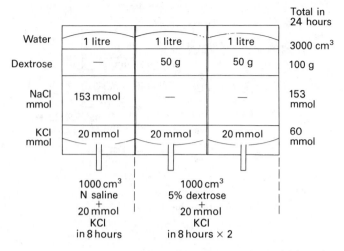

Fig. 17. Regime A: 2 litres of 5% dextrose saline and 1 litre of normal saline in 24 hours.

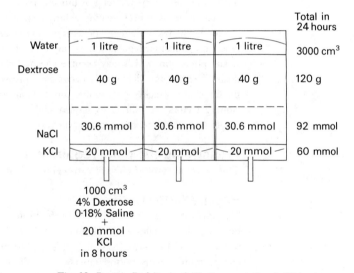

Fig. 18. Regime B: 3 litres of 4% dextrose saline in 24 hours.

Modified requirements

In certain circumstances the above basic regimes have to be modified and this is done to give one of the following:

1 Less fluid in 24 hours.
2 More fluid in 24 hours.
3 More sodium chloride.

4 More potassium.
5 Intensive therapy.

1 Less fluid

In the first 24 hours postoperatively the metabolic response to the trauma of surgery causes increased aldosterone and increased antidiuretic hormone release. This causes both salt and water retention and because of this some surgeons or anaesthetists prefer to give less fluid and no salt in the first 24 hours, e.g.

Prescription   5% dextrose 1 litre 12-hourly (Fig. 19).

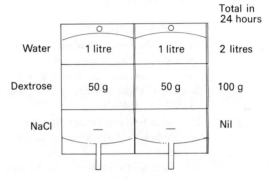

			Total in 24 hours
Water	1 litre	1 litre	2 litres
Dextrose	50 g	50 g	100 g
NaCl	—	—	Nil

Fig. 19. 5% dextrose 1 litre 12-hourly.

This is then followed by regime A or B (above) on day 2.

A lower fluid intake may also be indicated in patients with renal failure or cardiac failure, and also in small patients (including children). In that case the total volume to be given in 24 hours is decided and then prescribed in 500 cm^3 units. It is then necessary to check the overall salt and potassium load and adjust it according to requirements.

Example. To give 2 litres in 24 hours prescribe 500 cm^3 every 6 hours. If dextrose saline only is used, 60 mmol of sodium will be given during the day. This may not be enough and extra sodium and chloride may be given by substituting 500 cm^3 of normal saline for 500 cm^3 of dextrose saline. Potassium could also be added to each unit as required.

2 Extra fluid

Extra water is required when the patient is pyrexial, when the weather is hot and dry, or when the patient is dehydrated. An intake per day of 3000 cm^3 does cover some increased losses as commonly required by postoperative patients. If more is required it is simply necessary to increase the rate at which each litre is given (e.g. 1 litre every 6 hours = a total of 4 litres/day). It is then necessary to recalculate the salt and potassium being given and modify this accordingly. Less salt is given by substituting 5% dextrose for units containing sodium chloride and more salt by substituting normal saline.

3 Extra salt

Extra salt (sodium chloride) is required when the patient is suffering from losses of fluid rich in salt. This occurs in vomiting, diarrhoea and intestinal fistulae. The volume lost should be replaced as normal saline. Extra potassium will also usually be required.

4 Extra potassium

Most of the body potassium is in the cells and the serum potassium is not a good guide to overall depletion. The serum potassium may only fall when a large deficit has occurred. Those patients who may require extra potassium include the following:

(a) those receiving certain diuretics;

(b) those with large volumes of gastric aspirate or prolonged vomiting;

(c) those with a fistula from the biliary tract or small bowel;

(d) those with diarrhoea (e.g. ulcerative colitis or villous adenoma).

The amount of potassium required depends on the volume lost. For every 500 cm^3 of gastrointestinal loss, give an extra 5–10 mmol of potassium.

5 Intensive therapy

More intensive intravenous fluid therapy is required in the dehydrated or ill patient, especially if an operation is imminent. Any regime for such a patient is 'tailor-made' to suit their calculated deficit as judged by the history, the clinical state and the biochemical results. It may be necessary to infuse, for instance, normal saline at a rate of 1 litre/hour for a limited period. Clearly the state of the patient's kidneys and heart will dictate how safely such rapid replacement can be given. In these cases the decision about what should be given will have to be made by the registrar or consultant.

Special cases

Children and the elderly

These groups obviously need less fluid. The management of

babies and very small children is undertaken jointly between the surgeons and the paediatricians. This is not discussed further here.

The elderly patient on intravenous fluids requires close monitoring because of the risk of precipitating left ventricular failure. Ideally he is given a regime with less volume and no more sodium than is necessary, e.g.

Prescription

0.9% saline
  1 litre + 40 mmol KCl in 12 hours
5% dextrose
  1 litre + 20 mmol KCl in 12 hours

This gives 2 litres of fluid/day with 153 mmol of sodium and 60 mmol of potassium. He may need more fluid if he becomes dehydrated. Many elderly patients are on diuretics or digitalis and therefore a close eye must be kept on the electrolytes.

Haemorrhage

Blood loss should ideally be replaced by blood and after a certain point this is vital to maintain the oxygen-carrying capacity. However, while blood is being cross-matched, the circulating volume may be maintained with a colloid, e.g. dextran 70, Haemaccel or plasma protein fraction.

Burns

The main loss in burns is plasma and therefore plasma proteins are prescribed (see Burns, Section 12.5).

Acute renal failure

Here intravenous fluids must be severely restricted but must still replace the necessary constituents. The volume usually prescribed covers the daily insensible fluid loss plus the previous day's urinary output. Fluids may be written by the hour in this situation to allow closer control, e.g. 30 ml/hour plus the previous hour's output. The electrolytes must be watched carefully and usually the urinary electrolyte loss is measured twice a day. Sodium is replaced in proportion to the previous day's urinary loss. Potassium must not be given as it is usually retained.

Monitoring the effect of therapy

Whatever regime is chosen the effects must be constantly monitored. Assess the following parameters.
1 Pulse, blood pressure, JVP.
2 State of hydration: skin, tongue, mucous membranes.
3 Urine output: the minimum acceptable urine output is

720 ml/day or 30 ml/hour (ideally it should be in excess of 1500 ml/day).

4 Fluid balance (i.e. input compared with output). Check the totals on the observation charts. It is the houseman's duty to ensure that the nursing staff keep these records accurately and up to date.

5 Measurement of the urea and electrolytes: these are usually performed every two days.

6 CVP measurement: this gives a good indication of the degree of filling of the venous side of the circulation. It also provides information about cardiac function. A central venous pressure line is generally required in any patient requiring intensive fluid and electrolyte replacement therapy.

Central venous pressure (CVP)

Operation: setting up a CVP line

The objective is to place a long intravenous cannula or catheter with its tip in the superior vena cava. A strict aseptic technique is used and the patient is placed slightly head down. The skin of the selected entry site is cleaned and isolated using sterile towels. A bleb of local anaesthetic is inserted at the puncture site. Various entry points can be used as follows:

(a) *The basilic vein* in the ante-cubital fossa.

(b) *The subclavian vein beneath the clavicle*: the introducing cannula is inserted at a point 2 cm below the middle of the clavicle aiming at the centre of the suprasternal notch. The needle is kept horizontal and advanced while maintaining suction on the syringe. Blood appears in the syringe as the vein is entered. A catheter is then inserted through the lumen of the introducing cannula and threaded down the correct distance. This may be judged by marking the cannula previously.

(c) *The subclavian vein above the clavicle*: the introducing cannula is inserted just laterally to the insertion of the clavicular head of sternomastoid. The direction is at 45° in each plane. When blood is aspirated, sufficient catheter is inserted to leave the tip in the superior vena cava.

(d) *Internal jugular vein*. The vessel is cannulated just behind the sternocleidomastoid muscle in the neck. The vein can be fixed by grasping the muscle and elevating it slightly. The needle is inserted half-way between the mastoid process and the head of the clavicle and directed deep to the medial border of the clavicle. This approach is easier in the anaesthetized patient.

With any of these access sites the catheter may be tunnelled for some distance under the skin. This procedure decreases the chances of infection at the puncture site but should be carried out in the main operating theatre to allow the use of a thoroughly aseptic technique.

Once in place the catheter should be fixed with a suture or adhesive tape and the entry site dressed with antiseptic spray and dry gauze. The catheter is attached to a three-way tap. One limb of the tap is attached to a manometer and the other to a saline infusion. The meniscus should fluctuate with respiration. Also check that blood will run back up the line. The saline is run slowly at a rate sufficient to keep the vein open (e.g. 1 litre over 16–24 hours).

A chest X-ray is always taken to confirm that the catheter tip lies in the superior vena cava, and to check that there is no pneumothorax.

Complications of this technique include the following:

1 *Pneumothorax.* This may follow the cannulation of internal jugular or subclavian veins by any approach. Patients should be observed for dyspnoea and chest pain following the cannulation.

2 *Hydrothorax.* This occurs if the catheter lies in the pleural cavity.

3 *Phlebothrombosis.*

4 *Infection* of the catheter tip and *septicaemia.* If symptoms of septicaemia occur with no other known primary infection, the catheter should be removed and the tip cultured.

5 *Air embolus.* Accidental disconnection of a CVP line in an upright patient will lead to air entrainment. Lie the patient flat whenever making connections.

Measurement of the CVP (Fig. 20)

The scale of the manometer is set to a fixed reference point on the patient, usually with the aid of a spirit level. Two points used are the mid-axillary line and the sternal angle. Mark the point clearly on the skin and use it for all subsequent readings. The patient should be in the same position each time.

Having set the zero of the manometer scale to that level, continue as follows:

1 fill the manometer with fluid;

2 connect the manometer tube to the patient, closing off the saline infusion;

3 the meniscus should move up and down with respiration. Initially it will drop steadily until the meniscus is moving above and below a mean pressure. The lowest reading to which the meniscus falls is recorded;

4 reconnect the saline infusion isolating the manometer.

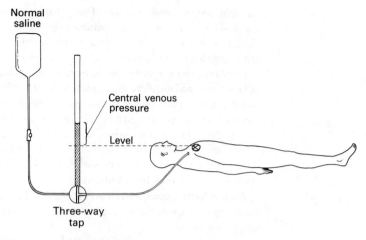

Fig. 20. Measuring the CVP.

For normal values in the supine patient, see Table 5. The reading is elevated if there is any right-sided cardiac failure or if the patient is being ventilated. It will be low in the hypovolaemic patient. A series of readings is more valuable than a single measurement. Due to the variation in venous tone in the normal patient, a trend will give a more accurate estimate of the venous filling of the heart and its response to therapy.

Table 5. Normal values in the supine patient

Reference point on patient	Pressure
Angle of Louis	-4 to $+4$ cm
5 cm posterior to angle of Louis (mid-axillary line)	$+1$ to $+9$ cm

Removing the line
Cut the holding suture, apply pressure over the entry point into the vein, and withdraw the line. Using a no-touch technique, cut off the tip and send it for culture.

Intravenous feeding
The following patients may require intravenous feeding.
1 Any patient who is unable to eat or drink for more than 4–5 days, e.g. after major surgery or a prolonged ileus (especially if he was chronically ill before operation).
2 Those with severe burns or multiple injuries.
3 Those with intestinal fistulae.

4 Those with malabsorption, e.g. bowel resection or Crohn's disease.

Most of these patients are catabolic and the aim is to reverse this catabolism by giving the patient protein and sufficient energy derived from non-protein sources, e.g. carbohydrate or fat. This is to ensure that the protein given is used for protein anabolism and is not itself broken down to provide a substrate for energy. Each gram of nitrogen prescribed needs 200 kcal of non-amino acid energy.

As a basic plan, a surgical patient needs 12−16 g nitrogen/day (80−90 g protein) and 3000 kcal. The kilo-calories may either be given as concentrated dextrose (4.5 kcal/g) or as fat, e.g. Intralipid (9 kcal/g).

Intravenous feeding is used either partly or wholly in place of a standard intravenous fluid regime as suggested above. When intravenous feeding is given, the requirement for fluids and electrolytes must be included in the overall calculations.

The fluids used are hypertonic and acid and so need to be given through a central vein. They are given slowly as they may be toxic to the heart. Intravenous feeding needs to be monitored by daily measurement of the urea, electrolytes and blood sugar. The liver function tests (protein) and haemoglobin are measured every third day. Patients on total intravenous feeding will also require trace elements and vitamin supplements.

Parenteral feeding is a complex subject and has been summarized very briefly here. There are many preparations and intravenous regimes available and each hospital will have its own accepted regime.

In those patients with an intact intestinal tract, an alternative to parenteral feeding is assisted enteral feeding, using a fine-bore nasogastric tube and continuous infusion into the gut. This is easier and carries less risk of infection. However, it may be difficult to control and absorption may be incomplete. Another alternative is combination feeding, giving the calories via the gut and the amino acids intravenously.

2.2 Prescribing Drugs for Surgical Patients

How to write a prescription

Prescribing drugs for patients is the houseman's responsibility. It is most important that the prescription should be written clearly and correctly. You will have to prescribe both those drugs the patient was taking before coming into hospital, and also any others that are to be given during admission.

Prescriptions will generally be written on the drug chart or on a specially designed form (EC 10). They may, however, be written on any headed notepaper. A specimen suitable for outpatient prescribing is shown in Fig. 21.

There are certain requirements which must be observed when prescribing drugs.

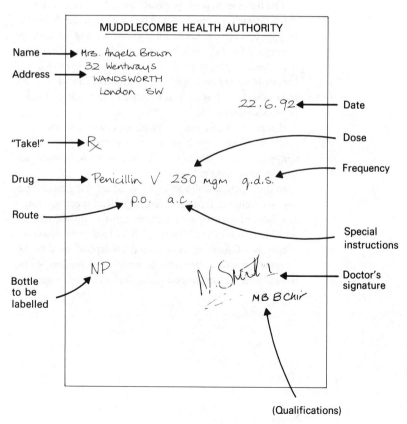

Name → Mrs. Angela Brown
Address → 32 Wentways
          WANDSWORTH
          London SW

MUDDLECOMBE HEALTH AUTHORITY

Date — 22.6.92

"Take!" → Rx — Dose

Frequency

Drug → Penicillin V 250 mgm q.d.s.

Route — p.o. a.c.

Special instructions

Bottle to be labelled → NP

Doctor's signature

MB BChir

(Qualifications)

Fig. 21. A specimen prescription (for abbreviations see p. 100).

1 *Identify patient.* The prescription must be clearly labelled with the patient's name, address, hospital number and date of birth. If there are two or more patients with the same name, then extra care is needed to avoid confusion.

2 *Date.*

3 *Drug.* Use the approved name of the drug and not its trade name.

4 *Dose.*

5 *Route.*

6 *Rate* or frequency of administration.

7 *Duration* of treatment with that drug or maximum number of doses.

8 *Signature* of a qualified doctor. This is a legal requirement. In addition it is usual to put your registered qualifications when you are prescribing on headed notepaper rather than the usual prescription form. Outpatient prescriptions require the doctor's address.

Controlled drugs

Drugs such as narcotic analgesics, because they are open to abuse, are controlled by the Misuse of Drugs Regulations (1973). These are known as 'controlled drugs'. The regulations state that the prescription must be made in ink by a qualified doctor in his own handwriting. The quantity and dose must be stated in words and numbers and the rate of administration stated exactly. It is illegal to prescribe a controlled drug on an 'and repeat' basis.

Review

While a patient is in hospital the drug chart should be reviewed every day and any drugs that are no longer required should be crossed off (e.g. antibiotics). Other drugs may need changing, e.g. from a stronger to a weaker analgesic.

Discharge

When the patient is discharged from hospital he must be given sufficient drugs to last him until he can obtain more from his own doctor. Usually hospital pharmacies will supply drugs to last the patient a maximum of 2 weeks. It is important to tell the general practitioner as soon as possible what drugs the patient has been given to take home. Point out any new drugs given for the present illness and how long they should be prescribed. Also note any change made to the patient's previous therapy. This is best done by a note sent to the GP (with the patient if this is possible) on the day of discharge.

Abbreviations

Those which may be used in writing a prescription are shown in Table 6.

Table 6. Abbreviations used in prescribing

Symbol	Latin/Meaning	Translation
R_x	Recipe	Take
Site		
p.o.	per os	by mouth
p.r.	per rectum	by rectal administration
i.m.	intramuscular	by intramuscular injection
i.v.	intravenous	by intravenous injection
s.c.	subcutaneous	by subcutaneous injection
s.l.	sublinguum	sublingual
Frequency		
stat.	statim	immediately
o.d.	omni die	every day (once a day)
b.d./b.i.d.	bis die/bis in die	twice a day
t.d.s.	ter die sumendus	to be taken three times a day
q.d.s.	quater die sumendus	to be taken four times a day
o.m.	omne mane	morning
o.n.	omne nocte	evening
s.o.s	si opus sit	if there is need, if necessary (usually a single dose)
p.r.n.	pro re nata	occasionally, when required Add the maximum frequency as well, e.g. p.r.n. 4-hourly (usually used for multiple doses)
Other terms		
a.c.	ante cibum	before food
p.c.	post cibum	after food
iu		international unit
tab.	tabletta/tabella	a tablet
mist.	mistura	a mixture
gtt.	guttae	drops
supp.	suppositorium	a suppository
tr./tinct.	tinctura	a tincture
ung.	unguentum	ointment
n.p.	nomen proprium	the proper name (usually means the dispenser should label the prescription with the proper name)
BNF		British National Formulary
BP		British Pharmacopoeia
BPC		British Pharmaceutical Codex

Drug management

The following are short notes on the use of analgesics, antibiotics, and sedatives in surgical practice.

Analgesics

Adequate pain relief after operation is important as it helps the patient to move and cough and thus lowers the risk of thrombo-embolism and pulmonary collapse. A patient will not always complain when he is in pain and you should enquire about this rather than wait for him to ask for drugs. Also ask him if the pain killers he has been given are adequate. Occasionally patients do not like to take pain killers at all and feel they should be able to do without them. They need firm reassurance that no harm will come from the drugs and indeed they will benefit from using them. If analgesia is written up 'p.r.n.' (as required) the patient should be informed of this so that he can ask for it when required. Analgesia must be sufficient to allow the patient to cough with the minimum of discomfort.

Analgesia can be achieved by:
1 local analgesics;
2 systemic drugs.

Local analgesics

In modern surgical practice, with the advent of long-acting analgesics such as bupivacaine (Marcaine), local analgesia has become the method of choice for analgesia after many surgical procedures. Excellent analgesia can be achieved for 8–10 hours. It may be given:

(a) By local infiltration of the wound at the time of surgery. This can be useful in the smaller operations such as removal of skin lumps, hernia repairs and so forth;

(b) by regional nerve block. Examples include intercostal nerve blocks for abdominal and thoracic operations, and ring blocks of toes and fingers. Epidural analgesia may be used, but requires high-dependency nursing. (Opiates may also be given epidurally.)

If regional local anaesthesia is used for day-case surgery, warn patients that they can damage the area anaesthetized without realizing it, and should be careful to avoid such damage.

Systemic analgesic drugs

There are many analgesics and these notes include examples of the ones commonly used.

Relief of acute pain

1 Severe pain

Opiates are the drug of choice.

These are all strong analgesics and narcotics. The controlled drug rules apply (see p. 99). Omnopon is a mixture of opiates, about 50% of which is morphine. Pethidine is a weaker analgesic than morphine. All three are very effective in the short term. Dependence and tolerance do develop, although this is never a problem in the patient immediately after surgery.

(a) Papaveretum (Omnopon) (10−20 mg i.m., orally, or i.v. 3−4-hourly). A normal dose for a 70 kg man with an abdominal incision would be 15−20 mg 4-hourly.

(b) Morphine (10−20 mg i.m./i.v. 3−4-hourly). Occasionally it is useful to give a small dose (e.g. 5 mg i.v. 2−3-hourly) so as to provide analgesia but avoid the side-effects seen soon after the administration of a larger 4-hourly dose. A normal dose of morphine for a 70 kg man with an abdominal incision would be 10−20 mg i.m. 4-hourly.

(c) Pethidine (75−100 mg i.m./i.v. 4-hourly). The normal dose for a 70 kg man would be 100 mg i.m. 4-hourly.

Intravenous infusions of these drugs may give improved pain control. These infusions may be either continuous at a rate adjusted to analgesic effect by nursing or medical staff, or intermittent boluses on demand (the patient presses a button on a patient-controlled analgesia system (PCAS)).

There are many side-effects. The following are of importance in the surgical patient.

1 Nausea and vomiting. All may require an anti-emetic (e.g. prochlorperazine (Stemetil) 12.5 mg i.m. This is a drug of the phenothiazine group).

2 Respiratory and cough suppression. This also occurs, but is less marked with pethidine.

3 Constipation (less with pethidine).

4 Biliary tract spasm, particularly closure of the sphincter of Oddi. This occurs with all three drugs, though less so with pethidine.

Remember that these drugs cause miosis (though this is minimal with pethidine) so avoid using them for patients with a head injury. If narcotic analgesia is required in these cases, pethidine should be given.

Contraindications

1 Respiratory disease − narcotics may precipitate respiratory failure.

2 Hepatic failure — small doses may precipitate hepatic encephalopathy.

3 Hypothyroidism, hypopituitarism, Addison's disease — use of narcotics may lead to coma.

4 Raised intracranial pressure — again narcotics may lead to coma.

5 Patients on monoamine oxidase inhibitors — these drugs potentiate narcotics.

2 Moderate pain

For example, somatic pain from the wound after the first 2−3 days.

(a) Dihydrocodeine (DF118) (25−50 mg i.m. 4−6-hourly; 30−60 mg orally 4−6-hourly).

Dihydrocodeine is midway between morphine and codeine in potency and its main side-effect is constipation. With prolonged use the patient may require laxatives.

(b) Pentazocine (Fortral) (30−60 mg i.m. 3−4-hourly; 25−100 mg orally 3−4-hourly).

Pentazocine is an opiate antagonist with an agonist action. It can precipitate withdrawal in addicts. It provides good analgesia but its oral absorption is unpredictable with a high first-pass metabolism in the liver. Parenteral administration is therefore preferred. It may cause an increase in systemic and pulmonary blood pressure. It should be used with caution in patients with cardiac failure. It must not be used with other opiates as it will antagonize them. Dysphonia is not uncommon.

(c) Codeine. This is an analgesic which is partly converted to morphine in the body. It has only one-quarter to one-sixth of the analgesic power of morphine and the side-effects are even less. Dependence does not usually occur. It is used for the relief of moderate pain (dose: 10−60 mg orally 4-hourly).

3 Mild pain

Fashions vary widely in the drugs which are popular at any one time for relief of mild pain. Some suggestions follow.

(a) Aspirin (300−600 mg (1−2 tabs) orally 4−6-hourly). The use of this drug is contraindicated in patients with a past history of stomach disorders.

(b) Paracetamol (0.5−1 g (1−2 tabs) 4−6-hourly). This is a good analgesic with very little in the way of side-effects.

(c) Distalgesic (1−2 tabs 4−6-hourly). Each tablet of Distalgesic contains 32.5 mg dextropropoxyphene (related to methadone) and 325 mg paracetamol. There is a known incidence of side-effects and toxicity (respiratory and cardiac depression) due to the dextropropoxyphene and its metabolite norpropoxyphene. It is an opioid analgesic and dependence is believed to occur. One or two cases of addiction have been reported. Although few trials have been done there is little evidence that it is superior to paracetamol in its analgesic effect.

It is contraindicated in patients with poor renal function due to the accumulation of norpropoxyphene.

Most mild analgesics must be given orally. Consider rectal preparations if the oral route is contraindicated. Diclofenac may also be given intramuscularly.

Control of chronic pain

The control of chronic pain is a speciality in itself. A few points can be noted here.

1 In a patient with incurable disease the aim is to prevent the pain, not to treat it once it occurs. Prevention is not only better for the patient but requires less analgesia. It is kind to leave the patient with some tablets by his bedside at night in case he wakes up with pain.

2 Opiates are usually required. In a terminally ill patient the danger of dependence is unimportant. However, tolerance develops, so the dose will need to be increased as time passes. The priority is to keep the patient free of pain.

3 Attempt, if possible, to control pain with oral drugs to save the repeated discomfort of injections. Some examples of drugs used are the following:

(a) Oral morphine/diamorphine, e.g. 10 mg 4-hourly and increase as required. An anti-emetic should be prescribed and a laxative may also be required.

(b) 'Brompton's cocktail' is an elixir made of morphine, chlorpromazine and cocaine. It has mixed analgesic and tranquillizing effects and can be very useful. Many hospital pharmacies have their own version of this cocktail and so ask them for advice as to the dose prescribed.

(c) Levorphanol (1.5−4.5 mg 1−2 times daily). This is a synthetic morphine-like drug which is well absorbed orally and causes less sedation than morphine.

(d) Oxycodone (Proladone) suppositories. These contain 30 mg of oxycodone pectinate. This is an opiate. One is useful at night as the drug is longer-acting than morphine. The effect is equal to 20 mg of morphine orally and it lasts about 8 hours.

(e) Buprenorphine (Temgesic, dose 400 µg 6−8-hourly). This is a long-acting analgesic and has both agonist and antagonist properties with opiates. It therefore must not be used with other opiates. It may be given sublingually.

Hypnotics and sedatives

Surgery, however minor, is always associated with anxiety. While drugs can be no substitute for gentle reassurance and explanation by both the housesurgeon and nursing staff, hypnotics and sedatives do have a use. The more rested and relaxed a patient is, the better he will tolerate operation. It is a good idea to prescribe night sedation for every patient, to have if required. The patient must be told that this is available. He may require reassurance that he will come to no harm by taking sleeping tablets for a few nights.

The following are short notes on some of the drugs commonly used.

1 *Diazepam (Valium)* (2 mg, 5 mg or 10 mg orally or i.m.). This drug is a benzodiazepine and is a tranquillizer and muscle relaxant. It can be used to relieve general anxiety during the day, often in small doses (e.g. 2 mg 8-hourly). It can also be used as an adjunct to pain killers for relief of pain from an abdominal wound when this pain is due to muscle spasm. It may be taken orally or intramuscularly. It is a very safe drug, although drowsiness and confusion can occur, especially in the elderly patient.

2 *Nitrazepam (Mogadon)* (5–10 mg orally nocte). This is also a benzodiazepine and is marketed as a hypnotic. It is safe and effective although it does cause a slight 'hangover' the next day and may well cause confusion in elderly patients.

3 *Temazepam and flurazepam* (hypnotics). These are two other benzodiazepines which are used as hypnotics (dose temazepam 10–30 mg nocte, flurazepam 15–30 mg nocte). Both have shorter half-lives. Temazepam, in particular, causes less 'hangover' and is suitable for the elderly.

All benzodiazepines can cause respiratory depression and are contraindicated in patients with chronic respiratory disease.

4 *Dichloralphenazone* (Welldorm, 1.3–1.95 g (2–3 tabs) nocte). This is a useful hypnotic, related to chloral hydrate, and is less likely than nitrazepam to cause confusion in the elderly patient. It is a safe drug, although it does interact with oral anti-coagulants, displacing them from their binding proteins. This increases their effect and their rate of elimination.

5 *Chlormethiazole edisylate (Heminevrin)*. This is a useful second-line drug for the relief of insomnia and is particularly good for agitation in the elderly patient: for insomnia, 2 capsules nocte; for sedation, 1 capsule 3-hourly (each capsule contains 192 mg of chlormethiazole in arachis oil).

Antibiotics

Antibiotics are used in a surgical patient for the following purposes.

1 Acute infections, e.g. bronchopneumonia, urinary infection, cholecystitis.

2 Prophylactic cover, for operations with a high risk of infection, e.g. colonic surgery.

3 Prophylactic cover where a prosthesis will be inserted and infection would be disastrous (e.g. hip prosthesis, arterial prosthesis).

4 Medical conditions requiring cover, e.g. valve disease, congenital heart disease and patent ductus arteriosus.

Table 7. Antibiotics for acute infections

Condition	Likely organism	Initial antibiotic therapy
Wound infection		
Indurated, localized	? *Staphylococcus*	Flucloxacillin 250 mg 6-hourly p.o.
Plus cellulitis	? *Streptococcus*	Penicillin, e.g. phenoxymethyl penicillin 500 mg 6-hourly p.o.
Foul-smelling	? Anaerobes	Metronidazole, e.g. 400 mg 8-hourly p.o. or 1 g supp. 8-hourly p.r.
Infected drip site	*Staphylococcus*	Flucloxacillin 250 mg 6-hourly p.o.
Chest infection		
Pneumonia	*Pneumococcus*	Penicillin 1 mega unit q.d.s., i.v.
Chronic bronchitis and pneumonia	*Haemophilus influenzae*	Ampicillin 500 mg 6-hourly, or cephalosporins* i.v.
Urinary tract infection		
Uncomplicated		Augmentin 375 mg 8-hourly or trimethoprim 100 mg 12-hourly p.o.
Severe, i.e. fever over 38.5°C, rigors, acute pyelonephritis		Gentamicin** 80 mg 8-hourly i.m. or i.v. initially (24 hours), then ampicillin, trimethoprim 100 mg 12-hourly p.o. or continued cephalosporin*
With indwelling catheter (mild)		See p. 432

See p. 432

* The following cephalosporins may be suitable.
Cefotaxime   1–2 g three to four times daily by severity.
Cefuroxime   750 mg – 1.5 g t.d.s.
Cephazolin   1 g q.d.s.
Cephamandole 1 g q.d.s.
Cefoxitin   1 g q.d.s. (does not need metronidazole accompaniment as anti-anaerobic).
** Patients on gentamicin are at risk from renal damage if levels rise too high. Levels should be measured twice weekly. The dose must be lowered if there is renal impairment.

Acute infections

The antibiotic used will depend on the infection to be treated and thus on the predicted organism. Confirmation of the causative organism and its antibiotic sensitivity will be obtained when a bacteriological culture has been performed. Specific surgical infections (e.g. acute cholecystitis) are discussed in the appropriate section.

In Table 7 some common surgical infections are shown, together with the possible initial antibiotics to use.

Antibiotic prophylaxis

Prophylactic antibiotics are timed to be present in wound fluids when the patient is most at risk from infection. Usually this means the peroperative period and the antibiotics are given just before the operation. The choice of drug is usually made by the consultant as part of his routine management. Some suggestions are shown in Table 8 although it is realized that these will rapidly become out of date. The reader may then wish to fill in the drugs that are at present used in his unit for his own future reference.

Medical conditions

See pp. 10, 23, 106–108.

Anti-coagulants

The usual drugs used for anti-coagulation are heparin and warfarin.

Heparin

Initial treatment is with heparin given intravenously in a dose of 100–150 iu/kg body weight immediately. This dose is repeated every 6 hours. A suitable regime for most adults would be 10 000 units intravenously stat., followed by 30 000–40 000 units per day. The drug is given by continuous intravenous infusion. The level of anti-coagulation should be monitored with daily partial thromboplastin times (PTT) and these should be kept at 1.5–2.5 times the normal level.

Warfarin

Depending on the nature of the thrombosis, anti-coagulation may be maintained with warfarin after 3–7 days heparinization. This drug takes 48–72 hours to take effect and therefore a loading dose is given while the patient is still on heparin. A suitable regime is as follows:

1 Prescribe a loading dose of warfarin. This is usually 10 mg/day orally given at 6.0 p.m. for 3 consecutive days. A

Table 8. Prophylactic antibiotics

Procedure	Organism	Prophylaxis
Large bowel surgery*	Anaerobes, coliforms, *Streptococcus milleri*	Gentamicin 80 mg i.v., metronidazole 1 g p.r., benzylpenicillin 1 mega unit i.v., all at induction (or with premed.) or cephalosporins (see footnote Table 7)
Appendicitis	Anaerobes	Metronidazole 1 g p.r. 2–3 hours preop.
Vaginal operations	Anaerobes	Metronidazole 1 g p.r. 2–3 hours preop.
Biliary surgery	Coliforms	Cefotaxime 2 g i.v. with premed. or ampicillin 500 mg and/or gentamicin 80 mg i.v. at induction
Arterial surgery	*Streptococcus* or *Staphylococcus*	Gentamicin 80 mg and flucloxacillin 500 mg i.v. at induction
Amputations	*Clostridium* (gas gangrene in stump)	Benzylpenicillin 1 mega unit 6-hourly 5 days i.m. or i.v. or metronidazole 500 mg i.v. Then 200 mg 8-hourly p.o. 5 days
Urinary tract surgery	*Escherichia coli, Proteus,* faecal *Streptococcus, Pseudomonas, Klebsiella,* enterobacter	Choice depends on urine culture
Insertion of hip prosthesis	*Staphylococcus aureus, Staphylococcus epidermidis*	Flucloxacillin 1 g i.m., gentamicin 80 mg i.m. 2 hours preop., or cephalosporin and metronidazole (see footnotes Table 7 and 8)

* N.B. (1) If faecal contamination has occurred then continue a 3–5-day course of medication.

(2) Metronidazole may also be given as 500 mg i.v. at induction of anaesthesia for colonic surgery.

(3) If gentamicin or cephalosporin resistance is common in your unit, ciprofloxacin (200 mg b.d. i.v. or 500 mg t.d.s. orally) may be a suitable alternative for procedures where gentamicin or cephalosporin is recommended, but will still need whatever penicillin or metronidazole accompaniment is recommended.

lower dose may be required for patients with a low body weight, or the elderly, or those with hepatic disease.

2 Stop the heparin infusion at midnight after the third loading dose (day 3). This will be about 54 hours after warfarinization has been commenced.

3 On the morning of day 4, test the coagulation time. A thrombotest or prothrombin time is used to assess the effect of warfarin. The thrombotest is now expressed as the INR or International Normalized Ratio. The INR times should be 2.5 to 4.5. Less than 2.5 denotes under-anti-coagulation and more than 4.5 over-anti-coagulation.

4 Prescribe further warfarin on the basis of this test and recheck the clotting values 1–2 days later. The dose to be given varies with the value of the thrombotest and is shown in Table 9. The blood test is taken in the morning and the warfarin is prescribed in the evening.

5 Further doses of warfarin are given on the basis of the second thrombotest.

Table 9. Dosage of warfarin to be given after result of INR test on day 4

	Suggested doses (mg)		
INR	Day 4	Day 5	Day 6
>4.5	Nil	Test	
4.5–3.5	1	Test	
3.5–2.8	3	3	Test
2.8–2.3	4	4	Test
2.3–1.9	5	5	Test
1.9–1.7	6	6	Test
1.7–1.5	7	7	Test
1.5–1.3	8	8	Test
<1.3	9	9	Test

The main side-effect is over-anti-coagulation and haemorrhage, particularly into the urinary and alimentary tract. The urine should be tested for blood regularly. If haemorrhage occurs, the drug should be stopped and a thrombotest performed. If bleeding is significant, fresh frozen plasma 2–4 units should be given. Phytomenadione (vitamin K_1) (10–20 mg i.v.) also reverses warfarin but takes some hours to work and prevents re-anti-coagulation for 7–10 days.

N.B. Many drugs and conditions affect the activity of warfarin and the patient's concurrent drug therapy must be reviewed regularly.

1 Some drugs displace warfarin from plasma proteins, increasing the anti-coagulation effect, e.g. aspirin, phenylbutazone and clofibrate.

2 Liver disease potentiates warfarin activity.

3 Low vitamin K (in association with jaundice or antibiotic treatment) also increases warfarin activity.

4 Liver enzyme induction, e.g. by chronic alcoholism or phenobarbitone therapy increases the rate of metabolism of warfarin and a higher dose is required. The dose must be reduced when the inducing agent is withdrawn.

Anti-coagulation is contraindicated if there is a recent history of haematemesis, peptic ulceration, ulcerative colitis, haematuria, cerebral haemorrhage or hypertension and in women in the first trimester or last 4 weeks of pregnancy. These contraindications are not absolute and the risks must be balanced against the benefits.

Thrombolytic therapy

Thrombi, once formed, may be dissolved using thrombolytic agents such as streptokinase or tissue plasminogen activator (TPA). These are dealt with on p. 60.

Bowel preparation

The aim of preparing the bowel before abdominal surgery is to clear the colon of exogenous material and lower the number of infective organisms. Such bowel preparation is essential before a colonic resection.

Emptying the bowel

The patient is started on a low residue diet and nutritious fluids and then given clear fluids only for 24 hours pre-operatively. The contents of the bowel are evacuated using laxatives and/or enemas. The following agents can be used.

1 *Osmotic laxatives.* These work by increasing the fluid content of the bowel, causing an osmotic diarrhoea. They include magnesium sulphate and lactulose elixir. Both are suitable for bowel preparation. Lactulose also lowers the pH in the bowel lumen, thereby inhibiting the growth of some microorganisms.

2 *Bulk-forming drugs and faecal softeners.* Drugs that increase faecal bulk stimulate peristalsis. Examples are bran, Isogel, Normacol and methyl cellulose. Faecal softeners lubricate the faeces and these drugs include liquid paraffin or dioctyl sodium sulphosuccinate (Dioctyl forte). Dioctyl forte also operates by affecting intestinal secretion and promoting motility.

3 *Stimulant laxatives.* These drugs promote defaecation by directly stimulating intestinal motility. Commonly used drugs include bisacodyl (Dulcolax), sodium picosulphate (Picolax), danthron (Dorbanex) and senna preparations (X-prep, Senokot).

4 *Mechanical procedures* to clear out the bowel include enemas and washouts. If a colostomy is present, then the distal limb may be irrigated. Lubricants, softeners or intestinal stimulants may be given rectally, e.g. glycerin suppositories or bisacodyl.

Antibiotics

Antibiotics used for bowel preparation are those which are poorly absorbed and have a broad spectrum. Examples are neomycin (1 g 6-hourly) or phthalylsulphathiazole (1 g 12-hourly). Metronidazole suppositories may also be given (1 g 12-hourly).

Suggested regime

Always check the regime with your consultant. Details are usually left with the ward sister. A typical regime is outlined below.

(a) Admit 2−3 days before operation.

(b) *Diet*. Low residue from admission; nutritious fluids, e.g. Clinifeed, 2 days before operation; clear fluids, e.g. jelly, clear soup, etc., 1 day before operation.

(c) *Laxatives*. Picolax 1 sachet/day for 1−2 days, 2 sachets the day before operation.

(d) *Washouts*. Rectal enemas or washouts are given the day before operation if required.

In addition, Dioctyl forte (100 mg 12-hourly) can be used to soften constipated hard faeces preoperatively. It is given from 3−4 days before operation as part of the above regime.

The patient may lose a lot of fluid and electrolytes during bowel preparation and in the elderly it may be necessary to replace these intravenously. Keep a daily check on plasma electrolytes.

Neomycin 1 g 6-hourly or phthalylsulphathiazole 1 g 12-hourly orally, with or without metronidazole 1 g 12-hourly rectally, may be given from admission.

2.3   Sutures and Drains

Sutures

It is useful to be familiar with the various types of suture,
their uses and their effect on the management of wounds.
Generally, a suture may be either absorbable or non-
absorbable, and has either a braided, twisted or monofilament
structure. New varieties of suture material are constantly
being developed.

Types of suture

Absorbable sutures are broken down in the body tissues over a
varying number of days either by enzymes or by hydrolysis
by the tissue fluid. It is important to differentiate between
the times of loss of tensile strength and of disappearance of
the material as these are not necessarily the same.

Non-absorbable sutures remain in place for some years
unless they are removed.

Braided sutures (where the strands are plaited together)
and twisted sutures (where the separate strands are twisted
round each other) are very flexible and therefore easy to
handle and knot. The knots usually hold and are secure.
The disadvantage of these types of suture is that fluid can
seep between the strands (capillarity) and microorganisms
can get into the interstices of the yarn, giving rise to long-
term infections. Most braided sutures are proofed or coated
in an attempt to prevent this.

Monofilament sutures, on the other hand, consist of only
one strand of material. They tend to be less flexible and
more 'slippery'. They are therefore less easy to handle and
knot, and the knots need more throws to be secure. The only
nidus provided for infection is within the interstices of a
knot.

Examples

*Several of these names are company trade marks and the
companies involved are then known.

Absorbable

Catgut − plain, chromic
Collagen − plain, chromic
Polyglycolic acid (Dexon, Davis & Geck)

Polyglactin 910 (Vicryl, Ethicon)
Polydioxanone (PDS, Ethicon)

Non-absorbable
Silk
Linen and cotton thread
Nylon
Polyester
Prolene (Ethicon)
Stainless steel wire

Notes on different types of suture material

Absorbable sutures
Their uses are as follows.
1 Tying off small arteries and veins near the skin.
2 Stitches in the ureter, urinary tract, or biliary tract (where permanent sutures form a focus for stone formation).
3 Closing off tissue spaces, e.g. subcutaneous space.
4 Occasionally for closing the skin in children, where it is an advantage not to have to remove the stitches.
5 In small bowel anastomosis or stomach mucosal anastomosis (non-absorbable sutures in the stomach can cause long-term ulceration).
The following are different types of absorbable suture.

Catgut. This is made of strands of collagen from the submucous part of sheep or cow intestine which is dried out and sterilized. It is absorbed by cell and tissue proteases. Plain catgut loses its strength in about 3 days. Chromic catgut is catgut soaked in potassium dichromate, which delays its breakdown. It retains its strength for 5–7 days. Both cause a tissue reaction but this is less with chromic catgut.

Collagen sutures. These consist of pure collagen fibrils from cow flexor tendons. They have a smoother surface and are more homogeneous than catgut. They can either be plain or chromic and cause minimal tissue reaction with good knotting properties. They are absorbed by proteases and are used in ophthalmic surgery.

Other absorbable sutures are synthetic and braided in structure. Their tensile strength lasts for longer than catgut or collagen.

Polyglycolic acid (*Dexon*, Davis & Geck). This is a homopolymer of glycolide and is braided. The material loses 50%

of its effective tensile strength in 20 days but is not absorbed for between 100 and 120 days.

Polyglactin 910 (Vicryl, Ethicon). This is a synthetic absorbable suture made of a copolymer of lactide and glycolide. It is braided and non-antigenic and causes minimal tissue reaction. It has good knotting properties. It loses 60% of its effective tensile strength in 20 days. The sutures are absorbed by slow hydrolysis in 60–90 days.

Polydioxanone (PDS, Ethicon). This is a synthetic monofilament absorbable suture. It is absorbed by hydrolysis and causes minimal tissue reaction. There is very little harbouring of infection. Its loss of tensile strength is slower than other absorbable materials. At 28 days 50–60% of its strength remains. It is completely absorbed in about 180 days. PDS is beginning to replace nylon for the main closure of abdominal wounds (see below).

Non-absorbable sutures

Silk. This is a strong, flexible material which handles easily and knots very securely. It is of two main types — a braided thread which has a rough surface, and floss silk which is very loosely twisted and allows cellular infiltration and the deposition of collagen. Although classified as non-absorbable, it loses 80% of its tensile strength in 80 days and is absorbed over about 2 years.

It is used for tying off large vessels and to provide a strong suture layer for intestinal and vascular anastomoses.

Dermal suture. This is a suture of twisted silk fibres coated in a non-absorbable layer of tanned gelatin or other protein. It is very strong. It is used to suture skin under tension and the coating prevents cellular infiltration that could interfere with its removal.

Linen and cotton thread. These sutures are made of twisted flax and cotton fibres. They are similar to silk but not as strong, although cotton fibres gain tensile strength when wet. Like all braided sutures they may become infected and can give rise to persistent sinuses. Their uses are the same as for silk, although the latter has now virtually replaced them.

Nylon. Nylon is a polyamide polymer and sutures can either be multi-filament (braided) or monofilament. The most commonly used is a monofilament nylon which is extremely strong and inert in the tissues, although it does degrade very slowly at about 15% per year. Knots can be unreliable unless tied with a double 'surgeon's knot' (see Fig. 22).

Nylon sutures are used for the following.

1 Stitching the skin. The minimal tissue reaction causes less scarring.

2 Closure of the abdominal muscles. A double monofilament nylon suture provides very good immediate wound strength.

3 Ophthalmology and microsurgery. At 11/0 it is the smallest suture made.

Polypropylene (Prolene, Ethicon). This is a synthetic polymer of polypropylene extruded into a monofilament suture. It is strong and inert causing minimal tissue reaction (it is the most permanent, non-absorbable suture) and it looks like nylon. It is, however, more flexible and has better knotting properties. It has a slippery surface and slides through the tissues well.

Prolene is popular for closure of the skin, particularly for subcuticular sutures. It is widely used in arterial surgery and some surgeons use it for large bowel anastomosis and bile duct surgery.

Polyester fibre sutures (Mersilene, Ethicon). This is a braided, multi-filament suture of polyester, another synthetic polymer. It is strong and well tolerated in the tissues.

Another type (*Ethibond*, Ethicon) is braided polyester coated with polybutylate — a surgical lubricant. This travels very smoothly through the tissues and knots securely. It is very inert with good tensile strength maintained over a long period. It is used in cardiovascular surgery for vessel anastomosis and attachment of prostheses.

Stainless steel wire. This material is popular with a few surgeons. It is difficult to use but is extremely strong and

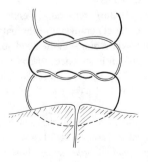

Fig. 22. A surgeon's knot.

non-reactive. Over a period of years it does fragment and therefore lose its tensile strength.

Some surgeons use stainless steel wire for closing the abdominal muscles. It is also used in orthopaedic surgery to wire bones together and in thoracic surgery for rejoining the sternum.

Sizes of sutures

Suture size is expressed on the scale given in Table 10.

Table 10. Sizes of sutures

Size	Metric scale (= mm x 10)	Diameter (mm)
4	6.0	0.6
3	5.5	0.55
2	5.0	0.5
1	4.0	0.4
0	3.5	0.35
2/0 (00)	3.0	0.3
3/0 (000)	2.0	0.2
4/0 (etc.)	1.5	0.15
5/0	1.0	0.1
6/0	0.75	0.075
7/0	0.5	0.05
8/0	0.4	0.04
9/0	0.3	0.03
10/0	0.2	0.02

These sizes only apply to synthetic materials. Natural collagen tends to be slightly larger. Size 0 silk is used for tying off arteries of about 5 mm in diameter. Size 6/0 is a very fine suture used in arterial surgery. Size 10/0 is only just visible to the naked eye and is used in micro-vascular surgery.

Suture removal

The time of suture removal depends on the site of the incision and the general state of the patient.

1 *Head and neck.* Wounds in the head and neck heal rapidly. A cosmetic result is also needed and therefore early suture removal is an advantage. Sutures in this area are generally removed within 3–5 days, e.g. thyroid scar 3 days, face scar 4 days.

2 *Abdomen and thorax.* Transverse or oblique incisions 5–7 days. Vertical incisions 7–10 days.

3 *In patients who are cachectic,* i.e. those with carcinomatosis, on steroid therapy, with severe infection, or with hepatic or

renal failure, the tissue healing can be delayed and therefore the sutures must be left longer (10−14 days or longer).

Needles

Needles are either curved or straight; eyed or atraumatic; round-bodied, taper-cut or with a cutting edge (see Table 11).

Table 11. Needles

Curved	Small — used with needle holders
Straight	Large — hand needles
Eyed	Suture material must be threaded through the eye
Atraumatic	The suture material is built into the end of the needle and the needle puncture therefore causes only a minimally larger hole than the suture itself
Round-bodied	The needle has a round shape and is only sharp at its tip. Used for suturing the peritoneum, fat, bowel, liver, etc.
Taper-cut	The needle also has a round shape but is sharpened on several sides towards the tip, giving it cutting properties. This type of needle is useful for passage through tough tissues where it is important to keep the needle track size to a minimum
With cutting edge	These are flattened and 'sword-like' and cut through the tissues as they are passed. They can be used on tough fibrous tissue (e.g. breast) or the skin, but may cause haemorrhage by cutting neighbouring blood vessels

Drains

Drains are put in by the surgeon to allow any fluid or air collecting at the operation site or in the wound to drain to the surface while allowing the main wound to heal. Fluids to be drained include blood, pus, urine, faeces, bile or lymph.

Drains may be:

1 superficial, i.e. in the wound;
2 deep:
  (a) intraperitoneal, e.g. covering an intestinal anastomosis,
  (b) in a hollow organ or duct, e.g. a T-tube in the bile duct,
  (c) in an abnormal channel, e.g. a fistula,

(d) to drain a deep cavity, e.g. an abscess or haematoma.

In addition drains may be:

1 open, i.e. draining into a dressing or bag open to the air;
2 closed, i.e. draining into a sterilized air-tight tube and container. The drainage system may be:

(a) on free drainage, e.g. drainage of ascites by gravity;
(b) on suction, e.g. Redivac drains;
(c) controlled by a one-way valve, e.g. an underwater seal or chest drains (see p. 231).

Types of drains and their uses

Open drains

Corrugated rubber drain (Fig. 23a). Rubber causes a tissue reaction and the drain track caused by this material persists longer than when inert materials are used. The drain is fixed by a suture at the end of the wound and a safety pin must be placed through the end to prevent the drain slipping inwards. Corrugated rubber drains can be used either for the wound or for deep drainage.

Yates' drain (Fig. 23b). This is a corrugated drain made of a series of capillary tubes joined side to side. It is generally made of polyethylene which is less reactive than rubber. The drain site, therefore, tends to close more quickly once the drain has been removed. Its uses are similar to corrugated rubber drains and it is secured as described above.

Penrose drain. This is a drain fashioned out of thin-walled rubber tubing and a gauze wick is threaded through the centre of the tube. Fluid can then either drain down the track once the tube is removed or through the centre whilst it is in place.

Closed drains

Redivac drain (Fig. 23c). This is a fine tube, with many holes at the end, which is attached to an evacuated glass bottle providing suction. It is used to drain blood beneath the skin, e.g. after mastectomy or thyroidectomy, or from deep spaces, e.g. around a vascular anastomosis.

'Shirley' wound drainage. This is a suction drain with an intake tube supplying air to the bottom of the main tube. This allows continuous suction and the flow of air prevents the tube getting blocked.

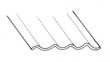
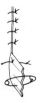

(a) Corrugated rubber drain

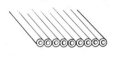

(b) Yates' drain

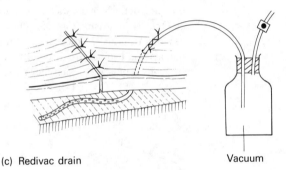

(c) Redivac drain   Vacuum

Fig. 23. Various types of wound drain.

Silastic tube drain. Silastic is a polymeric silicone and incites little tissue inflammation. Once this type of drain is removed, therefore, the track closes rapidly. A Silastic tube drain can be used to provide closed drainage to deep anastomoses, e.g. of the bowel (Fig. 24).

Red rubber tube drain. This causes an intense tissue reaction and fibrosis. The track will, therefore, persist for some time after the drain is removed. This feature can be useful for drainage of chronic abscess cavities such as an empyema or hepatic abscess.

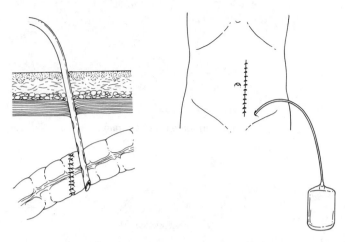

Fig. 24. Deep closed drainage of a colonic anastomosis.

T-tube drains. After bile duct surgery a T-tube is inserted in the bile duct, which allows bile to drain while the sphincter of Oddi is in spasm (Fig. 25). Once this relaxes the bile can drain normally down the common bile duct into the duodenum. T-tubes are made of a variety of materials and surgeons vary in the design they prefer.

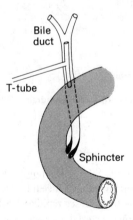

Fig. 25. A T-tube allows bile to drain if the sphincter of Oddi is in spasm.

Removal of drains
A drain is removed as soon as it is no longer required. Hence it is necessary to know the purpose for which it was inserted and you should ascertain this from the surgeon at the time of operation. The following are general guidelines:

1 Drains put in to cover perioperative bleeding and haematoma formation, can come out after 24−48 hours.

2 Drains put in to cover serous collections can come out after 3−5 days.

3 Where a drain has been put in because the wound may later become infected, it should be left for 1−5 days.

4 Drains put in to cover intestinal anastomoses should not be removed until after 5−7 days.

5 A T-tube can be removed after 6−10 days. Before this is done, a T-tube cholangiogram must be performed to make sure that there is distal patency in the common bile duct (see p. 291). Some surgeons clamp the T-tube for 24 hours before it is removed.

6 Chest drains − see management of thoracotomy (p. 234).

2.4 Relatives, Discharges, Deaths and Documents

Dealing with relatives

It is an important part of the houseman's job to answer enquiries from relatives as to the nature of the disease, the type of operation that is intended, and the prognosis. The relatives will view any operation as a very major undertaking and will often be dreading the outcome. Keeping them informed is not just a humanitarian exercise. If the relatives are happy about a patient's management, they will pass on this confidence to the patient and this can be a great help to you as his doctor. It is worthwhile setting aside two periods a week when you will be available on the ward for any relatives to come and see you. Tell the nursing staff when these will be.

The personal touch

It is better if only one person deals with the relatives. Otherwise misunderstandings may arise. This is occasionally difficult to achieve where a system of cross-cover is operated and the on-call houseman looks after patients on other wards as well.

Continuity is important because only you know what you have already told the relatives. If you know that they are visiting one evening, stay on the ward until you have seen them. This often takes less time than repairing the damage caused by an interview with someone who does not know the case.

If you are asked to see the relatives of a patient on another ward about whom you know nothing, start by asking them what they have been told so far and apologize that the doctor they normally see is not available. Before the interview look at the notes, not only to find out about the case, but also to see if any record has been made of previous conversations.

Documentation

After you have spoken to a patient about a diagnosis that may cause concern, or spoken to a patient's relatives, write down what you have told them in the notes and comment on any difficulty or reaction from those listening. For example, 'Mother told that her son has a malignant growth on the leg. Very upset. Has requested that the son should not be told. She is coming tomorrow with husband and would like to be seen again. Would also like an appointment with the consultant in the next clinic.' Tell the senior members of your surgical unit about the interview.

Patient discharge

When discharging a patient you must give them instructions on the following:

1 *Stitches*. When and how stitches are to be removed if this has not been done already.

2 *Activity*. How active he can be in the postoperative period and when he may go back to work. This depends on the nature of his job. Guidance on this topic is given in the 'codes' for individual operations later in this book.

3 *Drugs*. The patient should usually be given the drugs which he was on when he came into hospital together with any others which may be necessary as part of his present treatment. He should be told clearly how long he needs to take these. His GP must be informed of the therapy as soon as the patient is discharged from hospital. This is best done by giving him a note to take home.

4 *Follow-up*. When is the patient to be seen again?

Discharge summary

A summary of the patient's admission should be completed as soon as possible after the time of discharge and sent to the patient's GP. A copy is filed in the notes. It should include concise relevant information under the following headings:

Patient details (name, registry number, GP, address, date of birth)

Admission details (ward, date, emergency/elective, etc.)

Diagnoses

Reason for admission

Investigations (summary of inpatient results)

Operation details

Non-operative treatment

Postoperative details (problems, complications)

Information given to patient/relatives

Method of discharge (home, transferred, died, etc.)

Drugs and other discharge treatment

Follow-up arrangements

Other comments

In modern surgical units this summary is often produced by a computer from data entered on a proforma or a terminal for the purposes of surgical audit (see p. 131).

Dealing with death

The houseman often has the task of telling relatives that a

patient is going to die or has died. He is also responsible for the care of these terminally ill patients. This is a delicate job and each individual doctor will develop his own methods. Below are written some ideas, aimed to help you formulate your own approach.

Informing the relatives that a patient is going to die

The relatives will need to be told if the patient is likely to die. This is best done by taking them into a quiet room and explaining that nothing further can be done usefully to prolong life. Arrange not to be disturbed.

It is often best to start by asking the relatives what they feel is going to happen. Using this as a guide, the patient's situation must be explained honestly, clearly and slowly. Generally it is important to be absolutely truthful. There are very few situations, if any, where hiding the truth from the relatives is the more appropriate course of action. Try to be positive, rather than negative, emphasizing what you can still do to help the patient. Often the one comfort that you can give is to say that their relative will be given sufficient analgesia to stay free of pain. Point out what the relatives can do themselves to help the patient, i.e. to remain cheerful and positive rather than to show sadness.

A situation has become increasingly common where there are the means to keep a patient 'alive' although this would clearly be inappropriate (i.e. in cases of brain death). This may be difficult to explain to relatives. You may have to explain the hopelessness of the situation and the loss of dignity that keeping a patient 'alive' with brain death entails. Usually the relatives will understand and agree that the right thing to do is what is suggested.

When the relatives remain worried and further guidance is needed, arrange for them to see your consultant. In this situation he is likely to wish to see them anyway.

Care of the terminally ill patient

A terminally ill patient also needs to know what is going on. Choose a time to talk privately. Again it is better to be totally honest in what you say, although in this case there are a few situations where hiding the truth is more appropriate. Patients are not always ready to face the prospect of death and may have to be brought gently round to this over several interviews. A few patients make it clear that they never wish to discuss the possibility of death and you must be sensitive to this and respect their wishes.

Once the patient has accepted that death is imminent,

they will often ask, 'How long do I have, doctor?' It is best to be truthful and tell them that you do not know. If they persist, talk in terms of 'a matter of days, weeks or months' as seems appropriate. You will usually be wrong.

The everyday care of a dying patient is a nursing speciality, requiring great sensitivity and skill. The houseman must make certain that the pain relief is adequate. Added sedation at night is often necessary. Otherwise the purpose of treatment is the control of symptoms with the minimum of discomfort. The patient should still be seen regularly, especially when they are dying. Most patients know the situation and take a lack of visits by the houseman as evidence that they have been forgotten and are already regarded as deceased.

Confirming death

A doctor is required to verify death. The four signs to confirm are as follows.

1 No pulse.
2 No heart sounds.
3 No breath sounds.
4 Pupils fixed and dilated.

Sufficient time must be spent listening for heart and breath sounds to confidently exclude a very slow cardiac rate or intermittent breathing. Be particularly careful if the patient has taken an overdose or has been on sedative drugs.

If you are uncertain (for example in an obese patient in a deep coma, in whom you might not be able to feel the pulse or hear the heart sounds anyway), do the following:

1 Look in the optic fundi − the blood in the retinal veins becomes separated when circulation stops.
2 Perform an ECG or an electro-encephalogram (EEG).

As you leave the patient and are approached by the relatives, you must be absolutely certain whether or not death has occurred.

Informing the relatives of a patient who has died

The death may be expected or unexpected. Telling relatives about an expected death is usually straightforward. Giving information about an unexpected death often results in great distress and is a difficult situation to handle.

Again privacy is important when talking to the relatives. Leave your bleep outside and ask not to be disturbed. Speak clearly, slowly and truthfully and usually the best line to take is to tell them of the death early and then talk a little about the reasons of why and how it happened. Offer comfort where possible, saying, for example, that the patient died peacefully and was not in pain. Relatives will usually demand to know why the death has occurred and ask, 'What has gone wrong?' Try not to be defensive about the care the patient has received and make the seriousness of the patient's illness clear. Emphasize that prolonged suffering has been avoided if this is the case. After that it is useful to sit briefly in silence allowing the relatives to take it all in. Where appropriate, physical contact like grasping a hand does more good than ten minutes' talking.

It is a help to ask a senior nurse to come in and arrange for refreshments to be brought. However much the surgical team may have done for the patient, at that moment the relative sees you as the conveyor of bad news, and there may come a point when it is best to leave the relative in the company of a nurse who can sit, talk quietly and comfort them.

The post-mortem

Post-mortems are performed for two reasons. Firstly, all cases referred to the coroner undergo a post-mortem unless he is fully satisfied about the cause of death. This is done as a routine and is a legal requirement.

Secondly, post-mortems are performed to obtain information about a death, information which may be of value in treating other patients later. An autopsy should ideally be performed on all patients dying in hospital. Such a post-mortem is requested by the consultant responsible for the case and requires the relatives' permission. You may have to obtain this. It is best to tell the relatives that post-mortems are usually done on patients who die in hospital and ask for their permission, pointing out that the information obtained will benefit other patients. Most relatives understand the need but they do not wish to discuss details at a time of great distress. They also wish to be reassured that the funeral arrangements will not be delayed.

The housesurgeon must then send the case notes, any relevant investigations, the form of consent and usually another form with a brief synopsis of the patient's history and progress while in hospital, down to the post-mortem room. It is worth while finding out when the post-mortem is to be held so that you can attend. Often you are the only member of the surgical team who is able to do so.

Death certificates, the coroner and cremation forms

Death certificates

When one of your patients dies, you are legally required to fill in a death certificate and send this to the Registrar of Births and Deaths. The information is used to prepare national statistics about causes of death.

You can only fill in the death certificate if you attended the deceased before death. If you see the body for the first time after death you are not qualified to sign the certificate. It cannot be signed by someone else on your behalf either. Any medical practitioner who signs a death certificate must be registered. Provisional registration entitles a housesurgeon to sign death certificates only in cases arising out of his duties in an approved hospital while working for a fully registered practitioner.

Ideally a certificate should be issued for all deaths, even those that are also being referred to the coroner. In this case Box A on the back of the certificate must be initialled informing the registrar that he must wait for the coroner's decision before allowing the body to be buried or cremated.

In addition, a separate form must be signed and given to the informant saying that the death certificate has been issued. The informant, usually a relative of the deceased (other persons entitled to perform this role are listed on the back of the death certificate), is legally required to take the death certificate sealed in an envelope to the registrar within 5 days (8 days in Scotland). The informant will also be required to state certain particulars relating to the deceased's life. A counterfoil is filled in to be kept by the hospital.

The death certificate starts by stating the patient's particulars. There then follows a section where the housesurgeon is required to state whether he saw the body after death. This is not a legal requirement, although it is a sensible thing to do in order to avoid cases of mistaken identity.

Statement of cause of death

This is in two parts.

Part One records the sequence of conditions and diseases that led to the patient's death. This is written in sequential order, starting with the condition that actually caused death, and going on to the underlying disease. This sequence must be causally linked. Each condition entered at the top of the list should occur as a consequence of the condition written immediately below it, eventually ending up with the underlying cause.

For example, a patient with chronic peptic ulceration who dies of peritonitis a few days after an operation for perforation of a duodenal ulcer would be entered as follows.

(a) Peritonitis, due to

(b) perforation of duodenal ulcer [operation date], due to

(c) peptic ulcer of the duodenum.

The terms used must be precise. Words like 'pulmonary oedema' or 'coma' are not accurate enough. Words like 'cirrhosis' imply alcohol toxicity and, whether or not this is true, the registrar will refer the case to the coroner. If the condition was infectious, the site, causal organism and duration of infection must be stated. If a tumour occurs in the list, state the histology and whether it was malignant or benign, the anatomical site, and whether it was primary or secondary. If it was a secondary tumour, indicate the site of the primary and whether this had been removed or not.

Part Two records other conditions that may have contributed to the death, but are not related to the causal sequence of disease described in Part One.

For example, the above patient's form might be completed with 'Part Two: Chronic bronchitis'.

Other examples are available for guidance in the book of death certificates. There is also a list of unacceptable terms.

On the back of the death certificate there are two boxes. Box A has already been described. Box B is a box that must be initialled by the practitioner if he is still awaiting results of laboratory tests which may aid the diagnosis that he has put on the certificate.

It is most important that this death certificate is filled in legibly and correctly. Otherwise it will be rejected by the registrar and delay the arrangements for burial or cremation. There is no significant variation in the form of death certificate in Scotland, Wales or Ireland.

If you feel that the patient's death is unexplained, you cannot sign the death certificate and the case must be referred to the coroner.

Referral to the coroner

The role of the coroner is to investigate death. He does this in order to ensure that the cause of death was natural and to identify deaths where further enquiry is necessary. Such deaths include those where a crime may have been committed, where there is an accusation of negligence on behalf of the police authorities or medical profession, or where claims for compensation might follow. All the facts necessary to answer any such enquiry must be available before the disposal of the body.

Cases that need reporting

Below is a list of circumstances where a death should be reported to the coroner. The Registrar of Births and Deaths is under a statutory obligation to report such cases. Medical practitioners, however, are not, although in practice it saves time and establishes a close working relationship between the medical profession and the coroner's office if they do so. It is also the duty in Common Law of anyone to report such cases, although this is not enforceable.

1 Where the cause of death is unknown.

2 Where no doctor has treated the deceased in their terminal illness, or where the deceased's medical practitioner did not attend the patient within 14 days of death.

3 Where death is associated with medical treatment, e.g. deaths occurring during an operation or during recovery from a general anaesthetic. Generally, any death occurring in the 24 hours after an anaesthetic is reportable, although there is some variation with different coroners. Also, cases where any form of medical treatment, including drug therapy, has contributed to a patient's death should be reported.

4 Sudden, unexplained or suspicious death. This includes death occurring within 24 hours of emergency admission to hospital.

5 Death from industrial accident or disease, road traffic accidents, domestic accidents (e.g. death following a fall causing fractured neck of femur), deaths from violence or neglect, death following abortion, death from poisoning (including alcohol), and cases of suicide.

6 Any case where, following death, there is a definite or suspected claim for negligence either against the doctors or nursing staff. In such a case medical practitioners must not only inform the coroner but also inform their defence union immediately and give no verbal or written statement to the injured party until this is done.

7 Death while a patient was in legal custody. For instance, you might be involved in treating a case which has been brought in from police custody, having been found unconscious.

In cases where you are uncertain whether or not you ought to report the case to the coroner, always telephone him or his officer and discuss it. After hearing your story he may well give permission for you to write a death certificate.

The coroner has three courses of action in dealing with the case. Firstly, he may, after considering the facts, be satisfied that the cause of death was natural and no post-mortem is required. He will then allow a death certificate to be issued.

Secondly, he may require that a post-mortem be carried out, usually by a coroner's pathologist. If the result shows that the death was from natural causes then there is no need for an inquest and the death certificate can be issued.

Thirdly, he may feel, following a post-mortem, that an inquest should be held. This includes all criminal cases, suicides, death from accidents or industrial mishap, deaths in custody and deaths where claims of negligence have been put forward. In cases where negligence is claimed against a medical practitioner, he must be legally represented by his defence society.

The system in Scotland and Ireland is broadly similar, although in Scotland the role of the coroner is performed by the procurator-fiscal.

Cremation forms

Once the registrar has received the death certificate and approved it and providing that no further evidence is required from the body, he authorizes its disposal and issues a certificate for this. This may be by either burial or cremation. Cremation is under very strict control. This ensures that medico-legal evidence is not destroyed and that cremation is not performed against the wishes of the relatives or of the deceased.

The cremation form is in two parts, each signed by a separate doctor. These doctors must not be related and should not be partners of the same practice. In hospital the two doctors should not belong to the same 'firm'.

The first part ('Form B') is signed by the doctor who issued the death certificate. In this case the doctor is legally required to examine the body after death and give details of the mode of dying, in addition to the clinical diagnosis and cause of death. It also asks if the patient has a cardiac pacemaker. If this is present it must be removed before cremation because of the risk that the mercury batteries might explode.

The second part ('Form C') is signed by a doctor who must have been fully registered for at least five years. He must not be related to the deceased. He must also see the body after death and question the doctor signing Form B.

The purpose of this procedure is that both doctors must certify the cause of death, confirm that it is natural, and agree that further examination or enquiry is unnecessary.

Other medical certificates and legal statements

A doctor may be required to provide statements on a patient's health for insurance companies, for employment or to be used as evidence by the police. In the latter case, house-surgeons must discuss the case with their consultant, who is ultimately responsible for that patient. In casualty, statements are commonly required on victims of assault and the house officers are often the only people who have seen and treated the patient concerned. In this case they must write the report themselves. Any such statement should be factual and truthful. Keep to the medical facts and avoid laying the blame on anyone. Try to include measurements and figures where possible when describing injuries. In cases of difficulty the doctor's defence union will be able to advise.

Surgical audit

Carrying out a regular audit of medical activity is now a requirement for all units in the United Kingdom. You will be partly responsible for collecting data for this.

Data may be collected:

(a) manually − from what has been recorded in the notes and discharge summary, or

(b) into a computer − data are collected using a proforma or entered directly into the machine from a keyboard. This is often combined with the process of discharge summary production.

The data required for audit will include details of the following.

Patient: address, GP, date of birth, sex, etc.

Admission: emergency/elective, consultant, ward, source, etc.

Diagnosis: find out who is supposed to choose diagnoses and what system of verification (if any) is in use.

Operation: enough details are required to allow this to be coded for later analysis.

Complications: record anything which has been a problem during admission.

The data will subsequently be used for presentation at regular audit meetings when the total workload and any problems arising from it will be reviewed and discussed. You can make this process considerably easier by making sure accurate and relevant data are recorded *during the patient's admission*. Trying to ascertain facts after the patient has left the hospital is much more time-consuming.

Find out what system is in use on your unit. Keep up with the work by clearing notes each day. A huge pile of notes awaiting processing after patient discharge can become a depressing burden.

Coding

In order to allow accurate analysis, the diagnosis, the operation and often the complications will need to be coded. This may be done in two ways.

(a) *Manually*: a form of words is chosen by the medical team and then coded (using a code book such as ICD9) either by medical staff, secretaries or coding clerks.

(b) *By computer*: the diagnosis is selected from some kind of predetermined list, either of diagnostic terms or of codes. In the best computer programs the choice is in words and the coding is done by the machine.

Whatever system is used it is important to choose the diagnoses accurately, and it is the doctor's responsibility to do this. If a term has to be ill defined (e.g. diagnoses of abdominal pain of unknown cause), record the possible diagnoses considered (e.g. ?constipation, ?diverticular disease). When in doubt about what diagnosis to choose, ask your registrar or consultant.

3   The Head and Neck

3.1 Lumps in the head and neck
Introduction
Cervical auricle
Lumps in the parotid region
Lumps in the submandibular region
Lumps in the anterior triangle of the neck
Cervical rib

3.2 Cervical lymphadenopathy
Enlarged lymph nodes and lymphatic conditions
Malignant lymphoma
Cystic hygroma

3.3 Lumps in the thyroid gland and goitres
General assessment of thyroid lumps
Goitres
Solitary thyroid nodule
Cysts and adenomas
Carcinoma of the thyroid
Thyroglossal cyst

3.4 Parathyroids
Hyperparathyroidism
Multiple endocrine adenomas

3.5 Conditions of the mouth
Cleft lip and palate
Cysts in the mouth
Benign tumours of the mouth
Malignant tumours of the mouth
Tumours of the jaws
Malignant disease of the tonsil

3.6 Conditions of the tongue
Chronic superficial glossitis
Ulceration of the tongue
Neoplasms of the tongue
Carcinoma of the tongue

3.1 Lumps in the Head and Neck

Introduction

An important early step in the diagnosis of lumps in the head and neck is to decide whether the lump is in the skin or deep to the skin.

Lumps in the skin include those peculiar to this area, such as cervical auricle (see below), and others common anywhere in the skin such as sebaceous cysts, dermoids, lipomas, fibromas, basal cell carcinomata and squamous cell carcinomata. The latter are dealt with in Section 10.

If the lump is deep to the skin you will have to decide in which anatomical region it belongs and particularly whether it is behind, beneath or in front of the sternomastoid muscle. The important anatomical regions are the parotid, the submandibular, the pretracheal area, and the anterior and pos-

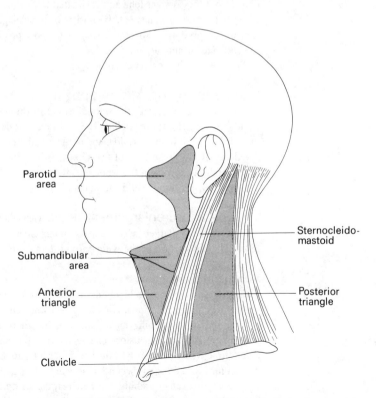

Fig. 26. Some important anatomical areas in the head and neck.

135

terior triangles of the neck (see Fig. 26). Lumps in these regions are dealt with on the following pages.

Parotid (pp. 136–140)
Submandibular (pp. 140–143)
Anterior triangle
    Branchial sinus (p. 143)
    Branchial cyst (p. 144)
    Carotid body tumour (p. 146)
    Pharyngeal pouch (p. 147)
Posterior triangle
    Cervical rib (p. 149)
    Cystic hygroma (p. 155)
Pretracheal area
    Thyroid (pp. 157–172)
    Parathyroid (pp. 173–177)
All areas
    Cervical lymphadenopathy (p. 151)
    Malignant lymphoma (p. 153)

Cervical auricle

This is an accessory ear lobe and is situated low in the neck anterior to the sternomastoid. It consists of a cartilaginous skeleton covered with skin, and is easy to diagnose providing the clinician is familiar with it.

Treatment is by cosmetic removal.

Lumps in the parotid region

You must be familiar with the normal extent of the parotid gland (see Fig. 26). If the swelling is in this area and deep to the skin, then it is in the parotid gland until proved otherwise. Swellings of the parotid are of two kinds.

1 Generalized, involving the whole gland.
2 Localized, i.e. lumps within the gland.

1 Generalized enlargement of the parotid

The parotid is enlarged secondary to either inflammatory disease or obstruction of the main parotid duct.

Viral parotitis – mumps

This disease is common in children and causes bilateral parotid swelling. Occasionally it may affect only one side. The parotid duct opening looks inflamed, but there is no pus. There is usually a history of contact with the disease about three weeks previously. Check whether the patient has had mumps in the past as second attacks are very rare. The virus may also cause orchitis and pancreatitis. In doubtful cases, two mumps virus antibody titres taken one week apart may be helpful. No specific treatment is required and the swelling usually resolves over 7–10 days.

Bacterial parotitis

The condition   Acute bacterial parotitis used to be common in surgical wards. The condition is usually secondary to obstruction of the duct by viscid secretions. Embolization during septicaemia has also been implicated. The condition is much rarer nowadays but may be seen occasionally. The usual organisms are *Staphylococcus, Streptococcus* or *Pneumococcus.*

Recognizing the   *The patient*
pattern   It occurs in dehydrated patients postoperatively, particularly in the elderly.

The history
This is of a dull throbbing pain and swelling on the side of the face. The pain is worse on speaking or eating.

On examination
Examination of the inside of the mouth may show pus extruding from the opening of the parotid duct. The whole gland becomes acutely inflamed and very tender and the patient looks toxic and ill.

Management   A pus swab is taken for culture and antibiotic sensitivity. The treatment is with antibiotics (ampicillin and flucloxacillin). The patient must be adequately rehydrated, and the mouth kept clean. Occasionally an abscess forms and may require drainage.

Auto-immune parotitis
Auto-immune disease usually affects both the other salivary glands and the lachrymal glands, causing symmetrical, painless progressive enlargement. Mikulicz's disease is enlargement of the salivary glands and lachrymal glands associated with a dry mouth. Sjögren's disease is similar but the syndrome also includes dry eyes and arthritis. The diagnosis and management of these conditions are beyond the scope of the book.

Obstruction of the parotid duct
The condition   Obstruction of the parotid duct due to stones is unusual as the parotid secretion is watery and the duct is wide. It is more often due to stenosis of the opening of the parotid duct. This may occur due to trauma of the inside of the cheek secondary to ill-fitting dentures.

The history

The patient is usually adult and complains of painful swelling
of the parotid gland during meals.

On examination

Inspection of the opening of the duct opposite the second
upper molar tooth may reveal the stenosis.

**Proving the
diagnosis**

A sialogram may be helpful in excluding the presence of
stones and may also show 'sialectasis'. This is dilatation of
the ducts within the gland due to chronic obstruction and
previous inflammatory episodes.

Management

This is usually conservative and the patient is taught to 'milk'
the duct contents forward by massaging the cheek and thus
preventing stasis in the duct. If the stenosis is severe, it may
be dilated using lachrymal duct dilators under a local
anaesthetic. Antibiotics are given if infection is present.

2 Localized lumps in the parotid

Causative lesions

Sixty per cent of parotid lumps eventually prove to be mixed
tumours (pleomorphic adenomas, see below).

An adenolymphoma (also called Warthin's tumour)
is benign but may be bilateral or multiple. This tumour
accounts for 10% of parotid neoplasms. The tumour is soft
and may feel cystic.

Other tumours are less common and include the muco-
epidermoid tumour and acinic cell tumour. Both of these are
benign but may recur locally and occasionally undergo malignant change.

The adenoid cystic carcinoma (cylindroma) is a malignant
lesion and has a tendency to spread along nerve sheaths.

Carcinoma of the parotid is a highly malignant lesion
which may arise from a mixed cell tumour. By the time it
presents there may already be extensive local infiltration with
or without nerve paralysis.

The most common non-neoplastic solitary nodule is a
cyst.

Mixed tumours of the parotid

The condition

Mixed tumours are so called because they contain adenoma
cells surrounded by pools of mucin, which look like cartilage
on histological sections. These tumours are benign but have
an incomplete capsule and consequently have a high rate of
local recurrence if incompletely removed. There is also a

risk of malignant change in the long term. Because of these factors it is very important to excise the tumour with a good margin.

Recognizing the pattern

The history
This is a slowly growing painless swelling on the side of the face. The patient is more often male and may be of any age beyond the teens.

On examination
There is a hard, smooth lump in the parotid area, usually in the lower anterior part of the gland just above the angle of the jaw. This may appear to be quite superficial, but careful examination will show that the skin moves over it. Establish that the lump is indeed in the parotid gland and not attached deeply to bone or muscle. Look for extensions inside the mouth or pharynx, and check whether the facial nerve is involved by observing facial movements. Look for involved lymph nodes on both sides of the neck. If any of these are found the lesion may be malignant.

Proving the diagnosis

The diagnosis is proved by excision biopsy, which is described below.

Management

A suspected mixed tumour of the parotid should be removed by superficial parotidectomy.

Preoperative management
The patient should be warned of the slight possibility of a facial weakness postoperatively, although this is usually transient. A nerve stimulator may be required during the operation and theatre should be informed of this.

Operation: superficial parotidectomy
A long incision is made behind the mandible and extended deeply beneath the external auditory meatus to identify the trunk of the facial nerve. The nerve and its branches are then traced forwards in the parotid gland and all tissue superficial to them excised together with the tumour. If the tumour is deep to the facial nerve it can be excised by displacing the nerve branches. The wound is usually drained using a suction drain.

Codes
Blood . . . .   0 . . . .
GA/LA . . . .   GA . . . .
Opn time . . . .   2−3 hours . . . .

Stay	3−5 days	....
Drains out	24−48 hours	....
Sutures out	3−5 days	....
Off work	2−3 weeks	....

Postoperative care

Check and record the movements of the facial muscles supplied by each individual branch of the facial nerve, i.e. temporal, orbital, buccal, mandibular and cervical. If there is any weakness, note whether it is partial (in which case full recovery is certain). If it is complete, recovery is also likely unless a nerve is known to have been divided at operation. Recovery takes 6−8 weeks.

The clips or sutures are removed, leaving those in any unhealed area until the last. If the tumour is malignant, radiotherapy will probably be given. Occasionally radiotherapy is also given to mixed tumours of the parotid, particularly if the margin of excision is close. With mixed tumours of the parotid, regular follow-up is advisable.

Management of other parotid lumps

Because of the possibility of neoplasia, these lumps will usually be excised to establish an exact diagnosis. If the lump is obviously malignant then biopsy and radiotherapy may be the only possible treatment. For lesions of unknown aetiology, however, biopsy alone is not advisable as it may result in local implantation of a neoplasm. Most lesions of the parotid are, therefore, removed by superficial parotidectomy.

Lumps in the submandibular region

The submandibular salivary gland measures about 4 cm × 3 cm and is situated beneath the angle of the jaw. Its superficial portion is in the neck outside the mylohyoid muscle and its deep portion lies in the floor of the mouth deep to the mylohyoid. Its duct drains from the deep part of the gland forwards to the floor of the mouth beneath the tip of the tongue (Fig. 27).

As in the parotid, enlargements are either generalized or localized.

Generalized enlargement of the gland is commonly secondary to stone formation. It also occurs in auto-immune syndromes (as in the parotid gland).

Localized enlargements are of the same aetiology as those already described for the parotid gland (p. 138).

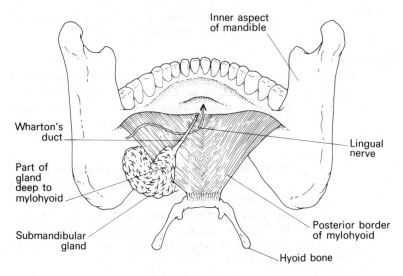

Fig. 27. The anatomy of the submandibular gland. The floor of the mouth viewed posteriorly (tongue removed).

Submandibular stones

The condition

The secretion of this gland is more viscous than that of the parotid and the duct is narrower, so stone formation and obstruction are relatively common. Secondary infection (usually with *Staphylococcus*, *Streptococcus* or *Pneumococcus*) is dangerous because of the risk of swelling and oedema in the floor of the mouth and consequent respiratory obstruction (Ludwig's angina).

Recognizing the pattern

The patient
The condition can occur at any age and is common in young adults.

The history
The history is of intermittent painful swelling beneath the jaw occurring with meals. The patient may also have noticed 'gravel' in the mouth.

On examination
The gland is palpable and tender during these episodes. A stone may be palpable in the duct in the floor of the mouth beneath the tongue.

Proving the diagnosis

These stones are radio-opaque and will be seen on a plain X-ray of the floor of the mouth. A submandibular duct sialogram will also confirm the presence of the stone, and detect any sialectasis within the gland (p. 138).

Management

In a few patients the stone will pass spontaneously. If it has been giving symptoms for 3 or 4 weeks, it can be removed from the duct using a local anaesthetic. Where the condition has become chronic, where stones are recurrent, or where the stone is situated in the gland itself, removal of the submandibular gland is preferable.

Operation: removal of stone from submandibular duct
Local anaesthetic is infiltrated in the floor of the mouth and a silk suture is passed around the duct proximal to the stone. This prevents the stone slipping back into the main gland. The buccal mucosa and the duct are incised over the stone and the stone removed. The wound in the floor of the mouth is not sutured.

Codes
Blood . . . . 0 . . . .
GA/LA . . . . LA (GA if the stone is small and will be difficult to find) . . . .
Opn time . . . . 30 minutes . . . .
Stay . . . . Day case . . . .
Drains out . . . . . . 0 . . . .
Sutures out . . . . . 0 . . . .
Off work . . . . 1 day . . . .

Postoperative care
Mouthwashes should be given.

Operation: removal of submandibular gland

Preoperative management
No special preparation is necessary. Warn the patient of possible transient weakness of the corner of the mouth (see below). A nerve stimulator can be useful at operation but it is not essential.

Operation
An incision is made 2.5 cm below the angle of the jaw over the gland. The mandibular branch of the facial nerve curves up over the jaw at this point, lying on the facial artery. It can be damaged if the incision is too high. It can also be damaged by retraction. This damage results in weakness of the corner of the mouth and care should be taken to avoid this.

When the deep portion of the gland is removed, care is

taken not to damage the lingual or hypoglossal nerves which lie deep to it. The wound is usually drained.

Codes

Blood	0 . . . .
GA/LA	GA or LA . . . .
Opn time	1–2 hours . . . .
Stay	48 hours . . . .
Drains out	About 48 hours . . . .
Sutures out	3–4 days . . . .
Off work	About 1 week . . . .

Lumps in the anterior triangle of the neck

These include the following.
Branchial sinus.
Branchial cyst.
Carotid body tumour.
Pharyngeal pouch.

Branchial sinus

The condition
During fetal life the second arch skin grows over the branchial clefts closing them off. If this closure is incomplete a fistula, sinus or cyst may result along the tract. A branchial sinus usually opens as a tiny hole in the lower part of the neck. Although the external opening may seem very small there is frequently a track running up the neck, which may go as high as the posterior pillar of the fauces in the pharynx (forming a fistula).

Recognizing the pattern
The patient
The patient is almost always a child, often in the first year of life.

The history
The sinus has usually been present from birth and the mother notices the discharge.

On examination
The opening is situated in front of the anterior border of the sternomastoid, one-third of the way up from the origin of the muscle. It discharges 'glairy' fluid intermittently.

Proving the diagnosis
The above history and signs are quite characteristic and no further investigation is necessary.

Management
The treatment is surgical removal of the whole sinus or fistula. The operation is best performed early in life before

the child's neck grows. In a baby it is often possible to excise even a long tract through one incision. The optimum time for operation is between the ages of 6 months and a year.

Preoperative management
With an older child the mother should be warned that more than one incision may be necessary to remove the whole tract. She will be surprised to hear this as the external lesion looks so insignificant.

Operation: removal of branchial fistula/sinus
The external opening is mobilized with an ellipse of skin. The tract is followed up in the neck using a lachrymal probe in its lumen as a guide. Some surgeons use methylene blue to outline the tract. The tract is dissected out as high as possible and then, if necessary, a second transverse incision is made, usually at about the level of the hyoid bone. The tract is then followed up between the internal and external carotid arteries until it reaches the pharyngeal epithelium. Frequently it peters out before this. The wound is usually drained.

Codes

Blood	Group and save serum . . . .
GA/LA	GA . . . .
Opn time	30–90 minutes depending on extent .
Stay	24–48 hours . . . .
Drains out	24 hours . . . .
Sutures out	3–5 days . . . .

Branchial cyst
A branchial cyst (Fig. 28) forms from an isolated remnant of a branchial cleft in the neck. Its wall contains lymphoid tissue and it may become inflamed in any generalized lymphadenopathy in the neck. Not infrequently the cyst contents become purulent and it may present as a cervical abscess.

Recognizing the pattern

The patient
The cyst usually makes its appearance in childhood or early adult life.

The history
It frequently appears as a swelling during an upper respiratory tract infection. It may be painful. The swelling persists once the infection has subsided. Abscess formation causes severe pain, which is worse on moving the head.

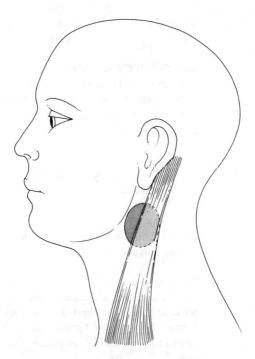

Fig. 28. A branchial cyst.

On examination
It is usually about 5–10 cm in diameter and lies deep to the sternomastoid muscle, appearing beneath its anterior border. It is frequently related to the upper third of this muscle behind the angle of the jaw (see Fig. 28). It fluctuates, but does not transilluminate as its contents are opaque.

Proving the diagnosis

The diagnosis is made on the history and the site of the swelling and no other tests are necessary.

Operation: removal of branchial cyst
A transverse incision is made over the lump and deepened until the cyst is encountered. It is then excised. Care is taken to avoid damage to the carotid vessels and internal jugular vein which usually lie deep to the swelling.

Codes
Blood . . . . 0 . . . .
GA/LA . . . . GA . . . .
Opn time . . . . 30–60 minutes . . . .
Stay . . . . 24 hours . . . .
Drains out . . . . . . 24 hours . . . .

Sutures out	3–5 days	
Off work	3–7 days	

Carotid body tumour

The condition

This tumour is a chemodectoma arising from the cells in the carotid body. It grows very slowly over many years and may finally metastasize. Histologically it is a non-chromaffin paraganglionoma.

Recognizing the pattern

The patient
The patient is usually aged over 50, although the condition can present earlier.

The history
He may notice the lump himself or it may be found at a routine medical examination.

On examination
The lump is hard and transmits pulsation rather than being pulsatile itself. It is situated at the carotid bifurcation and appears as a tumour beneath the anterior border of the sternomastoid. It is mobile from side to side but not up and down.

Proving the diagnosis

A carotid angiogram may be helpful both in defining the extent of the tumour and in establishing that there is an adequate collateral through the opposite carotid artery.

Management

The tumour is usually removed. It can, however, be safely watched for many years and this course may be preferable in the elderly, frail patient.

Preoperative management
The hairs over the upper neck should be shaved up to the mastoid process. Some surgeons may require the use of a carotid shunt (see p. 500).

Operation: removal of carotid body tumour
A vertical incision anterior to the sternomastoid is usually employed. The lesion is enucleated from around the carotid artery and this can be a very haemorrhagic procedure. Alternatively it can be excised and a graft placed between the common and internal carotid arteries. A suction drain is used. The wound is closed with clips or sutures.

Codes

Blood	4 units . . . .
GA/LA	GA . . . .
Opn time	90–120 minutes . . . .
Stay	5–7 days . . . .
Drains out	24–48 hours . . . .
Sutures out	5 days . . . .
Off work	3–4 weeks . . . .

Postoperative care

See carotid artery surgery (p. 500). The blood pressure should be monitored regularly and may tend to fall lower than preoperatively. This should be maintained by transfusing blood as necessary.

Pharyngeal pouch

The condition

A pharyngeal pouch is a pulsion diverticulum of the pharyngeal mucosa, probably arising as a result of a relative obstruction at the level of the cricopharyngeus muscle. There is frequently a previous history of heartburn and reflux due to hiatus hernia and it is possible that the obstruction is due to hypertrophy in an attempt to prevent overspill of refluxing gastro-oesophageal contents into the larynx. The mucosa protrudes through Killian's dehiscence (see Fig. 29).

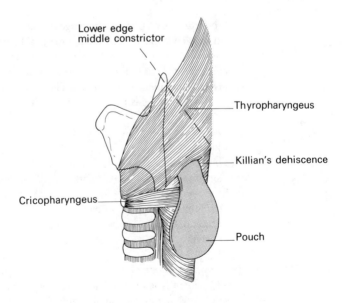

Fig. 29. The anatomy of a pharyngeal pouch.

Recognizing the pattern	*The patient* The condition occurs in elderly patients and it is more common in males.

The history

The story is one of dysphagia. Characteristically the first mouthful is easily swallowed but thereafter the pouch fills up with food and obstructs the upper oesophagus. The patient is then unable to swallow further food and will regurgitate the contents of the pouch. A swelling is present in the neck in about one-third of cases. Inhalation of regurgitated contents, especially at night, causes fits of coughing and episodes of pulmonary infection.

Proving the diagnosis

The pouch is easily demonstrated on a barium swallow. Ask the radiologist to look specifically in the upper neck.

Management

The management is to excise the pouch and release the crico-pharyngeal spasm.

Preoperative management

The patient should be put on fluids only for 24 hours preoperatively. Antibiotics may be given with the pre-medication (ampicillin and flucloxacillin). The patient is warned that he will not be able to swallow immediately postoperatively.

Operation: excision of pharyngeal pouch

An incision is made at the level of the hyoid bone usually on the left side. The mucosal pouch is found and excised and the mucosal defect closed. The crico-pharyngeus muscle is divided longitudinally (myotomy). The wound is drained and a nasogastric tube is passed down into the stomach.

Codes

Blood	0
GA/LA	GA
Opn time	1–2 hours
Stay	5–7 days
Drains out	5–7 days
Sutures out	5 days
Off work	3 weeks

Postoperative care

The patient is fed through a nasogastric tube and a barium swallow is performed on the fifth day. If this shows no leakage, normal feeding can be instituted. If leakage is demonstrated feeding continues with a nasogastric tube until a repeat barium swallow shows the pharyngeal wound has healed.

Cervical rib

The condition

In approximately 1 in 200 people the costal element of the seventh cervical vertebra over-develops to a varying degree. The result is a cervical rib which, when fully formed, is bony and attached to the first normal rib. It may, however, be nothing more than a fibrous strand. In half the cases the condition is unilateral, usually on the right side. The subclavian artery and first thoracic nerve pass over the cervical rib to gain access to the upper limb. The artery may be narrowed over the rib and dilated distally. In the latter case mural thrombus may form and give rise to distal emboli. The first thoracic nerve can also be damaged by direct pressure. Very often a thin fibrous strand causes more symptoms than a fully formed cervical rib.

Recognizing the pattern

The patient
The condition may occur in either sex and symptoms usually begin in the late teens when the neck extends and the shoulders droop.

The history
The patient may notice a swelling or tenderness in the neck on the affected side. There may be pain due to vascular insufficiency. This is worse on exercise, especially if the arm is elevated. There may be distal ischaemia with a cold pale hand and occasional numbness or even trophic changes in the fingers. More rarely the patient may complain of neurological symptoms, which include numbness and paraesthesiae in the forearm and weakness of the hands.

On examination
Palpation of the neck may reveal the abnormal rib. There may be signs of ischaemia or emboli in the hand. The radial pulse may disappear if the arm is fully elevated. Look for wasting in the hypothenar or thenar muscles and interossei and sensory changes in the first thoracic nerve distribution. There may be a bruit over the subclavian artery.

Proving the diagnosis

An X-ray of the cervical spine will demonstrate the presence of a bony cervical rib or an enlarged anterior tubercle of the seventh cervical vertebra (associated with a fibrous band).

Arteriography may demonstrate a constriction and post-stenotic dilatation in the region of the cervical rib, especially if the angiogram is taken with the arm elevated.

Management

A cervical rib causing neurological symptoms may be managed conservatively with physiotherapy to improve the muscles that elevate and support the upper limb girdle. A cervical rib causing vascular problems or well-marked neurological problems should be treated surgically.

Operation: removal of a cervical rib
The cervical rib is approached through a skin crease incision and removed, including its periosteal covering. If this covering is not removed there is a danger of recurrence. A fibrous band may also be excised. In some cases it is only necessary to split the scalenus anterior to relieve the pressure.

Codes
Blood . . . . 2 units . . . .
GA/LA . . . . GA . . . .
Opn time . . . . 1−2 hours . . . .
Stay . . . . 3−5 days . . . .
Drains out . . . . . . Suction 24 hours . . . .
Sutures out . . . . . 4 days . . . .
Off work . . . . 2−3 weeks depending on occupation .

Postoperative care
The postoperative course is usually uncomplicated. The patient should have a chest X-ray in the first few hours to exclude a pneumothorax.

Cervical Lymphadenopathy

Enlarged lymph nodes and lymphatic conditions

The condition
Enlarged cervical lymph nodes are the most common palpable lumps in the head and neck. The nodes may be enlarged due to either inflammatory or neoplastic processes and the precise node involved depends on the site of the primary pathology. It is therefore important to know which areas of the head and neck drain to the various lymph nodes (see Fig. 30 and Table 12).

Inflammatory causes of enlarged lymph nodes may be acute or chronic. Acute inflammations are common in chil-

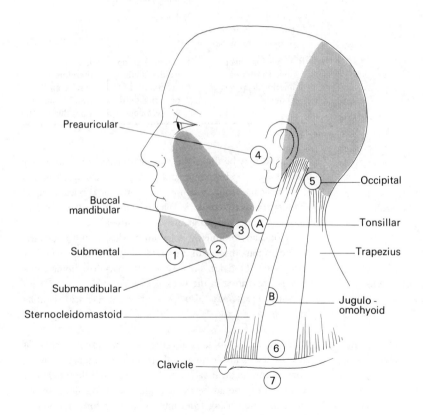

Fig. 30. The cervical lymph nodes and their areas of drainage. See Table 12 for key.

Table 12. The cervical lymph nodes and their areas of drainage

Name	Area of drainage
1 Submental group	Tip of tongue, anterior end of lower lip, floor of mouth and lower gum, bilateral drainage
2 Submandibular group	Submental group, centre of forehead, nose, paranasal sinuses, front of neck, lips, anterior two-thirds of tongue
3 Buccal and mandibular group	Cheek, lower eyelid
4 Preauricular group	Temple, vertex, eyelids, orbit, external acoustic meatus
5 Occipital group	Back of scalp, posterior edge of pinna
6 Supraclavicular group	Occipital nodes, axillary nodes, breast, body wall
7 Infraclavicular group	Lower neck, pre-axial border of upper limb, body wall, breast
A Tonsillar node (anterior superior deep cervical node)	Subcutaneous nodes, tonsil
B Jugulo-omohyoid node (posterior inferior deep cervical node)	Submental group, submandibular group, posterior third of the tongue ⎫ These nodes therefore receive all the lymph drainage from the tongue ⎭

dren and may be due to viruses or bacteria. The latter may progress to pus formation and present as a cervical abscess.

A typical chronic inflammatory cause of cervical lymphadenopathy is tuberculosis. These lymph nodes become very indurated and tend to give rise to sinuses.

Neoplasms producing enlarged cervical lymph nodes include primary disease of the lymphatic system and secondary neoplasms. Hodgkin's disease is a primary lymphoma commonly presenting in the neck.

Sarcoidosis may also present as a cervical lymphadenopathy.

Making the diagnosis

It is important to look for the possible primary sites of disease. Look inside the mouth, including the fauces, tonsils, tongue and teeth. Ideally a full ear, nose and throat (ENT) examination should be carried out. Nodes low down in the neck may be arising from intrathoracic or intra-abdominal pathology (Virchow's node). Look for enlarged nodes elsewhere and hepatosplenomegaly.

A battery of screening tests is indicated in any lymphadenopathy and this includes a full blood count, erythrocyte sedimentation rate, infectious mononucleosis screening, Wassermann reaction and chest X-ray. The final arbiter in diagnosis of cervical lymphadenopathy is a biopsy of the lymph nodes and histological examination.

Operation: biopsy of cervical lymph node

An incision is made over the enlarged node and it is removed. If the node is very large or infected a drain may be used. Remember to send part of the node for bacteriological culture, including tuberculosis, as well as for histological examination.

Codes

Blood	0 . . . .
GA/LA	LA or GA . . . .
Opn time	15–45 minutes: depends on size and adherence of node . . . .
Stay	Depends on cause . . . .
Drains out	24 hours . . . .
Sutures out	5 days . . . .
Off work	Variable . . . .

Postoperative care
The cause of the lymphadenopathy will have to be treated.

Acute inflammatory lymphadenopathy
The correct treatment in the first 24 hours is antibiotics, but once pus formation occurs (after 48 hours) drainage becomes necessary. Treating a cervical abscess with antibiotics leads to a chronic swelling (antibioma).

Tuberculous lymphadenitis
Modern treatment is with antituberculous therapy and excision of lymph nodes if they fail to settle.

Hodgkin's disease
The management of Hodgkin's disease is discussed below.

Malignant lymphoma

The condition
Lymphomas are malignant neoplasms of lymphoid tissue. They are divided on a histological basis into Hodgkin's disease and non-Hodgkin's lymphoma. Further subdivisions of lymphomas are made on histological and immunological criteria. These subgroups have different prognoses and may require different approaches to treatment.

A lymphoma typically presents with asymptomatic lymph-adenopathy which may or may not be localized. Some patients have systemic symptoms which may include fever, weight loss and night sweats (Type B symptoms). Other symptoms include malaise, pruritis and alcohol-induced pain. The diagnosis is confirmed by biopsy of an enlarged node. It is essential to send fresh unfixed material to the laboratory.

Staging the disease

Once the diagnosis has been made, further investigation is performed to stage the disease. This is done to determine what type of treatment is required and to predict the prognosis. The staging is as follows:

Stage I   A single group of nodes involved.

Stage IE   A single extralymphatic organ or site, e.g. skin (rare).

Stage II   Two or more lymph node sites are involved on the same side of the diaphragm.

Stage III   Lymph node sites are involved on both sides of the diaphragm. This includes involvement of the spleen.

Stage IV   Extralymphatic organ involvement (e.g. liver, bone marrow or lung).

Each stage is subdivided into A or B depending on the absence (Type A) or presence (Type B) of symptoms.

Investigations

The patients are usually 'worked up' on a medical or haematological unit. The investigations may include the following.

1 Full blood count, erythrocyte sedimentation rate (ESR), liver function tests and plasma proteins.

2 Chest X-rays.

3 Computerized axial tomography of the chest or abdomen.

4 Bone marrow biopsy.

5 Lymphangiogram — this is now rarely used.

6 Bone scan and/or liver and spleen scan.

7 Liver biopsy. This is done if there is significant hepatomegaly (more than 3.5 cm). A positive result means Stage IV disease and makes laparotomy unnecessary.

8 Staging laparotomy. This used to be carried out to look for abdominal spread if the above investigations failed to show definite Stage IV disease. It has since been outdated by improved imaging techniques.

9 Magnetic resonance scanning may be useful for imaging glands in the high cervical region and assessing node involvement.

Management	Lymphomas may be treated by radiotherapy, combination chemotherapy or both, the choice depending on the stage of the disease and histological subtype, and whether the patient has significant symptoms.

Radiotherapy may be given either to the group of involved nodes (involved field) or to wider areas (extended field, e.g. 'mantle' or 'inverted Y').

Chemotherapy is given systemically either with a single drug or more usually with a combination of drugs. The choice depends on the stage of the disease, the patient's age, the ESR, the bulk of the disease and the histological grading. The present principles of treatment are outlined below.

Stages IA and IIA: these categories of Hodgkin's disease are treated with radiotherapy (involved field or extended field). Adjuvant chemotherapy is increasingly used, even in limited stage disease.

All other stages are treated with combination chemotherapy.

Non-Hodgkin's lymphomata are treated on similar lines, although chemotherapy is introduced at an earlier stage, with combination chemotherapy for the higher histological grades and single agents for lower grade lymphomata. Radiation may be used to control local sites of disease.

Cystic hygroma

The condition

This is a congenital lesion made up of lymph-filled spaces which arise from an embryonic remnant of the jugular lymph sac. Its correct name is a cavernous lymphangioma. It occurs in the base of the neck, both in the posterior triangle and anteriorly. It may extend up to the jaw, over the anterior chest wall, and down into the axilla. Very occasionally it may occur in the axilla alone.

Recognizing the pattern

The patient
The lesion occurs in young children and is often noticed at birth.

On examination
There is a soft, cystic and compressible lump just beneath the skin, superficial to the neck muscles. It transilluminates brilliantly, tends to vary in size and may have a lobular surface.

Management

In the past, attempts have been made to obliterate this lesion in various ways, including the injection of hypertonic or boiling fluids. However, the lesion is best treated by surgical excision.

Preoperative management

The patient or parent should be warned of the slight possibility of damage to branches of the brachial plexus and that some of the lesion may have to be left behind in order to avoid this. If that turns out to be the case, there will be a possibility of recurrence.

Operation: excision of cystic hygroma

Removal of a large lesion can be tedious as it may ramify amongst the branches of the brachial plexus. It should be removed completely if possible, or it will recur. Occasionally a cystic hygroma extends into the axilla and in that case a separate incision is needed to remove it.

Codes

Blood	1 unit in babies, otherwise group and save . . . .
GA/LA	GA . . . .
Opn time	Depends on extent: 1−2 hours . . . . . .
Stay	2−5 days . . . .
Drains out	2−5 days . . . .
Sutures out	3−5 days . . . .

Postoperative care

This is usually uncomplicated. The main problem is that fluid and blood tend to collect at the site of the cystic hygroma and the suction drains therefore need to be left for a long time. If fluid continues to collect after they are removed, it will have to be aspirated until the cavity heals completely. The length of hospital stay depends on the extent of the lesion.

Solitary lymph cyst

This is a variant of the cystic hygroma in which only one cyst is present. It is treated by simple excision.

3.3   Lumps in the Thyroid Gland and Goitres

General assessment of thyroid lumps

Faced with a lump in the pretracheal region of the neck, you have to decide on the following:

1 Is it in the thyroid?
2 Is it solitary or generalized?
3 Is the patient toxic, euthyroid or myxoedematous?

1 Is the lump in the thyroid gland?

The thyroid gland is situated behind the pretracheal fascia and, as this fascia is attached to the larynx, the gland moves up and down on swallowing. This feature, together with their midline situation, makes the diagnosis of thyroid swellings easy. The patient is given a glass of water and asked to raise his chin. The clinician first observes the lump from in front and then feels it standing behind the patient. The patient is asked to swallow and the movement of the lump is noted.

2 Is it solitary or generalized?

Is the enlargement of:
(a) the whole gland (a goitre)? This is dealt with on p. 158;
(b) or a nodule within the gland (solitary nodule)? This is dealt with on pp. 164–170.

3 Thyroid status

The patient may be:
(a) thyrotoxic;
(b) euthyroid, i.e. normal;
(c) myxoedematous.

Thyrotoxicosis

Patients with an over-active thyroid gland have symptoms of tiredness, weight loss, anxiety, tremor, palpitations and amenorrhoea, and tend to prefer cold to hot weather.

On examination there is nervousness and agitation, a tachycardia of over 100, fine tremor of the fingers, and lid lag. There may also be exophthalmos. A bruit is often audible over a toxic goitre.

Myxoedema

Myxoedematous patients are slow in thought, speech and

157

movement, are overweight, have thickened skin, and tend to lose their hair. They have a slow pulse rate. They prefer warm weather.

Investigations for thyroid lumps

The following tests are used to investigate thyroid lumps.

1 *Serum tri-iodothyronine and tetra-iodothyronine (T3 and T4).* These are raised in thyrotoxicosis.

2 *Thyroid stimulating hormone (TSH).* This gives an indication of the activity of the pituitary in stimulating the thyroid. There is a feedback mechanism whereby TSH is raised when the thyroid hormone level is below normal. An elevated TSH therefore confirms hypothyroidism. In hyperthyroidism it is depressed, but most assay methods are not accurate enough to detect this.

3 *Thyrotrophin releasing hormone test (TRH test).* In this test thyrotrophin (TSH) levels are measured after a dose of TRH (200 µg in 2 ml i.v.). Normally this produces a rise in TSH by 20 minutes and levels fall again by 60 minutes after the injection. No such rise occurs in thyrotoxicosis because the pituitary is suppressed by the high T4 level. The rise is exaggerated in primary hypothyroidism.

4 *Thyroid antibody estimation.* (See Hashimoto's disease, p. 159.)

5 *X-ray of thoracic inlet and chest X-ray.* The important points to look for are whether the trachea is deviated by the nodule and whether it is narrow in either its anteroposterior or lateral diameter. On the chest X-ray look for a retrosternal extension of the thyroid lump.

6 *Thyroid scan.* The patient is given radio-active technetium to drink and the tissue uptake over the thyroid gland is plotted. A toxic gland shows a markedly increased uptake of radio-active tracer over the normal. This increased uptake may be generalized, as in Graves' disease, or focal (a 'hot nodule'), as in a toxic autonomous nodule. A cold (inactive) nodule suggests possible malignancy.

7 *Ultrasound scan.* This shows if the lump is solid or cystic and may show if it is solitary or part of a multinodular goitre.

Goitres

There are four main types:
(a) physiological,
(b) nodular,
(c) inflammatory,
(d) toxic.

Physiological goitre

A physiological goitre occurs at puberty, during pregnancy and in conditions of iodine deficiency. Apart from the latter state, no treatment is necessary.

Nodular goitre

A nodular goitre is a benign enlargement of the thyroid gland with areas of hyperplasia and involution. No treatment is necessary, unless:

(a) the patient becomes thyrotoxic;

(b) there is compression of other neck structures, resulting in dyspnoea or dysphagia;

(c) the patient is particularly worried by the cosmetic appearance of the goitre;

(d) a focal increase in size or the development of hoarseness (due to recurrent laryngeal nerve palsy) suggests malignant change.

In any of these cases subtotal thyroidectomy may be indicated (see below).

Inflammatory goitre

The usual causes of diffuse inflammation of the thyroid gland are Hashimoto's disease and De Quervain's thyroiditis. Riedel's thyroiditis is very rare.

Hashimoto's disease

The condition

In this condition antibodies are produced against thyroid components.

Recognizing the pattern

The patient is usually a middle-aged female who presents with a goitre and is usually at first thyrotoxic and later myxoedematous. The gland is diffusely enlarged initially, but later becomes replaced by a small fibrotic remnant with a characteristic bosselated surface.

Proving the diagnosis

The diagnosis is proved by finding thyroid antibodies in the serum.

Management

In Hashimoto's disease operation should be avoided as this will hasten the onset of thyroid deficiency. Patients should be warned that they may eventually require thyroid hormone replacement. If they are already myxoedematous, this should be instituted (thyroxine 0.15−0.25 mg/day). Thyroidectomy is occasionally required to relieve pressure symptoms, for cosmetic reasons, or to establish a diagnosis.

	De Quervain's thyroiditis
The condition	This is a non-suppurative inflammation of the gland due to a viral infection. The usual organism is the Coxsackie virus.
Recognizing the pattern	A patient of either sex (more commonly female) presents with an acutely swollen, tender gland, often preceded by a sore throat and mild constitutional upset. The patient becomes pyrexial and transiently thyrotoxic.
Proving the diagnosis	There may be a lymphocytosis and a raised ESR. Typically the T4 may be elevated in the acute state but the uptake of radio-active iodine by the inflamed gland is diminished. There are no thyroid antibodies in the serum.
Management	Mild analgesia is usually sufficient. More severe cases may be treated with three courses of prednisolone (10−20 mg/day). The condition settles spontaneously but may recur. Hypothyroidism is very unlikely.

Riedel's thyroiditis

Riedel's thyroiditis is a rare condition of the thyroid in which the gland becomes hard and enlarged with infiltration of scar tissue, which then involves the surrounding tissues. It results in hypothyroidism, recurrent laryngeal nerve palsy and stridor. Because of these features, it mimics carcinoma of the thyroid. It often has to be biopsied in order to establish the diagnosis. The management, once the diagnosis is established, is to leave well alone and treat with thyroxine if the patient becomes myxoedematous.

Toxic goitre (thyrotoxicosis or Graves' disease)

The condition	Thyroid hormones regulate the basal metabolic rate. Their own level is controlled by the thyroid stimulating hormone (TSH) released by the pituitary.

Graves' thyrotoxicosis is now thought to be an autoimmune disease. Auto-antibodies against the TSH receptor on thyroid membrane have been isolated, and these stimulate the gland. Long-acting thyroid stimulator−protector (LATS−P) is a human-specific immunoglobulin found in almost all patients. LATS itself is not human specific and is found in fewer patients. The TSH levels are abnormally low.

The condition has a familial incidence, and there is an association between it and other auto-immune diseases (e.g. myasthenia gravis, pernicious anaemia, Addison's disease). There is diffuse enlargement of the gland with hyperplasia and hypertrophy. There may be a lymphocyte and plasma cell infiltration. In a proportion of patients the disease is self-limiting.

Recognizing the pattern

The patient
Females are more often affected than males and the disease usually occurs between the ages of 15 and 45. Thyrotoxicosis may, however, occur in both younger and older patients. The symptoms of toxicity are described on (p. 157).

On examination
In a toxic goitre the gland is smoothly enlarged and the patient shows signs of thyrotoxicosis. The skin over the gland may be warm and there is often a systolic bruit. Thyrotoxicosis may also be associated with exophthalmos or pretibial myxoedema.

Management

There are three possible forms of management available for the thyrotoxic patient. These are as follows.
1 *Medical treatment.* This is the first-line treatment of Graves' disease in patients younger than 25, providing the goitre is not too large.
(a) The production of thyroid hormones can be blocked using drugs such as carbimazole (5–10 mg 8-hourly) or propylthiouracil (100 mg 8-hourly). The drugs are stopped after 18–24 months. If the patient relapses, then surgery should be considered.
(b) Propranolol gives symptomatic relief, particularly of tachycardia, palpitations, tremor, sweating and nervousness. The usual dose is 80–120 mg/day in divided doses. It is used in the preoperative preparation of the patient (see below), in the control of a 'thyroid crisis', and in patients who need to have their own production of thyroid hormones monitored (e.g. following ^{131}I therapy).
2 *Radio-active iodine treatment.* Because of the slight risk of late malignancy, radio-active iodine is contraindicated in younger patients and is reserved for those with thyrotoxicosis over the age of 50. It is also used for recurrent thyrotoxicosis after thyroidectomy. The patient drinks radio-active iodine, which is concentrated in the thyroid, which thus undergoes self-destruction. A variable dose is required and it takes about three months to take effect. In that time propranolol is used to control symptoms. A second dose of radio-active iodine may be needed. Regular follow-up is required and at least 40% of patients become hypothyroid within 10 years, requiring replacement therapy.
3 *Surgical treatment.* This is subtotal thyroidectomy. It is indicated for patients:

(a) with large goitres which are causing pressure symptoms or are unsightly;
(b) who relapse after two courses of drugs;
(c) with nodular goitre;
(d) who do not want the inconvenience of prolonged medical treatment;
(e) who are planning a pregnancy.

Summary of management of thyrotoxicosis
Patients under the age of 50 are usually treated medically in the first instance. If they relapse following cessation of medical treatment, operation is indicated. Young patients developing thyrotoxicosis have a high relapse rate and many physicians refer patients under the age of 25 for surgery as soon as they have become euthyroid, rather than undertaking a trial of medical therapy.

Patients over the age of 50 are usually treated with radioactive iodine.

Preoperative management
It is dangerous to operate on a patient who is actively thyrotoxic. Manipulation of the gland during operation produces considerably raised blood levels of thyroxine and this can result in a 'thyroid crisis' (see p. 164). A crisis is prevented by adequate preoperative preparation. Two methods are possible.

Method 1: antithyroid drugs. The patient is made euthyroid by using carbimazole or some other antithyroid agent which blocks the production of thyroxine. This also causes the gland to become larger and more vascular. The treatment is therefore stopped 10 days before the operation is planned and changed to Lugol's iodine (0.5 ml 8-hourly) or potassium iodide (60 mg daily). The iodine is taken up by the gland, which becomes less vascular and firmer. Treatment is continued until the operation.

The iodine initially has a thyroid blocking action but beyond 10 days it begins to be mobilized into thyroxine and thyrotoxicity recurs. It is therefore essential to plan the operation to take place 10 days after the antithyroid agent is stopped and the iodine started.

Method 2: beta blockade. An alternative method of preoperative preparation is to give the patient large enough doses of propranolol to suppress the adrenergic toxic effects (dose = 40 mg 8-hourly, although more may be required). In this case the serum thyroxine remains raised, but is ineffectual in producing cardiac arrhythmias, tachycardia or hyperpyrexia. The patient may also be given Lugol's iodine as above, while continuing on propranolol.

The advantage of the second method is that the gland does not become large and haemorrhagic and is therefore easier to operate on. In addition, the preparation is much more rapid than with carbimazole. With the latter a preparation of 2 or 3 months is required but with propranolol the patient can be made ready for surgery within a week or 10 days.

The drug should be given on the day of operation and continued for a week postoperatively.

The vocal cords should be checked before the operation to make sure they are moving adequately.

The patient's serum must also be checked for antibodies as thyrotoxicity is not uncommon early in Hashimoto's disease and thyroidectomy may be contraindicated in this condition (see p. 159).

Operation: subtotal thyroidectomy

The thyroid is exposed by a 'collar' incision. Care is taken to avoid damage to the recurrent laryngeal nerves and also the parathyroid glands. Four-fifths of the thyroid gland is removed leaving remnants posteriorly on both sides of the trachea. The wound is drained with or without suction. A pressure bandage is usually applied over the wound.

Codes

Blood	Group and save serum . . . .
GA/LA	GA . . . .
Opn time	90−120 minutes . . . .
Stay	5−7 days . . . .
Drains out	24 hours . . . .
Sutures out	3−4 days (clips 2−3 days) . . . .
Off work	4−6 weeks . . . .

Postoperative care

The patient has a very sore throat and usually has a desire to cough. Cough suppressant analgesics such as Omnopon or codeine are of value. If the neck swells up rapidly due to haemorrhage, there is a danger of compression of the trachea. In this case the wound may have to be reopened in the ward to avoid asphyxia. A pair of clip removers should be kept close to the bed. When the neck has been decompressed, the patient is returned to theatre to restore haemostasis.

Postoperative stridor may be due to laryngeal oedema and unconnected with contained haemorrhage. The patient must be returned to the theatre and reintubated by an experienced anaesthetist. Failure to reinsert the tube will necessitate tracheostomy. The intubated patient is nursed in intensive care for 12 hours, and can usually be extubated without problem.

The vocal cords should be routinely checked to ensure that the recurrent nerves have not been damaged.

Hypocalcaemia is an occasional complication of operations for thyrotoxicosis. This may be due to accidental removal of parathyroid glands but is more often due to calcium being mopped up by the skeleton after the decalcification associated with the thyrotoxic state. If the serum calcium does fall, tetany may occur (see p. 177).

Treatment of thyroid crisis
This is caused by a sudden surge of thyroxine and may occur if surgery is performed on inadequately prepared patients. It may also be seen if the postoperative dose of propranolol is omitted in patients prepared on this drug alone. Signs include delirium, anxiety, tachycardia, cardiac failure, hyperpyrexia, abdominal pain and diarrhoea. It may result in adrenal failure and coma.

It is treated by a slow infusion of propranolol (5−15 mg) followed by oral administration of 40 mg 8-hourly. Intravenous fluids may be required and steroids may be given to cover adrenal failure. Chlorpromazine (100 mg i.v.) is useful.

Long-term follow-up
The patient should be reviewed regularly for signs of developing myxoedema. The serum T3, T4 and TSH are measured regularly. The serum TSH is usually raised after partial thyroidectomy but this does not matter providing the serum thyroxine remains in the normal range.

Solitary thyroid nodule
Lesions presenting as solitary thyroid nodules can be classified as follows:
1 Benign:
   (a) cyst;
   (b) adenoma;
   (c) a discrete nodule in a nodular goitre.
2 Malignant, primary:
   (a) thyroid adenocarcinoma;
   (b) malignant lymphoma;
   (c) medullary carcinoma.
3 Malignant, secondary:
   (a) direct spread;

(b) indirect spread from: (i) breast, (ii) rectum, (iii) colon, (iv) hypernephroma, (v) lung, (vi) lymphatic tumours.

Having decided that the lump is in the thyroid, determine whether the opposite lobe of the thyroid is also palpable and whether it is nodular. In this way you may be able to determine whether the nodule is truly solitary or part of a nodular goitre. The patient should also be fully examined to determine his thyroid status (as on p. 157).

All solitary nodules should be investigated by the following:
1 *Thyroid scan.* This determines whether the nodule is active ('hot') or inactive ('cold'). Cold nodules are more likely to be malignant.
2 *X-ray of thoracic inlet and chest X-ray.* This is done to look for signs of pressure on the surrounding structures, particularly the trachea. A chest X-ray may show a retrosternal extension of the mass.
3 *Thyroid hormones* (T3, T4, TSH). These determine the patient's thyroid status.
4 *Thyroid antibodies* — to look for evidence of thyroiditis.
5 *Ultrasound* to show if the lesion is solid or cystic.

Management

Cystic lesions may be aspirated. Most solitary solid thyroid nodules will require surgical removal and histological examination in order to exclude thyroid malignancy. This usually involves a hemi-thyroidectomy. This will first be described, followed by some notes on the individual lesions presenting as a solitary thyroid nodule.

Preoperative management
As for subtotal thyroidectomy, the patient's vocal cords are examined to make sure there is no pre-existing paralysis. The patient is warned of the slight danger of a husky voice following the operation.

Operation: hemi-thyroidectomy
The thyroid gland is explored through a 'collar' incision. The involved lobe is exposed and excised completely. In order to do this the recurrent laryngeal nerve must be exposed.

There are differing views as to what to do once the lobe has been removed. Some surgeons send it for frozen-section histology and may proceed to a full total thyroidectomy at the same operation if the lesion is malignant. Others will leave the contralateral lobe strictly alone and be prepared to come back and remove the other lobe later if necessary (see under management of individual thyroid carcinomas). The author's preference is for the second course.

Codes

Blood	Group and save serum . . . .
GA/LA	GA . . . .
Opn time	60−90 minutes
Stay	4−7 days . . . .
Drains out	24−48 hours . . . .
Sutures out	3−4 days (clips 2−3 days) . . . .
Off work	4 weeks . . . .

Postoperative care
This is as for subtotal thyroidectomy and is described on p. 163. Hypocalcaemia and hypothyroidism are not a problem if the other lobe has been left intact.

Operation: total thyroidectomy
In this procedure both lobes of the gland are removed. There is an increased danger of parathyroid deficiency postoperatively, although it is usually possible to leave at least one parathyroid on each side of the neck.

Codes

Blood	Group and save serum . . . .
GA/LA	GA . . . .
Opn time	2−3 hours . . . .
Stay	5−7 days . . . .
Drains out	24−48 hours . . . .
Sutures out	3−4 days (clips 2−3 days) . . . .
Off work	4−6 weeks . . . .

Postoperative care
The serum calcium is monitored daily and any hypoparathyroidism treated as on p. 177. The patient will require thyroid replacement therapy (up to 0.13 mg/day of thyroxine).

In the unlikely event of both recurrent laryngeal nerves being damaged at operation, the patient will develop severe stridor. Emergency reintubation is required and a tracheostomy may be necessary.

Cysts and adenomas

Thyroid cyst

The condition
This is usually a degenerative part of a nodular goitre although true thyroid cysts do occur. A common complication is haemorrhage into the cyst. When this occurs, there is rapid enlargement and the lump may be painful. There is a possibility that such rapid enlargement may compress the trachea.

Recognizing the pattern	*The patient* The patient is of any age and is euthyroid. There may be a history of rapid enlargement and pain.
Proving the diagnosis	The lump may be shown to be cystic on ultrasound examination.
Management	If the swelling is thought to be cystic and the rest of the gland is normal, some surgeons will aspirate the cyst. It tends to refill, however, and some carcinomas have cystic areas in them which may be misleading. We therefore tend to excise the cyst.

Thyroid adenomas

The condition　There are four types of thyroid adenoma. The names refer to the histological appearance. They are:
(a) papillary,
(b) follicular,
(c) embryonal,
(d) hurtle cell.

A few adenomas are functioning and may even produce thyrotoxicosis. Occasionally haemorrhage may occur into the tumour causing a rapid increase in size.

Management　The distinction from a carcinoma can only be made on histological examination. For this reason most adenomas are excised. If, however, the lesion shows as a 'hot' nodule on thyroid scanning, it may be possible to suppress it with thyroxine treatment. Otherwise the management is hemi-thyroidectomy as above.

Papillary adenomas are hard to differentiate from carcinoma and routine follow-up after excision is necessary.

Nodule of a nodular goitre

A solitary nodule often turns out to be part of a nodular goitre and not truly solitary. However, this may well be impossible to distinguish before operation and so the lump has to be excised to be certain. If this is in fact the diagnosis, no further treatment is necessary.

Carcinoma of the thyroid

There are five types of primary thyroid malignancy:
(a) papillary adenocarcinoma;
(b) follicular adenocarcinoma;
(c) anaplastic carcinoma;
(d) medullary carcinoma;
(e) lymphoma.

Each has a characteristic pattern of behaviour and response to treatment. They are all usually 'cold' on scanning, although very occasionally a 'hot' malignant tumour is seen. The latter are usually TSH-dependent.

Management The tumour is excised by hemi-thyroidectomy as above. In the case of anaplastic carcinoma this may not be possible, in which case the lesion is biopsied. Descriptions of the individual types of thyroid carcinoma together with their management, are given below.

Table 13 shows the main features of each type.

Table 13. The features of various types of thyroid cancer

Type	Age-group	Response to hormone therapy	Response to deep X-ray	Response to ^{131}I	Spread
Papillary (paediatric)	10–40	+ +	–	–	Lymph nodes
Follicular (forties)	40–60	+	–	+	Bloodstream
Anaplastic (aged)	50–60	–	+	–	Local and lymphatics

Papillary carcinoma

The condition Papillary carcinoma is of low-grade malignancy and rarely fatal. It occurs in the younger age-group, usually in children or young adults, and is more common in females. On histology there is hyperplastic epithelium in the follicles with very little colloid. The disease may be multifocal. It tends to spread to lymph nodes and these may appear before the primary growth is palpable. This was described in the past as a 'lateral aberrant thyroid'. There is an association with irradiation of the neck in childhood.

Treatment Papillary carcinomas are hormone sensitive. Following hemithyroidectomy the patient is started on thyroxine and maintained on this therapy for life. Some surgeons perform a total thyroidectomy for this lesion because of its multifocal nature. Others adopt a 'wait and see' policy and remove the other lobe of the thyroid gland if there is evidence of further disease. Direct suppression is achieved with thyroxine 0.3–0.4 mg per day. This tumour is usually not sensitive to radio-active iodine therapy and if metastases occur to lymph nodes locally they are usually treated by limited block dissection.

Follicular carcinoma

The condition   This tends to occur in slightly older patients, often middle-aged. Females are more affected than males. The growth spreads through the bloodstream and bony secondaries are common. The lesion may arise in a pre-existing nodular goitre. The tumour is radio-sensitive.

Treatment   Radio-active iodine is the treatment of choice for secondary disease. Metastases will not, however, take up the iodine if the rest of the thyroid is present and the gland has to be ablated by radio-active iodine or excised before they can be treated. Metastases can then be detected and treated by further radio-active iodine scanning. Patients with follicular carcinoma are also maintained on thyroxine suppression therapy.

Anaplastic carcinoma

The condition   This aggressive carcinoma occurs in elderly patients, particularly in women. It grows rapidly and infiltrates the tissues in the neck. Compression of the trachea is common. Cervical lymphadenopathy and evidence of distal spread are often apparent when the patient is first seen.

Treatment   Many anaplastic carcinomas are sensitive to radiotherapy and this is the treatment of choice, although there are special problems if the airway is compromised. Treatment with radiotherapy causes further swelling of the gland and this can prove fatal. A recent advance has been to give the patient helium and oxygen to breathe during the initial radiotherapy and this can allow ventilation to continue. Otherwise a tracheostomy is required. This can sometimes be carried out at the initial biopsy operation.

Medullary carcinoma

The condition   This carcinoma arises in the parafollicular cells. It is of moderate malignancy and spreads to lymph nodes. It may secrete calcitonin which can then be used as a tumour marker. There is a familial incidence and an association with adenomas elsewhere (see p. 177). The patient may be of any age and the tumour has an equal sex incidence. In these respects it is different from other thyroid carcinomas. It is also much less common.

Treatment	Medullary carcinoma is treated by total thyroidectomy and block dissection of lymph nodes if these are involved. Calcitonin can be regularly measured postoperatively to detect metastases.

Malignant lymphoma

The condition	There is much lymphatic tissue in the thyroid gland and lymphomas can arise there. They may also occur as secondaries from other sites. Lymphomas may occur in patients with Hashimoto's thyroiditis.
Treatment	They are treated in the same way as lymphomas elsewhere.

Thyroglossal cyst

The condition	The thyroid develops from the floor of the mouth. It migrates down from the foramen caecum of the tongue passing anterior to, and then behind, the hyoid bone, to eventually lie in the pretracheal space. As it descends it leaves a small canal connected to the tongue called the thyroglossal duct (Fig. 31a). Remnants of this duct may persist and give rise to a thyroglossal cyst.

The cyst lies in the midline anywhere between the chin and the thyroid isthmus. Fifty per cent lie over the hyoid bone. It may be connected to the tongue or the thyroid by fibrous remnants of the thyroglossal duct. Very occasionally these remain patent, forming either a sinus or a thyroglossal fistula.

Recognizing the pattern	*The patient* The patient may be of any age, although the condition is commoner between the ages of 15 and 30. Women are more often affected.

The history
The patient notices a painless lump in the neck. It may become infected, in which case it presents as a localized abscess which points to the skin.

On examination
There is a smooth, round, 1–3 cm diameter swelling lying in the midline of the neck, often near the hyoid bone. The skin moves over it unless it has been fixed by scarring following an episode of inflammation. The lump is of firm consistency and may fluctuate and transilluminate.

Ask the patient to open the mouth, steady the jaw, and then protrude the tongue. Characteristically the cyst will move upwards (Fig. 31b). This may be easier to feel than see

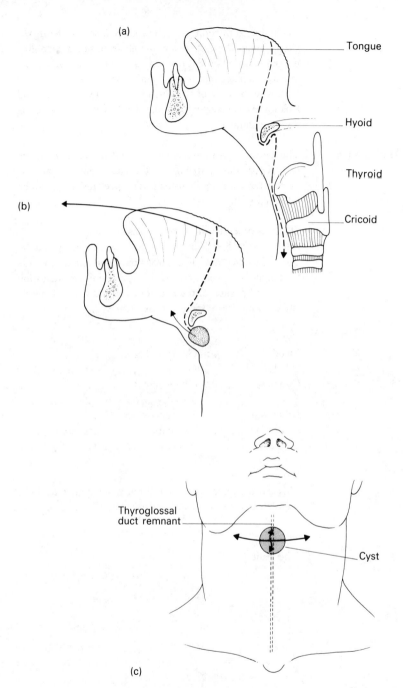

(a)

Tongue

Hyoid

Thyroid

Cricoid

(b)

Thyroglossal
duct remnant

Cyst

(c)

Fig. 31. (a) The descent of the thyroid − the track forms the thyroglossal duct. (b) As the tongue is protruded a thyroglossal cyst moves forwards. (c) A thyroglossal cyst is more mobile from side to side than up and down.

and is due to traction on the fibrous remnant of the thyro-glossal duct. The cyst is more mobile from side to side than up and down (Fig. 31c). It may also move on swallowing, due to its attachment to the hyoid bone.

Palpate the base of the tongue for any thyroid tissue and look for any sinus opening to the skin (usually just above the thyroid isthmus).

Management

The treatment is to excise the cyst and any remnant of the thyroglossal duct. Because of the latter, the operation is more extensive than the patient will expect and he should be informed of this preoperatively.

Operation: excision of thyroglossal cyst

A transverse elliptical incision is made over the lump and the cyst is dissected out. The fibrous track running up towards the tongue is also excised and this usually involves removing the central portion of the body of the hyoid bone. Similarly any downward extensions are also removed.

Codes

Blood	Group and save . . . .
GA/LA	GA . . . .
Opn time	60−90 minutes . . . .
Stay	3−5 days . . . .
Drains out	48 hours . . . .
Sutures out	4−5 days . . . .
Off work	2 weeks . . . .

Postoperative care

This is usually uncomplicated. If remnants of the track have been left behind, however, recurrent sepsis can occur.

3.4 Parathyroids

Hyperparathyroidism

The condition

The diagnosis and management of hyperparathyroidism rests on an understanding of the nature and physiology of the parathyroid glands and their secretion, parathormone. There are two glands on each side of the neck and they lie behind the thyroid gland. Each measures about $6 \times 2 \times 2$ mm. They consist of one main cell type, the 'chief cell', which has a 'water clear' appearance on microscopy when it is active.

Parathormone is a polypeptide hormone which regulates calcium metabolism. It has effects on the kidney, bone and gastrointestinal tract. Its secretion is controlled by the serum calcium level, being increased in hypocalcaemic states.

In the kidney it increases the reabsorption of filtered calcium, increases the excretion of phosphate, and stimulates the production of the active metabolite of vitamin D.

In bone parathormone increases the number and osteolytic activity of osteoclasts and osteocytes, thereby mobilizing both calcium and phosphate. Vitamin D metabolites are necessary for this process.

In the gut parathormone indirectly increases calcium absorption by increasing the production of 1,25-dihydroxy-cholecalciferol (the active metabolite of vitamin D).

Hyperparathyroidism may be primary, secondary or tertiary.

Primary hyperparathyroidism

The parathyroid glands may become over-active and secrete excess parathormone causing hypercalcaemia.

This is due to one of the following:
(a) a solitary adenoma (in 67% of cases of hyperparathyroidism);
(b) more than one adenoma (8%);
(c) generalized hyperplasia of all four glands (21%);
(d) carcinoma (2%): this is locally invasive and may metastasize via the bloodstream. Recurrence after removal is common.

Secondary hyperparathyroidism

This occurs as a physiological response to chronic hypocalcaemia (e.g. chronic renal failure).

Tertiary hyperparathyroidism

Occasionally one of the glands involved in secondary hyperparathyroidism may develop an autonomous adenoma. This is tertiary hyperparathyroidism.

Recognizing the pattern

The patient

Primary hyperparathyroidism is more common in women than men and is usually seen after the age of 40. There may be a familial history of multiple endocrine adenomas (see p. 177).

The history

The clinical features are very varied.

1 Renal stones. The patient presents with ureteric colic, haematuria or urinary tract infection. Three per cent of those with stones are shown to have primary hyperparathyroidism.

2 Renal disease. The kidneys are damaged by nephrocalcinosis, which predisposes to pyelonephritis and eventually chronic renal failure.

3 Bone involvement. This can cause vague rheumatic bone and joint pains. Pathological fracture is rare.

4 Hypercalcaemic symptoms, e.g. anorexia, weight loss, dyspepsia, polydipsia, polyuria, muscle weakness and tiredness. Hypertension and dyspnoea can occur.

5 Pancreatitis. There is a raised incidence of this condition with parathyroid over-activity.

6 Duodenal ulceration. This can occur in hyperparathyroidism and the latter is diagnosed when a serum calcium is measured as part of the general work-up.

On examination

There is rarely anything to find. There may be corneal calcification adjacent to the corneo-scleral margin. Bone disease can cause tenderness and swelling. It is very rare to feel an adenoma in the neck.

Proving the diagnosis

The following investigations may be undertaken.

1 *Serum calcium.* The specimen must be taken from a fasting patient with no cuff on the arm. Fifty per cent of the calcium is bound to albumin so a correction must be made if the albumin is low. The range of normality (which may vary slightly between laboratories) is 2.25−2.55 mmol/litre.

2 *Serum phosphate.* This is low in primary disease but may be increased if there is any renal impairment.

3 *Alkaline phosphatase.* This is raised if there is significant bony disease.

4 *Urinary calcium and phosphate clearance.* The 24-hour clearances of both calcium and phosphate are usually elevated but this is not consistent.

5 *Parathormone assay.* Parathormone can be measured by an immuno-assay (normal range 0.15—1.0 ng/ml). Patients with primary hyperparathyroidism occasionally have normal levels of parathormone, but this is still inappropriate in the presence of their high calcium levels. Hypercalcaemia from other causes will suppress parathormone production and the levels will be undetectable.

6 *Hydrocortisone suppression test.* This was useful before a reliable parathormone assay was available. A 10-day course of hydrocortisone (40 mg 8-hourly) lowers the serum calcium in all cases of hypercalcaemia except those caused by hyperparathyroidism. Three serum calcium levels are taken, then the 10-day course of hydrocortisone is started, and three further calcium samples are taken on days 8, 9 and 10.

7 *Radiology.* There are characteristic bone changes due to excess of parathormone, particularly seen in the skull and hands. X-rays also help in the differential diagnosis, e.g. carcinoma of the bronchus seen on chest X-ray or myeloma seen on a skull X-ray.

8 *Localization of an adenoma.* It is now possible to selectively cannulate the inferior thyroid veins and measure the parathormone levels. This can sometimes localize the source of excess parathormone production. Radio-scanning of the neck with thallium, and CAT scanning are also used but are of limited value.

Other causes of hypercalcaemia

Once hypercalcaemia has been detected, other causes of hypercalcaemia must be excluded. These include:

1 Carcinoma (bone metastases causing mobilization of calcium, or production of parathormone by a tumour).

2 Myeloma.

3 Vitamin D intoxication (due to excess intake of vitamin D-containing foods).

4 Milk alkali syndrome (due to ingestion of milk and alkalis for indigestion).

5 Thyrotoxicosis.

6 Sarcoidosis.

7 Addison's disease.

8 Paget's disease or osteoporosis (where the patient is immobilized).

Management

The management of primary or tertiary hyperparathyroidism is surgical.

Acute hyperparathyroidism. In this state the calcium level exceeds 3.75 mmol/litre. The patient is dehydrated due to vomiting and polyuria and complains of headache, weakness and thirst. There may be tachycardia and low blood pressure, and eventually coma. An ECG may show a short QT interval and evidence of dysrhythmia. This condition must be treated before operation can be undertaken, primarily by correcting dehydration. A saline infusion is given and potassium may be required. Intravenous therapy should be monitored by central venous pressure measurement as the mortality is high. Intravenous calcium chelators are available (e.g. intravenous phosphate or disodium edetate). These should only be used in specialized centres as they are not without risk (e.g. intravenous phosphate can precipitate acute renal failure). If the calcium level still remains very high after rehydration, dialysis should be considered.

Vocal cord check. The vocal cord movements should be checked both before and after operation.

Arrange frozen section facilities. Immediate histology is required during operation to identify parathyroid tissue.

Calcium estimations. It is worthwhile warning the laboratory that serial calcium estimations will be required postoperatively, particularly if this will be over a weekend.

Operation: exploration of the neck for parathyroid adenoma

The neck is opened with a transverse skin crease incision and the thyroid is exposed as in subtotal thyroidectomy. The thyroid lobes are mobilized and retracted forwards. A methodical search is made for each parathyroid gland. If an adenoma is found it is removed and the diagnosis confirmed on frozen section. Further adenomas must also be excluded.

When all four glands are hyperplastic it is usual to remove three and a half glands, possibly re-implanting the remnant into a forearm muscle for ease of subsequent access.

If carcinoma is found, a radical local excision is performed.

Codes
Blood . . . .   Group and save . . . .
GA/LA . . . .   GA . . . .
Opn time . . . .   2−4 hours . . . .

Stay	5–7 days	
Drains out	24 hours	
Sutures out	Clips or sutures 3–4 days	
Off work	1–2 months	

Postoperative care
As with thyroid surgery a pair of skin clip removers must be placed next to the bed in case acute haemorrhage should occur and cause tracheal compression.

Hypocalcaemia
This is common in the first 48 hours after operation and may be transient due to bruising of the remaining parathyroids, or permanent if they have all been removed. Serum calcium levels must be taken each day for the first 3 days after operation. The clinical features of hypocalcaemia are tingling of the lips, fingers and toes, followed by the development of spasm of the hands and feet (tetany). Incipient tetany can be demonstrated by Trousseau's sign (if the patient is hypocalcaemic, carpal spasm develops within 2 minutes of inflating a blood pressure cuff on the arm above systolic pressure) or Chvostek's sign (tapping of the facial nerve in the cheek causes a twitch of the corner of the mouth and side of the nose). Overt tetany is shown by carpo-pedal spasm, when the hand is flexed at the metacarpo-phalangeal joints with straight fingers and the thumb strongly adducted. The foot and toes are plantar flexed.

Treatment of hypocalcaemia in the short term is with intravenous boluses of calcium gluconate (10% 10 ml). If the calcium level does not return to normal over the next few days, long-term treatment with vitamin D is required. Often large doses are needed and it may take a week before it begins to work. The newer synthetic analogues (e.g. 1-α-hydroxycholecalciferol) work more quickly. Control can be difficult and often the levels need to be topped up with oral calcium preparations.

Multiple endocrine adenomas

Parathyroid adenomas may be associated with adenomas elsewhere in the APUD (amine precursor uptake and decarboxylation) cell system, e.g. the anterior pituitary, pancreas (insulinoma or gastrinoma), phaeochromocytoma, or medullary carcinoma of the thyroid. Such multiple endocrine adenomas often have a familial basis.

Those conditions of the mouth to be considered include the following:
Cleft lip and palate (p. 178).
Cysts in the mouth (p. 179).
Tumours of the mouth (p. 183).
Conditions of the tongue are dealt with on pp. 189–195.

Cleft lip and palate

The condition   The most common developmental abnormalities are cleft lip and palate. These occur when there is failure of fusion of the processes contributing to facial development (Fig. 32). Twelve per cent of cases are familial. The left side is more commonly affected than the right. Of those babies with abnormalities, one-quarter have a cleft lip alone and a further quarter a cleft palate alone. The other 50% have both lesions. Fifteen per cent of cleft lips are bilateral.

Making the diagnosis   All but the most minor abnormalities are seen at birth. The main problem is with sucking and therefore feeding. Speech and dentition are also affected when there is a cleft palate, while a cleft lip on its own leads to an abnormality of facial development. Fifty per cent of patients with cleft palates have some hearing loss due to oedema around the Eustachian tube.

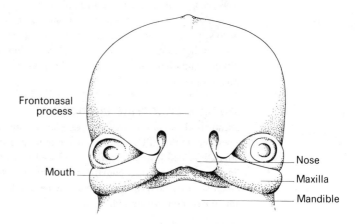

Frontonasal process

Mouth

Nose

Maxilla

Mandible

Fig. 32. Cleft lip and palate. The facial processes during development (7 weeks of gestation).

On examination

Note:

1 whether the condition is unilateral or bilateral;
2 whether the palate is involved;
3 how extensive the palatal lesion is.

Ten per cent of cases have other abnormalities so a thorough general examination should be undertaken.

Management

Treatment is surgical repair and is undertaken by a specialist plastic surgeon. In a cleft lip alone feeding is unimpaired and the lesion may be repaired at about the age of 6 months so that normal facial development may occur.

A cleft palate is associated with feeding problems and the baby will need to be either spoon-fed or fed with liquid dripped into the mouth. The lesion is usually repaired between 1 and 2 years of age to avoid significant speech impairment and dentition problems.

When both abnormalities exist together, the cleft lip is often repaired at the age of 8 weeks and the cleft palate at the age of 1 year.

Cysts in the mouth

Mucous retention cysts

The condition

When the duct of a mucous gland becomes blocked, mucus collects under the epithelium of the lip. Although these cysts may occur anywhere where there are mucous glands, they are usually on the lower lip or inside the buccal mucosa (Fig. 33).

Recognizing the pattern

The patient

The patient may be of any age and complains of a slowly growing lump which is painless. It may be accidentally bitten.

On examination

The cyst is a pale pink or blue colour with a glairy appearance. It usually measures between 0.5 and 2.0 cm in diameter and is not fixed to the underlying muscle.

Operation: removal of mucous retention cyst

Although the operation may be carried out under a general anaesthetic (in a particularly nervous patient or in a child), it is usually done with local anaesthetic infiltration (e.g. 1% xylocaine with 1/200 000 adrenaline). The lip is incised and the cyst enucleated or deroofed.

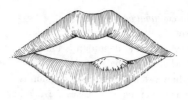

Fig. 33. A mucous retention cyst.

Codes

Blood	0 . . . .
GA/LA	LA . . . .
Opn time	15 – 30 minutes . . . .
Stay	Outpatient . . . .
Drains out	0 . . . .
Sutures out	5 days or absorbable . . . .
Off work	2 – 3 hours . . . .

Ranula

The condition

Ranula is Latin for a small frog. The term is used to describe a unilateral cystic swelling in the floor of the mouth formed either from a blocked mucous gland or from an accessory salivary gland.

Recognizing the pattern

The patient

The patient is usually a child or young adult of either sex who presents with a history of a swelling in the floor of the mouth. This develops over a few weeks and may fluctuate in size. There may be a past history of similar swellings. The lump is painless.

On examination

The swelling lies on one side of the floor of the mouth between the tongue and mandible. It is semi-transparent, grey, and up to 5 cm in diameter. It is smooth, spherical and cystic. It transilluminates. Rarely a ranula may possess a deep extension into the neck (possibly developing from the cervical sinus). The ranula is not attached to the overlying mucosa, mylohyoid or muscle of the tongue. The submandibular duct either overlies the lesion or is displaced to one side.

Management

Management is excision or marsupialization.

Operation: excision/marsupialization of ranula

Ideally the cyst is completely excised. This is occasionally difficult and in that case it may be marsupialized, the remains of the cyst now becoming the floor of the mouth. If there is deep extension of the ranula below the mylohyoid, the cyst must be completely removed and it is approached from the neck as opposed to the floor of the mouth.

Codes

Blood	0 . . . .
GA/LA	GA . . . .
Opn time	Proportional to extent and depth . . . . .
Stay	2−5 days . . . .
Drains out	0 . . . .
Sutures out	Usually absorbable . . . .
Off work	Variable . . . .

Dermoid cyst

The condition   This is a midline swelling on the floor of the mouth, originating during development by entrapment of ectoderm beneath the skin during fusion of the mandibular processes. It may be above or below the mylohyoid.

Recognizing the pattern

The patient
A patient of either sex usually presents between the ages of 10 and 25 complaining of a painless swelling under the floor of the mouth. This may cause a double chin appearance. It may occasionally become infected.

On examination
The swelling is in the midline in the floor of the mouth or beneath the chin. It is 2−5 cm in diameter and is spherical, smooth and cystic or 'putty'-like. The contents are opaque and it will not transilluminate.

Operation: excision of dermoid cyst in the mouth
The cyst may be approached from an external incision beneath the mandible or a small one can be removed from within the mouth.

Codes

Blood	0 . . . .
GA/LA	GA . . . .
Opn time	30 minutes, depending on site . . . . . .
Stay	Day case . . . .
Drains out	0−24 hours . . . .
Sutures out	Usually absorbable . . . .
Off work	1−2 weeks . . . .

Developmental cyst

The condition This is a cyst, which forms in the same way as a dermoid cyst but occurs within bone. The commonest is the globular maxillary cyst, which occurs in the upper jaw between the premaxilla and the maxilla, i.e. between the incisor and canine. The treatment is excision.

Dental cyst

The condition This is a cyst around the root of an erupted but decayed or infected tooth, which develops from epithelial cells of the enamel organ.

Making the diagnosis The patient may be of any age or sex and presents with a painless swelling, usually of the upper jaw. There is a history of dental caries. The cyst may become infected and therefore painful.

The diagnosis is confirmed by X-ray.

Management Treatment of dental cysts requires complete excision of the epithelial lining and is undertaken by an orodental surgeon. Obviously existing dental caries must also be treated.

Dentigerous cyst

The condition This is a cyst containing an unerupted tooth and usually develops around the upper or lower third molar.

The patient is usually a young adult who presents with a painful swelling.

On examination there is swelling of the jaw, usually near the upper or lower third molar and this may have damaged the outer table of the bone. There will be one tooth missing.

Proving the diagnosis The diagnosis is confirmed by X-ray.

Management The cyst is excised by a dental surgeon (as under Dental cyst).

Alveolar abscess

The condition This is an abscess formed around the root of a decaying tooth, often in a previous dental cyst. Under pressure the pus tracks out usually through the thinner lateral plate of the jaw, to form an abscess beneath the cheek or mandible.

Making the diagnosis

The patient

The patient is usually a child or young adult and presents with a dull, throbbing ache and swelling of the jaw. He may be generally unwell with a past history of dental caries.

On examination

The patient is pyrexial with a hot, tender, red swelling of the jaw, spreading either to the labial or buccal margin. When the patient still has his first dentition, either the upper or lower jaw may be affected. There is evidence of dental caries and there may be cervical lymphadenopathy.

Proving the diagnosis

The diagnosis is proved by X-ray.

Management

This consists of drainage and antibiotics. Advanced cases may be complicated by severe swelling of the floor of the mouth and the danger of incipient respiratory obstruction.

Benign tumours of the mouth

Epulis (localized swelling of the gum)

Fibrous epulis

This is a fibroma developing from the periodontal membrane and presenting as a localized lesion between the gum and the tooth. Malignant change may occur, forming a friable, bleeding mass.

The management is removal. Histology should be requested.

Bony epulis

This is an osteoclastoma causing the overlying gum to become locally hyperaemic and oedematous. It is also referred to as a giant cell tumour. Depending on its size, it may be curetted out or may require excision of a large amount of mandible and bone grafting.

Granulomatous epulis

This is a mass of granulomatous tissue forming around a chronically infected or carious tooth or ill-fitting denture. The treatment is tooth extraction and curettage of the granulomatous tissue, which should be sent for histology.

Mixed salivary tumour (accessory pleomorphic adenoma)

The condition

There are accessory salivary glands in the oral cavity, particularly lining the hard palate, where salivary tumours can arise. As in the parotid gland, a mixed salivary tumour is benign but has an incomplete capsule. This may result in recurrence after simple enucleation. Malignant change is more common in accessory salivary glands than in the parotid.

Recognizing the pattern

The patient
The patient may be of either sex and is usually elderly. The lesion presents as a slowly growing but progressively enlarging painless lump in the palate. Eventually it may interfere with eating and speaking.

On examination
There is a smooth, hard lump beneath the mucous membrane. The mucosa is usually mobile over it. Initially the lump is also mobile over the mandible but it may later become attached. Alteration or a rapid increase in size suggests malignant change.

Proving the diagnosis

The diagnosis is proved by excision biopsy.

Management

Management is by excision with a margin of normal mucosa. It is unusual to have to remove palatal bone.

Malignant tumours of the mouth

Adamantinoma

The condition

This is a locally invasive tumour of epithelial cells derived from the enamel organ and it resembles a basal cell carcinoma in both histological appearance and behaviour. It usually forms multi-loculated cysts.

Recognizing the pattern

The patient
The patient is usually a schoolchild or young adult, more commonly of African or Asian origin, who presents with a painless swelling of the jaw. There may be a past history of excision and recurrence.

On examination
There is swelling, usually of the molar region or the mandible, which may cause egg-shell cracking of the overlying bone.

Proving the diagnosis

The X-ray appearances are characteristic. There are large loculi in the bone, which has a honeycomb appearance. This differentiates it from the cysts described above.

Management	Local curettage is inadequate as the condition will recur. The tumour must be excised with a margin of normal bone either side and bone graft may be required postoperatively.

Carcinoma of the lip

The condition	This carcinoma is often called 'countryman's lip'. Histologically it is a keratinizing squamous cell carcinoma. Aetiological factors include pipe-smoking and long exposure to sunlight or severe weather. Ninety-three per cent of the lesions occur in the lower lip. Five per cent occur in the upper lip and 2% at the angle of the mouth. The lymphatic drainage is to the submental nodes if the lesion is in the lower lip and to the submandibular nodes if the lesion is in the upper lip. Blood-borne spread to the liver and lungs is late and rare. Lesions in the angle of the mouth have a worse prognosis due to the involvement of two lymph fields.
Recognizing the pattern	*The patient* Ninety per cent occur in men aged over 65. Most have led an active outdoor life or have been pipe-smokers. *The history* The history is of a chronic ulcer of the lip which enlarges and fails to heal. It may present as a warty growth or a fissure. More advanced lesions may be painful, become infected, and disturb eating. *On examination* The ulcer usually has a characteristic raised rolled edge with blood-stained slough in the base.
Proving the diagnosis	This is done by biopsy.
Management	An early lesion may be treated by either surgery or radiotherapy. Some of these lesions are small and can be treated as an outpatient procedure under a local anaesthetic. **Operation: wedge excision of carcinoma of the lip** A simple wedge resection is performed (see Fig. 34). There is marked bleeding from the marginal artery of the lip and this can be controlled by pressure on the lip while a suture is inserted. It is important to remove an adequate margin of normal tissue on either side. The cosmetic result is very satisfactory.

185 SECTION 3.5

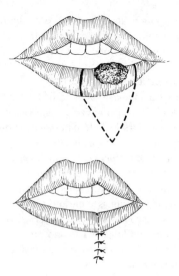

Fig. 34. Wedge excision of carcinoma of lip.

An alternative to surgery is radiotherapy. There is a 75% 5-year survival with either form of treatment.

A larger lesion will require resection and plastic reconstruction of the lip.

Codes

Blood	0 . . . .
GA/LA	GA or LA . . . .
Opn time	30–60 minutes . . . .
Stay	2–7 days . . . .
Drains out	0 . . . .
Sutures out	7–10 days . . . .
Off work	3 days to 2 weeks depending on the size of the lesion . . . .

Squamous cell carcinoma

Squamous cell carcinoma or anaplastic variants of it can occur at any site in the mouth where there is stratified squamous epithelium. Carcinoma of the tongue is an example (p. 192). The presentation and management of lesions elsewhere depends on the precise site and extent of the lesion. The mainstay of treatment is either radiotherapy or excision with or without reconstructive surgery.

Malignant melanoma

Malignant melanoma can rarely occur in any part of the lining of the mouth. Its treatment is considered in the section on skin conditions (p. 527).

Tumours of the jaws

These may be either primary or secondary and both are rare.

Carcinoma of the maxillary antrum

The maxillary antrum is lined by respiratory epithelium. The usual type of carcinoma occurring in this site is a squamous cell carcinoma, although adenocarcinomas are also seen. Carcinoma in the nasal sinuses occurs in woodworkers after a long latent period.

Making the diagnosis

The patient is usually male and elderly. The primary is usually undetected whilst it remains within the sinus and only becomes evident when it has invaded the surrounding structures including either the orbit, the nasal cavity or the hard palate and upper jaw. In these situations it presents as a mass or an ulcerated lesion. On examination the tumour is then fixed to bone.

Proving the diagnosis

The diagnosis is confirmed by X-rays of the skull and maxillary antrum.

Management

This consists of either radiotherapy, or excision and reconstruction.

Malignant disease of the tonsil

The condition

Malignant disease of the tonsil may be due to either a squamous cell carcinoma (85%) or a lymphosarcoma. The lymphoid tissue may also be involved in a more generalized lymphoma. A carcinoma of the tonsil spreads to adjacent structures such as the palate and base of the tongue and thence on to the deep cervical nodes.

Recognizing the pattern

The patient with squamous cell carcinoma is usually over the age of 60 and presents with pain in the throat which radiates to the ear. There is progressive enlargement of the tonsil causing dysphagia and 'thickening' of the speech. Eventually the growth ulcerates causing bleeding and marked fetor oris.

In contrast, lymphosarcoma occurs in slightly younger patients between the ages of 50 and 65 and the enlargement is usually painless. Ulceration and bleeding occur very late.

The ipsilateral deep cervical nodes may be enlarged due to secondary growth or due to infection secondary to a malignant ulcer.

Proving the diagnosis

The diagnosis is proved by biopsying the enlarged tonsil.

Management   Both types of tumour are treated by radiotherapy to the affected tonsil and the ipsilateral side of the neck. Large squamous cell tumours are occasionally treated by surgical resection combined with radiotherapy. Metastases in the cervical nodes may be treated by block dissection of the neck (see p. 194).

(see p. 194).

Conditions of the Tongue

Chronic superficial glossitis

The condition Chronic inflammation of the tongue is characterized by leucoplakia (white matt patches seen on the normal stratified squamous epithelium). The condition is premalignant. Macroscopically there is epithelial hyperplasia (hyperkeratosis), widening of the prickle cell layer (acanthosis) and a chronic inflammatory cell infiltrate. The presence of atypical cells, loss of polarity, local mucosal invasion, and nucleated cells appearing close to the surface indicate malignant change.

Classically the aetiological factors are the six Ss: smoking, spirits, spices, syphilis, sharp tooth, sepsis.

Syphilis was once an important factor although it is now very rare in this country. Pipe-smoking and chronic trauma due to bad teeth or ill-fitting dentures are now the most significant causes. Chronic superficial glossitis can also be 'idiopathic'.

Recognizing the pattern *The patient*
The patient is frequently an elderly male.

The history
The presenting complaint is usually that the patient or his relatives have noticed a change in colour of the tongue or a new irregularity. Otherwise it causes very few symptoms (unlike acute glossitis which is painful). There may be a past medical history of venereal disease or dental problems.

On examination
Typically it presents as patchy changes on the tongue and may be sited close to the cause (e.g. a sharp tooth).

There are four clinical stages.
1 A thin, grey, transparent film appears on the surface of the tongue.
2 Opaque white patches may develop (leucoplakia). With time these become yellow and may show cracks or fissures.
3 Further hyperplasia produces white nodules on the surfaces while desquamation in between leaves red, raw areas.
4 The development of a nodular or papillary growth may indicate carcinoma in situ.

The superficial and deep cervical lymph nodes should also be palpated.

Management

If there is any suggestion of malignant change, a biopsy of the lesion should be performed. If there is only a small patch of leucoplakia, it may be removed completely; at the same time any known cause must be remedied. A Wassermann reaction is done to exclude syphilis. If the lesion is too large to remove completely and there are no suspicious areas, it can safely be left and should improve once the cause has been removed. The patient must be reviewed regularly to detect any evidence of malignant change.

Ulceration of the tongue

Tongue ulcers may be:
(a) traumatic,
(b) aphthous,
(c) tuberculous,
(d) syphilitic,
(e) chronic non-specific,
(f) carcinomatous.

Traumatic ulceration

The condition

This is an ulcer on the side of the tongue caused by a sharp tooth or ill-fitting denture.

Recognizing the pattern

The patient
The patient is of any age and complains of a painful ulcer on the side of the tongue.

On examination
There is a chronic infected ulcer close to a cause such as a cracked tooth or an ill-fitting denture.

Management

When the cause is removed or remedied, the ulcer heals over a few days. A common cause of traumatic ulcer in the past was whooping cough, which damaged the underside of the tongue in the midline. This is now rare.

Aphthous ulceration

The condition

There are many causes of these small ulcers. In children both viral and fungal (*Candida*) infections are implicated. In adults this common type of ulcer is non-contagious and frequently shows a familial disposition.

Recognizing the pattern

The patient
The patient is usually an adolescent or young adult and the

condition is more common in women than men. The ulcers are very painful.

On examination
There is a small, round, white ulcer on the tongue, gums or inner aspect of the lips. The ulcers may be multiple.

Management
The patient should be reassured that the condition is not serious. The ulcer will heal on its own over a period of about 10 days. Healing can be hastened by topical hydrocortisone tablets. Oral salicylate gel gives symptomatic relief. If the ulcer fails to heal, then the diagnosis should be reviewed and if necessary a biopsy performed.

Tuberculous ulcer
The condition
This is a rare cause of tongue ulceration nowadays. It occurs in undiagnosed advanced pulmonary tuberculosis.

Recognizing the pattern
Multiple, very painful ulcers with undermined edges occur along the edges of the tongue.

Proving the diagnosis
The diagnosis of tuberculosis is proved on chest X-rays, sputum culture and microscopy.

Management
Treatment is antituberculous therapy.

Syphilitic ulcer
The typical lesions of the tongue are the chancre of primary syphilis, snail-track ulcers, Hutchinson's wart of secondary syphilis, and the gumma of tertiary syphilis.
   Treatment is with antibiotics (penicillin).

Chronic non-specific ulcer
This is a chronic ulcer which is usually situated on the anterior two-thirds of the tongue. No predisposing factor can be found. The lesion is usually painful. Syphilis and tuberculosis are excluded by investigation. The diagnosis is confirmed and the lesion cured by excision biopsy.

Neoplasms of the tongue
These may be either benign or malignant. Benign neoplasms of the tongue are rare. The following may occur:
(a) papilloma,
(b) angioma,
(c) lingual thyroid,
(d) neurofibroma,
(e) lipoma.

These are treated by excision. In the case of a lingual thyroid, it is important to be sure that there is other thyroid tissue lower down in the neck. A thyroid scan will give this information.

Carcinoma of the tongue

The condition This is usually a keratinizing squamous cell carcinoma. The aetiology is the same as that for chronic superficial glossitis and leucoplakia. The prognosis becomes worse the further back the lesion is on the tongue. Overall the 5-year survival is 25%.

Recognizing the pattern

The patient
The patient usually presents between the ages of 60 and 70. Carcinoma of the tongue used to be very much more common in men, but now, thanks to the declining incidence of syphilis and the disappearance of the clay pipe, the incidence in men and women is equal.

The history
There may be a past history of dental caries, pipe-smoking or venereal disease. More advanced carcinomas cause pain in the tongue, which may be referred to the ear. There may also be excessive salivation and defective tongue movement or difficulty with speech due to spread into the floor of the mouth. If the lesion becomes infected, fetor oris results.

On examination
The lesion may be one of the following.
1 A wart with a broad firm base and surrounding induration.
2 An ulcer with typical everted rolled edge and infected bleeding slough in the base.
3 A hard indistinct nodule.
   The patient may have had a pad of cotton wool in his ear for the pain and there may be evidence of secondary lymph node involvement.
   The extent of secondary spread must be assessed. The tip of the tongue and the posterior third have bilateral lymphatic drainage (see Fig. 35) so examine both sides of the neck. Blood spread occurs late and almost always from carcinoma on the posterior third of the tongue.

Proving the diagnosis The diagnosis is confirmed by biopsy. The differential diagnosis includes that of other ulcers of the tongue (see p. 190) and other solid lesions of the tongue (see p. 191).

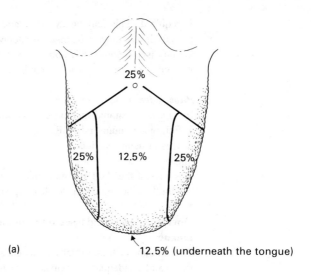

(a)

25%

25%   12.5%   25%

12.5% (underneath the tongue)

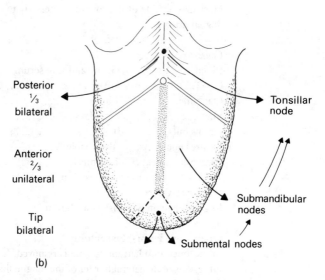

Posterior
⅓
bilateral

Tonsillar
node

Anterior
⅔
unilateral

Tip
bilateral

Submandibular
nodes

Submental nodes

(b)

Fig. 35. The distribution of sites of malignancy of the tongue.
(b) The lymphatic drainage of the tongue.

Management

Treatment is by excision and/or radiotherapy. The latter can be administered either as external irradiation or by radio-active implants. The choice of type of therapy and operation depends on the extent of the lesion.

A small lesion less than 1 cm in diameter may be excised locally. Larger lesions are initially treated by radiotherapy but, if the lesion does not respond or recurs, then operation is required. This may be extensive and consist of either a partial glossectomy, a hemi-glossectomy or subtotal glossectomy (see below). If lymph nodes are involved, a block dissection of the neck will be required.

Preoperative management
Investigations should include the following.
1 Full blood count and ESR.
2 Wassermann reaction.
3 Chest X-ray.
4 X-rays of the skull and mandible.
   Mouthwashes may help to clean up an infected lesion.

Operation: partial glossectomy for carcinoma of the tongue
The amount of tissue removed depends on the size of the lesion and an adequate margin is necessary. Bleeding may be profuse and the assistant can help to control this by compressing one side of the tongue posteriorly to compress the lingual artery.

Codes
Blood	Group and save serum ....
GA/LA	GA ....
Opn time	1 hour ....
Stay	3−5 days ....
Drains out	0 ....
Sutures out	Absorbable ....
Off work........	1 month ....

Postoperative care
Regular daily mouthwashes are given.

Operation: hemi-glossectomy
In this operation half the tongue is removed. It is performed for lesions of the lateral border of the tongue that are clear of the mandible. A submandibular dissection may also be required and sometimes this is combined with a block dissection of the neck on that side.

Codes
Blood	2 units ....
GA/LA	GA ....
Opn time	1−3 hours ....
Stay	10−14 days ....
Drains out	3−5 days ....
Off work........	4−6 weeks ....

Operation: block dissection of the neck

This operation is undertaken as part of an attempted radical cure of any lesion which has spread to the cervical lymph nodes. A long incision is made along the sternomastoid muscle and extended laterally beneath the jaw and along the clavicle. The block of tissue centred on the internal jugular vein is removed, together with the sternomastoid muscle.

Codes

Blood	2 units	....
GA/LA	GA	
Opn time	3−5 hours	
Stay	7−10 days	
Drains out	3−5 days	
Sutures out	7 days	
Off work........	4−6 weeks	

Operation: commando operation

In this procedure an extensive block dissection of the neck, mouth and pharynx is carried out, including a segment of the body or ramus of the mandible. The intra-oral defect is repaired, using a vascularized skin flap. The symphysis menti, geniohyoid and genioglossus muscles are disrupted, and the airway is in danger as the tongue is liable to fall back. Elective tracheostomy is required.

Codes

Blood	4 units	
GA/LA	GA	
Opn time	6 hours	
Stay	3−4 weeks	
Drains out	3−5 days	
Sutures out	7−10 days	
Off work........	3 months	

In all these operations an oropharyngeal pack is inserted and this must be inspected as it is removed. If blood has soaked right through it, there is a danger of aspiration and extra care should be taken to look for postoperative chest problems. In extensive procedures the airway may need to be maintained. A fine-bore nasogastric tube can be used for feeding purposes.

4 The Breast

4.1 Assessment of breast lumps and benign disease
Introduction
Methods of assessment
Benign mammary dysplasia
Cystic disease
Mammary duct ectasia
Fat necrosis
Benign neoplasms

4.2 Carcinoma of the breast
General management
Management of early carcinoma
Management of advanced carcinoma

4.3 Other breast presentations
Discharge from the nipple
Pain in the breast

4.4 Conditions of the male breast
Carcinoma
Gynaecomastia

4.1 Assessment of Breast Lumps and Benign Disease

Introduction

The most common presentation of breast pathology is a breast lump. Other presentations include a discharge from the nipple and pain in the breast. The latter are dealt with on pp. 222 and 224 respectively. Common causes of a breast lump are dealt with in Sections 4.2 and 4.3, and include the following:

1 benign mammary dysplasia,
2 benign neoplasms,
3 malignant neoplasms,
4 fat necrosis.

The normal breast

In order to understand the way breast lumps develop, it is necessary to know about both the normal anatomy of the breast and the cyclical changes which occur during the menstrual cycle. Normal breast tissue is in a continual state of change brought about by the changing hormonal profiles during the cycle.

The normal breast consists of about 12 lobes, each drained by a duct that opens at the nipple. The structure of each lobe is depicted in Fig. 36 and may be visualized as an inverted tree, the trunk representing the main duct.

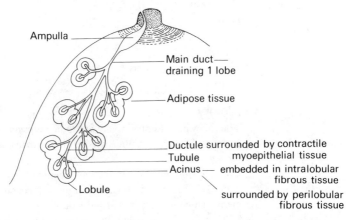

Ampulla

Main duct— draining 1 lobe

Adipose tissue

Ductule surrounded by contractile
Tubule   myoepithelial tissue
Acinus — embedded in intralobular
                      fibrous tissue
Lobule
surrounded by perilobular
fibrous tissue

Fig. 36. The anatomy of a breast lobe. There are 12–15 lobes in each breast. Each lobe is separated by fibrous tissue joining the pectoral fascia to the skin and thus supporting the breast (ligaments of Astley Cooper).

The secretory unit of the breast is the acinus, represented by the leaves. Each acinus drains into a ductule and several such units make up a lobule with its own duct. The ducts of all these lobes eventually join together to form the main duct.

There are two types of epithelium under hormonal control, the acinus containing glandular epithelium, and the duct containing ductal epithelium.

Surrounding all these glandular elements is the fibrous stroma. There is a loose hyaline layer around the ducts and acini and a more compact layer around the lobules. The rest of the breast is made up of adipose tissue interspersed with a rich network of blood vessels and lymphatics.

During the first half of the menstrual cycle, under the influence of oestrogens, there is proliferation of the duct system (the tree grows).

In the second half of the menstrual cycle under the influence of progesterone and luteinizing hormone, there is acinar hypertrophy (the leaves develop). At the time of menstruation all these changes regress (involution). There is also an increase in fibrous tissue. Involutionary changes are particularly marked after the menopause.

Methods of assessment

The woman presenting with this problem is almost always extremely anxious, and will be seeking reassurance. Her anxieties must be allayed and this can best be done by carrying out a thorough professional assessment. This will be described in detail here.

The following methods are used:
History.
Examination.
Aspiration.
Mammography (soft-tissue X-rays).
Biopsy.

History

The following essential points are to be determined.

1 *Age* of the patient. Lumps are very rarely malignant under the age of 30.

2 *Length of history*. Determine how long the lump has been noticed. What was the relationship of its appearance to the menstrual cycle? Has it changed in size?

3 *Pain*. Was the lump painful at onset and is it painful now?

4 *Menstrual history*. It is essential to determine the approximate date of the last menstrual period. Without this

information it is not possible to tell which phase of the menstrual cycle the breast is in.

Lumps which are present during the first two weeks of the menstrual cycle are more likely to persist than those which appear just before menstruation.

Even if the woman has had a hysterectomy, she may still have breast and abdominal symptoms which will allow you to determine the timing of her hormonal cycle.

5 *Does the lump vary in size* with the menstrual cycle?

6 *Nipple discharge.* Has there been any discharge? If so, was it bloodstained? Nipple discharges are dealt with on p. 22.

7 *Pregnancy and breast-feeding.* Has she had children and if so how old are they now? This will tell you how old she was when she conceived them and there is some evidence to suggest that pregnancy early in life is protective against malignancy. Were the children breast-fed or not and if so for how long?

8 *Family history.* Have any relatives had a mastectomy or breast disease?

9 Is the patient on any *medication* — in particular, the contraceptive pill or other hormonal treatment?

Examination

The patient must be examined in a good light as changes in the contour of the breast are critical in making a diagnosis and cannot be seen in poor light.

1 Ask her to sit up first and observe both breasts looking for masses or dimpling of the skin. Ask her to point to where she thinks the lump is.

2 Then ask the patient to raise both hands high in the air and look again. The pectoral skin is raised by this manoeuvre and any skin-tethering due to a mass in the breast tissue will become visible.

3 Observe the arms and decide if one is swollen or not. Look for any oedema of the skin over a lump.

4 Have the patient lie down and palpate each quadrant of each breast in turn, starting medially and working laterally, finishing with the upper and outer quadrant. Benign breast thickening is more common in this quadrant and it is useful to 'educate' the fingers to the more normal breast first. Palpate with straight fingers, and avoid digging into the breast with the fingertips.

5 Note the general turgidity and firmness of the tissue. With practice you will be able to tell whether the patient is premenstrual or not.

6 If a lump is found, the following must be determined.

    (a) Shape, i.e. rounded, irregular, flattened, etc.

(b) Size — in centimetres.

(c) Surface — smooth, irregular, lobulated.

(d) Edge — well defined, poorly defined.

(e) Consistency — soft, hard, cystic.

(f) Mobility — freely mobile within the breast or only mobile in continuity with the rest of the breast tissue.

(g) Attachments. (i) Attachment to the skin is best detected by careful observation as above. (ii) Attachment to the pectoral fascia — ask the patient to place her hand on her hip. Test the mobility of the lump both laterally and up and down while the patient remains relaxed. Ask her to press in hard on her hip. Test the mobility again. This contracts the pectoral muscle and the lump will become more fixed if it is attached to the pectoral fascia.

7 Finally look for metastatic spread. Examine the axillary and supraclavicular lymph nodes and also the chest and abdomen, particularly for hepatomegaly. The lymphatic drainage of the breast is shown in Fig. 37.

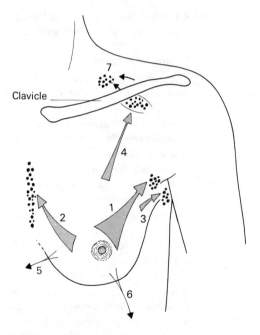

Fig. 37. The lymphatic drainage of the breast. 1, 2: Main routes of drainage, to the anterior axillary nodes and internal thoracic nodes. 3, 4: Minor routes; the axillary tail drains to the posterior axillary nodes and the upper and outer quadrant drains to the infraclavicular nodes. 5, 6: Potential routes of drainage, to the opposite breast, axilla, and the extraperitoneal lymphatics of the anterior abdominal wall. 7: Routes 1, 3 and 4 drain ultimately to the supraclavicular nodes.

Aspiration

Following a full history and examination, a decision must be made whether to aspirate the lump or not. This may well be decided by a senior surgeon. If aspiration is attempted, the lump is fixed between the thumb and forefinger and presented up to the surface. A 21-gauge needle attached to a 10 or 20 cm³ syringe is inserted into the centre of the mass. This manoeuvre alone often gives valuable information about the consistency of the lump, the 'gritty' feel of a carcinoma being easily recognized. When a cyst is entered, the surrounding tissue may be quite hard and there is a distinct 'give' as a cavity is entered and fluid, often under pressure, withdrawn. The further management of a cyst is discussed on p. 207.

Mammography

Mammography is a useful adjunct to clinical examination providing its results are not taken too seriously. This somewhat flippant statement contains much truth. While many carcinomas may show up as such on mammography, and a few show up even when no clinical lesion is felt, there is a significant false negative and false positive rate. Of these the false negative (where the X-ray is normal in spite of a cancer being present) is the most dangerous and anyone using mammography must keep this in mind. A mammogram may be used to reassure the patient but it should not be allowed to reassure the clinician.

The features on a mammogram suggestive of cancer are as follows.

1 The general crab-like shape with disruption of the normal structure.

2 Micro-calcification within the substance of the mass.

3 Thickening of the skin over the lesion due to early oedema.

Biopsy

This is the final arbiter in all persistent breast lumps. The biopsy may be carried out as follows.

1 By aspiration — this is done through a fine needle. Cells from the lesion are aspirated and sent for cytological examination. The accuracy of this method depends entirely on the skill of the cytologist available.

2 By cutting-needle biopsy — with this technique a small cylinder of the lesion is excised using a special needle. It may be difficult to accurately position such a needle if the lump is small. There is no evidence to suggest that either aspiration or needle biopsy of a cancer causes spread of the disease.

3 Open excision and biopsy of the lump.

Operation: biopsy of breast lump

Although it is possible to biopsy a lump in the breast under a local anaesthetic, this is generally not advisable. Once the breast tissue has been infiltrated with local anaesthetic the lump becomes very difficult to define and nothing is more tragic than an attempted breast biopsy which actually misses the important lesion and gives rise to incorrect reassurance.

The lump is marked preoperatively. It is fixed between finger and thumb and a skin incision is made over it in Langer's lines. Before the lump is reached the cut is extended underneath the two skin flaps thus isolating the lump centrally. The lump is then grasped with tissue forceps and excised with an adequate margin. The specimen should be carefully palpated to make sure the palpable mass is included in it. A long time should be spent obtaining adequate haemostasis within the biopsy cavity and the wound may also be drained.

Histology

Paraffin section. The tissue is first embedded in wax and allowed to set before sections are cut and stained. The process takes about 2–3 days.

Frozen section. The fresh tissue is frozen hard and cut immediately. A histological diagnosis is usually available in about 15–20 minutes. The quality of such sections is slightly inferior to paraffin sections.

Codes

Blood	Not needed for biopsy alone — will be required if mastectomy is a possibility . . . .
GA/LA	GA . . . .
Opn time	15–30 minutes . . . .
Stay	24 hours . . . .
Drains out	24 hours . . . .
Sutures out	5–7 days . . . .
Off work	Less than 1 week . . . .

Postoperative care

Following paraffin section, an outpatient appointment should be made for the next week so that she can hear the result and have the sutures removed.

Following frozen section for a lesion which has turned out

to be benign, the patient should be told the result as soon as she wakes up. Where the lesion has been found to be malignant the further management is discussed on p. 214.

Summary of the management of a breast lump
Fig. 38 summarizes the steps in the management of a lump in the breast.

The individual breast pathologies encountered will now be discussed.

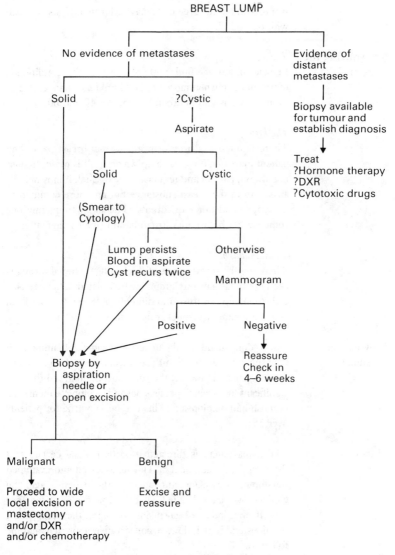

Fig. 38. The management of a breast lump.

Benign mammary dysplasia

The condition

This condition represents an aberration of the normal changes of hyperplasia and involution described on p. 200.

Various pathological terms are used to describe the changes which occur in the breast. Hypertrophy of the duct epithelium is referred to as epitheliosis. Hypertrophy of the glandular element in the acini is known as adenosis. Hypertrophy of the fibrous tissue is known as fibrosis.

During involution several acini may coalesce and form cysts. The degenerating epithelial cells draw in fluid due to osmosis and quite large cysts may be formed. Cysts are dealt with on p. 207.

Recognizing the pattern

The patient

Females of any age under 60 are affected. The condition is more common when more marked hormonal changes occur, as in the teens and between the ages of 40 and 60.

The history

There is often a history of premenstrual breast pain. The patient may then notice a lump which itself is often, though not always, painful and tender to touch. Such lumps may be anywhere in the breast substance but are more common in the upper and outer quadrants. The lump frequently becomes larger before menstruation and smaller thereafter.

On examination

There may be several areas of thickening scattered throughout both breasts or the lump may be isolated. Characteristically the lump is diffuse and difficult to define. It is not fixed and there is no skin-puckering. It may be tender.

Proving the diagnosis

This is done mainly on the history and signs. A mammogram may show characteristic diffuse thickening and no evidence of malignancy. However, the rule must be followed that any significant lump which persists beyond a complete menstrual cycle should be biopsied. This is especially true for patients over 35.

Management

The management is directed towards making certain that the lump is, in fact, benign. Having assessed and examined the lump, and taking into account the patient's age, the clinician will have decided what the chances of malignancy are. If the index of suspicion is high, the lump must be biopsied. If it is low, a conservative approach may be followed.

1 Where no lump is felt, the patient can be reassured. A decision is then made whether the breast should be reviewed once more in 6 weeks' time or not.

2 If a lump is present but felt to be benign, a mammogram is undertaken and the patient reviewed in 6 weeks.

3 If a lump is present and there is a suspicion of malignancy, it is biopsied.

4 When the patient is reviewed at the second appointment the lump may have disappeared, in which case full reassurance can be given. If the lump is smaller, a decision may be made to reassure completely or to review it once more. If the lump is persistent or larger, it must be biopsied.

Diffuse lumpiness of the breast

The patient with diffuse lumpiness of the breast presents a difficult problem. In these women it is impossible to follow the rule that any lump must be biopsied as there are simply too many lumps to do this. Such a patient must be reviewed regularly until the clinician is satisfied in his own mind that there is no enlarging mass. Any areas which are suspicious on mammography must be biopsied. It is useful to review the patient in the first two weeks of a subsequent menstrual cycle. Any area which remains persistently hard or seems to be enlarging must be biopsied.

If the patient is co-operative and sensible she should be shown how to assess her own breasts and told to attend at any time if she is worried that a new lump has appeared and persisted beyond menstruation, or if the previous one seems to be changing in character.

If this regime is not thought possible, then the patient should be regularly reviewed by the clinician and careful notes and diagrams made at each attendance.

Biopsying breast thickenings in young girls should be avoided as far as possible. This group is most unlikely to develop malignant breast disease and the scar provided by a breast biopsy can cause psychological harm. Also the scarred breast is more difficult to assess later on.

Cystic disease

The condition

The formation of cysts in the involuting breast has already been described. Cysts may be of any size and are frequently multiple. An isolated cyst is not, however, uncommon.

Recognizing the pattern

The patient

Breast cysts can occur at any age before the menopause

The history

The most characteristic history is that the lump has appeared suddenly, even though it is quite large. There is frequently pain at the onset. Occasionally the patient has also noticed that the lump has become smaller since it first appeared. There may be a previous history of other cysts.

On examination

Some cysts are very characteristic. They feel smooth and rounded and they may even be visible through the skin as the 'blue-domed' cyst. More often, however, the cyst arises in the centre of a block of fibrous tissue and is therefore less well defined. It is very unusual to have a breast cyst which fluctuates. More often the lump feels hard. Although the edge may be irregular, the overall shape of the mass is nevertheless rounded.

Proving the diagnosis

This is done by aspirating fluid from the cyst.

Management

It is quite safe to manage a breast cyst by aspiration and avoid biopsy providing the following rules are obeyed.

The area must be biopsied after aspiration if:

1 the fluid aspirated is bloodstained;
2 the mass does not disappear completely;
3 the cyst refills more than twice;
4 the lump is solid and aspiration fails.

If a good cytological service is available, the contents of the cyst should be sent for cytology. If malignant cells are found, then the lump will have to be excised. Negative cytology does not rule out biopsy if any of the criteria above are positive.

Once a cyst has been aspirated, it will be necessary to review the patient after 4 or 6 weeks to make sure it has not refilled. During this time a mammogram can usefully be carried out. Once the cyst has been emptied, however, the patient can be strongly reassured that this particular lump is not malignant. Being able, after aspirating a cyst, to reassure a patient who was sure that her life was in danger from malignancy of the breast is a rewarding experience.

Galactocoele

A galactocoele is a milk-containing cyst which arises during pregnancy. The diagnosis is made by aspirating milk from the cyst. This is also the treatment. It may recur, in which case repeated aspirations are necessary until it resolves.

Mammary duct ectasia

The condition

This lesion occurs as part of the involutionary problems occurring in and around the menopause. The ducts become full of hypertrophic epithelium, which then breaks down and causes duct blockage. The problem has been well described as the 'stagnant duct syndrome'. The duct may rupture and the stagnant contents exude into the surrounding breast tissue, where they cause a foreign body reaction. This reaction is characterized by the presence of plasma cells and the lesion is known as 'plasma cell mastitis'

Recognizing the pattern

The patient
She is middle-aged and in or around the menopause.

The history
There is a history of discharge from one or more duct orifices and the discharge may even be bloodstained (see p. 222). The patient may then develop a painful area in the breast with an associated lump.

On examination
The lump may be palpable and tender, and there may be surrounding inflammation.

Management

The problem here is to distinguish the lesion from a carcinoma as it occurs in the same age-group. Biopsy is frequently indicated.

Where there is a nipple discharge, a ductogram may be performed and this may show enlarged, dilated breast ducts, changes which give the lesion its name.

Having excluded carcinoma, no further treatment is necessary for this condition and the patient should be reassured. The inflammation settles in time.

Fat necrosis

The condition

The importance of this condition lies in the fact that it closely mimics the physical signs of carcinoma. It is rare. There is a clear history of injury and usually of marked bruising in the region of the breast. Beware, however, because patients with cancer often also claim a history of injury although the presence of bruising is unusual.

As the bruising settles and the haematoma resolves, a hard area remains in the breast and this eventually gives rise to scarring and consequent puckering of the skin over the lesion.

The patient
Patients of any age may be affected and large breasts are more often subject to fat necrosis than small ones.

On examination
The physical signs are of a hard lump with puckering of the skin over it.

Management

Because this lesion is difficult to distinguish from carcinoma of the breast, a biopsy is almost always necessary. The diagnosis is then proved on histology.

Benign neoplasms

These may arise from any of the elements in the breast but the most common are fibroadenomas. The only other tumour which is not rare is the lipoma.

Fibroadenomas

The condition

These constitute 75% of all benign breast neoplasms. Two types are described histologically and must therefore be mentioned, although in practice the distinction between them is not very marked. Intracanalicular fibroadenomas are more common in older women and in these the fibrous tissue predominates and projects into the lumen of the ducts within the adenoma. In pericanalicular fibroadenomas, small, rounded islands of adenoma tissue are encircled by whorls of fibrous tissue.

A third type of rare fibroadenoma is the giant fibro-adenoma (cystosarcoma phylloides, serocystic disease of Brodie). This occurs in women over the age of 35 and presents as a huge lobulated mass. The tumour must be removed in its entirety or it tends to recur locally. Malignant change can occur though it is rare.

**Recognizing the
pattern**

The patient
Fibroadenomas are common in women under the age of 35. Giant fibroadenomas occur in the older age-group.

The history
The patient almost always presents by noticing the lump, which is painless.

On examination
The fibroadenoma is described as a 'breast mouse'. It is small, hard and extremely mobile. It slips round the breast tissue underneath the examining fingers and is difficult to isolate.

Proving the diagnosis   A fibroadenoma shows up on a mammogram as a character-istic well-defined, rounded, lesion. The diagnosis is proved by biopsy.

Management   Fibroadenomas should be excised both to finalize the diagnosis and because they go on slowly enlarging if they are not removed. If the diagnosis is clear, there is no particular hurry for this procedure. However, beware of the 'fibro-adenoma' presenting in women aged between 35 and 50. This may well be a small carcinoma.

Carcinoma of the Breast

Cancer of the breast is the most common malignant disease in women in the Western world. Six per cent of women will develop the disease in the United Kingdom, an annual incidence of 50 per 100 000. The carcinomata are of various histological types, the commonest being the scirrhous tumour, in which there is a marked fibrous stromal reaction to the malignant cells. The malignant nature of the lump gives rise to the clinical features by which it is recognized. Infiltration into the surrounding lymphatics causes blockage and localized oedema of the skin overlying the lump. In severe cases this is clearly visible as 'peau d'orange'. Further infiltration leads to involvement of local lymph nodes and these may be palpably enlarged in the axilla or the neck. The fibrous component of the cancer may undergo contraction (as does any other scar tissue) and this results in the characteristic puckering and deformity.

Acute inflammatory carcinoma is a highly anaplastic growth occurring during lactation or pregnancy. Obstruction of the lymphatics and veins produces congestion, erythema and oedema of the skin, mimicking acute inflammation.

Distant spread of carcinoma of the breast typically involves the bones, lungs, brain and liver.

Recognizing the pattern

The patient
The patient is usually over the age of 30. Cancers developing in the elderly may grow very slowly and may present with extensive local lesions.

The history
The patient herself or her husband notices the lump or it is noticed at a routine medical examination. Occasionally cancers do present with localized pain in the breast before any lump appears and this symptom must always be taken seriously in the relevant age-group. Other presentations include a bloodstained nipple discharge (p. 222) and symptoms from metastases (e.g. bone pain). There may also be a positive family history of breast cancer.

On examination
The lump may be hard or soft and of any size. The size should be carefully recorded at the first examination. Puck-

ering of the skin over the lesion or deep fixation are the most reliable physical signs of malignancy although these signs may also be shared by areas of fat necrosis (see p. 209).

Proving the diagnosis

The diagnosis of carcinoma of the breast may be proved on mammography but as already mentioned a negative mammogram does not exclude malignancy. The features of malignancy seen on mammography are detailed on p. 203. A lesion suspected of being malignant must, however, be biopsied by one of the methods detailed on p. 203.

General management

A patient who is strongly suspected of having carcinoma of the breast should be fully investigated to establish the extent of the disease. Metastatic spread should be looked for, using the following investigations.

1 Liver function tests, particularly alkaline phosphatase and alanine transaminase (ALT).

2 Serum calcium.

3 Chest X-ray to look for any pulmonary deposits.

4 Bone scan or skeletal survey by X-rays.

5 Computerized axial tomography may become increasingly useful in detecting metastases.

Patients can become extremely worried by these screening procedures and you should explain to them that they are routinely done in every case under investigation and do not carry any particular significance for the individual patient.

As a result of this assessment, the tumour can be staged according to the internationally recognized tumour−node− metastasis (TNM) system (see Table 14).

On the basis of this staging a decision can be made on whether it is possible to attempt a cure (carcinoma involving the breast and axilla only with no further spread), or whether cure is impossible because of disseminated disease.

Paget's disease

The condition

Paget's disease is a description applied to an eczematous, scaling plaque which appears around the nipple. It is associated with intraduct carcinoma invading the lymphatics and the epithelium of the areola.

Recognizing the pattern

There is a red, scaly, weeping plaque involving part of the nipple and areola. The examination must include the breast and regional lymph nodes as described under 'methods of assessment' on p. 200. There may be a palpable lump beneath the areola.

Table 14. The TNM classification of breast cancer

Tumours	Nodes	Metastases
	0 No nodes	0 No metastases
1 0−2 cm, no skin fixation	1 Palpable mobile nodes (a) not clinically significant (b) clinically significant	1 Evidence of metastasis including skin beyond the breast, contralateral nodes, liver, bone, etc.
2 2−5 cm, skin distortion, no pectoral fixation	2 Palpable immobile axillary nodes	
3 5−10 cm, skin ulcerated over the lump, pectoral fixation	3 Supraclavicular nodes, oedema	
4 10 cm or more, breast skin involved beyond the lump, chest wall fixation		

Example $T_2N0\ M0$ = a malignant mass less than 5 cm in diameter causing puckering of the skin on elevation of the arm but no other abnormalities found.

Proving the diagnosis

A mammogram may show a lesion beneath the areola. The diagnosis is proved on biopsy.

Management

The lesion is managed as an early carcinoma of the breast. Because the carcinoma is superficial and presents early, the prognosis is good.

Management of early carcinoma

This is a carcinoma confined to the breast and regional axillary lymph nodes and therefore considered potentially curable. The management of early primary carcinoma of the breast is still a matter of controversy. Surgical treatment has been becoming steadily more conservative over recent years. The most conservative accepted therapy is wide local excision of the carcinoma followed by radiotherapy. Surgeons who feel this is inadequate treatment may perform a simple mastectomy or even a radical mastectomy. Wide local excision is not usually recommended where there are palpable axillary nodes, or where the disease in the breast is multifocal.

Where the lesion has been found on mammography and is impalpable, it will be necessary to arrange radiographic localization in the X-ray department immediately before operation.

Preoperative management

Whatever the form of definitive therapy, an initial biopsy will usually be carried out. This may either be done before a definitive procedure (aspiration biopsy, needle biopsy or paraffin section) or be planned at the same time (frozen-section biopsy). In the latter case it will be necessary for the houseman to inform the laboratory of the need for frozen-section facilities and of the probable time it is to be expected.

The consultant will have discussed the pros and cons of the various forms of surgery with the patient and reached an understanding of what is to be done. Find out what has been said. Ensure that the patient fully understands the procedure to be carried out and what forms of further therapy may be involved. The consent form must be signed to cover both the biopsy and any possible other surgery.

Operation: wide local excision

The lesion is removed together with a 2 cm margin of tissue all round. This may involve excising a complete quadrant of the breast. The axillary nodes may be sampled by extending the incision laterally, or through a separate incision. The histologist should be asked to check the completeness of the excision. A simple mastectomy may be required if the lesion reaches the edges of the specimen.

Codes

Blood	0
GA/LA	GA
Opn time	30 minutes
Stay	48 hours
Drains out	48 hours
Sutures out	7 days
Off work	2−3 weeks

Operation: simple mastectomy

In this operation the breast is excised through an elliptical incision centred around the lump. The nipple is included in the skin flap removed. It is possible to combine this operation with excision of the lowest axillary nodes either as a curative procedure or as a less extensive 'sampling' procedure. In the latter case information is gained about the spread of the growth by histological assessment of the lymph node. It is important to make sure that the laboratory realizes that axillary tissue has been removed and that they should examine it for lymph nodes.

Codes

Blood	2 units	. . . .
GA/LA	GA	. . . .
Opn time	90–120 minutes	. . . .
Stay	7 days	. . . .
Drains out	3–5 days	. . . .
Sutures out	7–10 days	. . . .
Off work.	3–4 weeks	. . . .

Operation: radical mastectomy

In this operation the breast is excised *en bloc* with the sternal head of the pectoralis major and pectoralis minor. An extensive dissection of the axillary nodes is also carried out. In the supraradical operation the anterior chest is opened and the internal mammary chain of nodes is also removed.

In Patey's operation, which is a modified radical procedure, the pectoralis major muscle is left *in situ* but the pectoralis minor muscle is excised from beneath it, together with a full dissection of the axillary nodes.

Codes

Blood	2 units	. . . .
GA/LA	GA	. . . .
Opn time	2 hours	. . . .
Stay	7–10 days	. . . .
Drains out	3–5 days	. . . .
Sutures out	7–10 days	. . . .
Off work.	3–4 weeks	. . . .

Postoperative care

The main problem after mastectomy is of serous collections underneath the skin flaps. These tend to collect late (around the seventh to fourteenth day). Their development can be partially prevented by good early drainage, and suction drains are useful for this. Some surgeons also apply external pressure by wrapping a crêpe bandage around the chest.

Swelling of the arm is a late complication of extensive axillary dissection. There is no really satisfactory treatment for this complication.

Adjuvant radiotherapy following mastectomy is a well-established practice. Some surgeons use it for all patients, others only for the patients whose lymph nodes are histologically involved. Three weeks after the operation, by which time the wound is satisfactorily healed, the patient is given a course of radiotherapy, which may include the bed of the breast, axilla, supraclavicular fossa and internal mammary chain.

Treatment with adjuvant systemic chemotherapy given at the time of primary treatment is more widely accepted, following the publication of numerous clinical trials. Cytotoxic chemotherapy is said to reduce the chance of death by 14% irrespective of age. In pre-menopausal patients the reduction is 22%. In post-menopausal women tamoxifen (an oestrogen receptor blocker) reduces the chance of death by 16%. There is no indication for adjuvant tamoxifen in premenopausal patients. It has a weak effect and does not affect prognosis.

Oestrogen receptors
The presence of oestrogen receptor sites on the tumour cells affects the response to hormonal therapy. Oestrogen receptors are cytoplasmic proteins which bind and transfer oestrogens into nuclei. The binding capacity is expressed as femtomoles of ^{3}H-oestradiol bound per mg of cytosol protein. Values greater than 10 are positive and less than 3 fmol/mg are negative. Fifty per cent of primary breast cancers are positive but less than 50% of metastases are positive. Ninety per cent of well-differentiated and lobular cancers are positive. In ductal cancer the positivity rate is 60%. Pre-menopausal women have a low rate of positive cancers (30%) and peri-menopausal women the lowest (<20%). Visceral metastases, especially hepatic, have the lowest rates of oestrogen receptor positivity. Oestrogen receptor-negative tumours have the highest proliferative rate.

Hormone therapy is effective in 50–60% of oestrogen receptor-positive tumours and in only 10% of oestrogen receptor-negative tumours. Progesterone receptors are found in 40% of oestrogen receptor-positive cancers.

At least 40% of patients fail to respond to hormonal treatment despite the presence of cytosol receptor for oestrogen.

Reconstruction of the breast
The loss of a breast is a severe psychological blow to the patient and can lead to symptoms of depression and anxiety, together with sexual and marital problems. Many patients will ask whether or not the breast can be reconstructed. This

can either be done at the time of mastectomy or 2–3 years later. The reconstruction can consist of a silastic implant placed either subcutaneously or under the pectoralis major. A myocutaneous flap may also be constructed, using lattisimus dorsi. Possible disadvantages of reconstruction are that the prosthesis may mask the detection of recurrent disease and the cosmetic result is not always successful. Many patients are entirely satisfied with an external prosthesis worn over the mastectomy scar. You should make sure that arrangements have been made for fitting such an external prosthesis when the patient is discharged from hospital.

Management of advanced carcinoma
If evidence of more distant spread is found the likelihood of cure is remote, and management is then aimed at prolonging survival as far as is possible and preventing undue suffering. Of the two, prevention of suffering is the more important. Forms of treatment which cause pain or other side-effects need strong justification.

Methods of management
These include the following:
Surgery
Radiotherapy
Hormonal therapy
Chemotherapy.

Surgery
There is a limited place for operative surgery in the treatment of advanced carcinoma.
1 The control of local disease is still important, although surgical procedures are usually as conservative as possible.
2 Suspected metastases may be biopsied.
3 Operation may be indicated to achieve palliation for pathological fractures or to decompress the spinal cord after a vertebral collapse.

Radiotherapy
Where the patient has advanced carcinoma of the breast, radiotherapy can be useful in the following ways.
1 To treat local skin recurrence or axillary node recurrence.
2 For the treatment of metastases in bones. A pathological fracture may be treated with orthopaedic fixation combined with radiotherapy and this will usually result in healing. Radiotherapy can be very effective treatment for the extreme pain that occurs with metastases in the spinal vertebrae.

3 In treating metastases that are causing symptoms.
4 In endocrine ablation therapy, as discussed below.

Hormonal therapy

Sixty per cent of breast tumours are sensitive to steroid hormones. Endocrine therapy is used to try and change the hormonal balance of oestrogens to androgens in an attempt to produce an environment hostile to tumour growth. This can produce effective remissions in one-third of patients and a partial response in a further third of patients. The type of treatment given depends on the age of the patient.

Patients who develop carcinoma of the breast before the menopause, in whom the malignant tissue is often dependent on oestrogen, frequently respond to therapy aimed at decreasing oestrogen levels.

Oestrogen production can be lowered by the following.
1 Surgical removal of the ovaries (see below).
2 Irradiation of the ovaries producing an 'irradiation menopause'.
3 Conservative treatment with androgens and prednisolone in an attempt to suppress the adrenal cortex and therefore the production of oestrogens.
4 Tamoxifen is a drug which blocks the oestrogen receptors in tissues and can be very effective in post-menopausal women, particularly in the first 15 years after their last period. Tamoxifen may be effective in younger patients, as second-line treatment, when remission has been successfully induced previously by ovarian ablation.
5 Aminoglutethamide can affect advanced breast cancer in two ways. It inhibits adrenal steroid production. Even though the adrenal itself produces no oestrogens it does normally secrete androstenedione, which is converted elsewhere into oestrone and oestradiol. Aminoglutethamide blocks this process when given in doses of 250–1000 mg per day. It also suppresses the conversion of cholesterol to pregnenolone in the adrenal itself. Patients will require glucocorticosteroid supplements, such as hydrocortisone (30 mg daily) or prednisolone (10 mg daily).

In a woman who is 10 years or more beyond the menopause, oestrogen, androgens and progesterones have all been found to be effective. The side-effects of oestrogens include withdrawal bleeding from the vagina, and sodium and fluid retention. Androgens cause masculinization.

Operation: bilateral oophorectomy

The pelvis is approached through a transverse lower abdominal incision and the ovaries are removed. The opportunity is also taken to look for other evidence of intra-abdominal disease.

Codes

Blood	2 units	. . . .
GA/LA	GA	. . . .
Opn time	1 hour	. . . .
Stay	About 1 week	. . . .
Drains out	0–24 hours	. . . .
Sutures out	5–7 days	. . . .
Off work	Variable	. . . .

The methods outlined above are the first phase of hormonal treatment and the patient's response is then measured. Patients who show no response are not considered for further more drastic hormonal therapy. They are treated with cytotoxic drugs (see below). In patients who do show a response but then relapse, further ablation may then be successful in the form of either adrenalectomy or hypophysectomy. Hypophysectomy is usually carried out by neurosurgeons or otorhinolaryngologists and will not be dealt with here.

Operation: bilateral adrenalectomy
The adrenals may either be exposed through bilateral loin incisions or more frequently through an upper abdominal transverse incision anteriorly. The exposure is difficult, particularly on the right side, and ligation of the right suprarenal vein as it drains into the vena cava may be hazardous.

Codes

Blood	4–6 units	. . . .
GA/LA	GA	. . . .
Opn time	2–3 hours	. . . .
Stay	Variable — at least 1 week	. . . .
Drains out	2–4 days	. . . .
Sutures out	7–10 days	. . . .
Off work	Variable	. . . .

Patients who respond to adrenalectomy or hypophysectomy but then relapse may still respond to cytotoxic therapy.

Chemotherapy — cytotoxic agents
Drugs may be used singly or in combination, and the treatment may be intermittent or continuous. The agents commonly used are doxorubicin (Adriamycin), cyclophos-

phamide, methotrexate, 5-fluorouracil and vincristine, all with or without prednisolone. Cytotoxic agents are used in patients who have disseminated disease and have not responded to endocrine therapy. Forty to sixty per cent of patients respond initially but the response is usually shortlived. Cytotoxic agents are usually more effective against soft-tissue metastases than those in bone. Side-effects of these drugs may be severe, particularly causing baldness, nausea and vomiting. Many patients refuse further treatment because of these side-effects.

Immunotherapy

This is still experimental and the results are very variable. Some tumours do show evidence of an immune reaction with lymphocytic infiltration around the tumour. If such a response is present, the prognosis is improved. Following this observation, attempts have been made to boost native immunity by non-specific vaccination with immunostimulants such as bacillus Calmette–Guérin (BCG).

Terminal care

When the patient is dying from carcinoma of the breast, there are a number of symptoms that require treatment, the most important of which is pain. Analgesia should be given frequently and in sufficient doses to keep the patient out of pain. Bone pain is often best treated with a prostaglandin inhibitor such as indomethacin or aspirin rather than opiates. Local radiotherapy can be useful. Breathlessness from a pleural effusion or lymphangitis carcinomatosa can be helped by corticosteroids and aspiration of the effusion. Symptoms from hepatic metastases (e.g. pain and anorexia) may also respond to corticosteroids. Cerebral metastases may cause severe headache and focal neurological deficits and these may respond to dexamethasone or radiotherapy. Lymphoedema of the arm following radical mastectomy or extensive radiotherapy can be relieved to some extent by elastic bandages and physiotherapy or pneumatic compression.

Other Breast Presentations

Discharge from the nipple

The condition

When the patient presents with a discharge from the nipple and a lump is found in the breast, the management is as for a breast lump and the discharge is of secondary importance.

When a patient presents with nipple discharge without a lump, the course to be followed depends on the type of discharge and whether one duct or more than one is giving rise to the fluid.

Milky or serous discharge occurs in early pregnancy and also occasionally in mammary dysplasia. It is nothing to worry about and reassurance can be given.

A coloured discharge (green, brown or yellow) which comes from several ducts is usually associated with mammary dysplasia. Providing it is not associated with a lump, reassurance can be given. If such a discharge comes from an isolated duct, it may be due to an intra-duct papilloma or mammary duct ectasia and very occasionally can even be due to a carcinoma. An isolated duct discharge of this type will require further investigation (see below).

A bloodstained discharge must always be taken seriously. Causes include the following:

1 Intra-duct carcinoma or a carcinoma invading a duct.

2 Intra-duct papilloma. This is a benign lesion a few millimetres in diameter, arising from duct epithelium.

3 Mammary duct ectasia (see p. 209).

Management

Investigations

1 If the discharge is coloured or bloodstained, a smear should be made and sent for cytology. If this shows the presence of malignant cells, a breast biopsy will be undertaken and a mastectomy is likely.

2 As in any other case where the patient is worried by change in the breast, it is sensible to perform a mammogram.

3 Where an isolated duct is involved, a 'ductogram' may be useful. A fine cannula is inserted by the radiologist into the offending duct and a small amount of contrast injected. An intra-duct papilloma may show up as a filling effect or as a blocked duct. Mammary duct ectasia may also be nicely demonstrated.

Preoperative management

If the discharge is from an isolated duct or bloodstained, then a carcinoma of the breast will have to be excluded by biopsying the breast tissue beneath the nipple. The site of the affected duct must be carefully noted because the discharge may not be visible when the patient is on the operating table. Note the segment of the breast which, on pressure, produces the discharge. This is described by its position on a clock face centred on the nipple. Once this has been determined, no further discharge should be expressed until the patient is in theatre. The patient should also be told to avoid expressing it herself.

Two operations are possible. A microdochectomy is indicated where the discharge is from a single, defined duct. A mammodochectomy is undertaken where a bloodstained discharge issues from several ducts or where the sites of the discharges have not been determined.

Operation: microdochectomy

The offending segment is pressed so that the discharge is visible. A fine probe is then passed down the involved duct. A peri-areolar incision is made and that side of the nipple raised. The duct containing the probe can then be identified underneath the skin and is excised up to its orifice at the nipple and down for two or three centimetres. The central end is marked with a stitch and it is sent for histology.

Codes

Blood	0	. . . .
GA/LA	GA	. . . .
Opn time	30−60 minutes	. . . .
Stay	2−3 days	. . . .
Drains out	1−2 days	. . . .
Sutures out	5 days	. . . .
Off work	1−2 weeks	. . . .

Operation: mammodochectomy

In this case the nipple is again raised off the underlying tissues by a peri-areolar incision. The main ducts underneath the nipple are then excised as a block and sent for histology.

Codes

Blood	Group and save	. . . .
GA/LA	GA	. . . .
Opn time	30−60 minutes	. . . .
Stay	3−4 days	. . . .
Drains out	2−3 days	. . . .

Sutures out	5–7 days
Off work	2–3 weeks

Postoperative care

Bruising and haematoma formation are the main complications of both operations. Histological examination of the specimen usually reveals the aetiology of the discharge. An intra-duct papilloma requires no further treatment. A carcinoma may be treated by mastectomy. In the rare case where no aetiology is found, the patient must continue to be followed up to make sure that no lump appears in the residual breast.

Pain in the breast

Breast pain may be due to one of the following:
1 mammary dysplasia,
2 carcinoma,
3 mammary duct ectasia and plasma cell mastitis,
4 breast abscess,
5 referred pain (e.g. cervical nerve root pressure).

Patients presenting with pain in the breast associated with a non-inflammatory lump have already been discussed. Very occasionally a breast cancer presents with pain alone in the absence of a lump. For this reason, any patient in the right age-group who has unexplained breast pain should be investigated. A mammogram should be undertaken and the patient followed up to make sure that a breast lump does not appear.

Mammary duct ectasia can also give rise to inflammatory disease in the breast due to extravasation of stagnant duct contents (see p. 209). Occasionally this may even progress to an abscess.

The usual cause of a breast abscess is secondary to a bacterial mastitis.

Breast abscess

The condition

Breast abscesses occur, usually in the lactating breast, secondary to infection which gains access through a crack in the nipple. Occasionally they occur in non-lactating breasts, often in association with an indrawn nipple or mammary duct ectasia.

Recognizing the pattern

The history

The patient complains of a gradual onset of pain in one segment of the breast.

On examination

The signs of inflammation are obvious. There is a hot,

tender swelling of the infected area. In the later stages this becomes very indurated and fluctuation may be elicited. If the mastitis has been treated with antibiotics the breast abscess may be surprisingly non-tender. The abscess is sterilized by the antibiotics and a chronic fibrous mass results which can persist for many weeks (antibioma).

Proving the diagnosis

The diagnosis of a breast abscess can be proved by aspirating pus from the mass. The pus should be sent for culture.

Management

Ideally a bacterial mastitis should be treated with antibiotics in the first 24 hours of the infection. In this way, abscess formation can be aborted. Unfortunately, many women present rather later than this when abscess formation may have already started. Antibiotics will then take away the pain and the inflammation but a mass persists.

If an abscess is present it should be drained.

Operation: drainage of breast abscess
The mass is incised and a corrugated drain inserted.

Codes

Blood	0 . . . .
GA/LA	GA . . . .
Opn time	15 minutes . . . .
Stay	24 hours . . . .
Drains out	3–4 days . . . .
Sutures out	0 . . . .
Off work	Not usually applicable . . . .

Postoperative care
The patient should continue feeding her baby from the opposite breast and expressing the milk from the affected breast manually. The milk can be boiled and given to the child. If an attempt is made to suppress lactation both breasts will become engorged and tender, and the situation may be made worse. It is usually possible to resume normal breast-feeding within a few days of draining the abscess.

If the patient presents with a chronic antibioma, this should be excised as it is unlikely to resolve on its own.

Mammillary fistula
Occasionally, when an abscess has been incised or drained spontaneously, a fistula occurs between the skin and the duct, and continues to discharge.

Treatment is to excise the fistula, using a peri-areolar incision to remove the duct which is blocked near the nipple.

4.4   Conditions of the Male Breast

Carcinoma

The condition   Approximately 0.6—1% of breast malignancies occur in males. Carcinoma may develop in pre-existing gynaecomastia, and there is an association with Klinefelter's syndrome. It has a worse prognosis than carcinoma of the female breast because it is often advanced at presentation. The male breast is smaller and the growth therefore tends to invade and metastasize sooner.

Recognizing the pattern

The patient
He is usually aged around 60 or over and notices a lump beneath the areola.

On examination
There is a fibrotic nodular mass beneath the areola. The overlying skin may become ulcerated. The lesion is usually painless. There may be palpable, involved, axillary lymph nodes.

Proving the diagnosis   The investigation, biopsy and staging are carried out as in the female.

Management   Early carcinoma is treated by mastectomy and/or radiotherapy.
    Advanced carcinoma is treated with hormonal therapy. Orchidectomy (see p. 441) gives good results with 60—70% of patients going into remission. If the condition relapses, some patients respond to oestrogen therapy.

Gynaecomastia

The condition   This is hypertrophy of the male breast. It may occur on one or both sides. There are many causes, the most important of which are listed in Table 15.

Recognizing the pattern

The patient
He may be of any age but the condition is most commonly seen at puberty or in the elderly (60—70) when it is often due to oestrogen treatment. The presenting complaint is of unilateral or bilateral swelling beneath the nipple. There may be some discomfort. It may be discovered as part of

more widespread disease, e.g. cirrhosis. It is important to take a careful drug history.

On examination
The whole breast tissue is enlarged and there is no fixity to the skin or underlying muscle. Inspect the testes for signs of an adenoma and look for evidence of liver failure or hyperthyroidism.

Table 15. Causes of gynaecomastia

1 Physiological	Neonatal Pubertal
2 Idiopathic	
3 Hormonal	Decreased androgens: hypogonadism Increased oestrogens: oestrogen therapy Tumour: testis, adrenal, liver Increased human chorionic gonadotrophin (HCG)
4 Cirrhosis	
5 Hyperthyroidism	
6 Drugs	Digoxin Spironolactone Cimetidine Isoniazid

Management

This depends on the cause. Pubertal gynaecomastia usually settles down within a year. The patient should be reassured. If after one or two years the condition continues to cause embarrassment, a subareolar mastectomy may be carried out. The management of other forms of gynaecomastia depends on the cause, which should be corrected if possible.

Operation: subareolar mastectomy for gynaecomastia
A semi-circular incision is made around the edge of the areola and the nipple raised as a skin flap. The enlarged breast tissue is separated from the skin and underlying muscle, and removed through the central incision. The wound is drained using suction. The excised breast should be sent for histology.

Codes

Blood	2 units	
GA/LA	GA	
Opn time	90–120 minutes	
Stay	5–7 days	
Drains out	5 days	
Sutures out	5 days	
Off work	3–4 weeks	

Postoperative care

Removal of the breast leaves a subcutaneous space which tends to fill with blood and serum. It is important to maintain suction drainage and external pressure sufficiently long for the cavity to heal. The cosmetic result is very good and after a few months the incision is barely visible.

5   The Chest

5.1   **Chest drainage and thoracotomy**
Chest drains
Thoracotomy
Tracheostomy

5.2   **Dysphagia**
Assessment
Impacted foreign body
Oesophageal perforation
Acute caustic stricture
Chronic benign stricture
Oesophageal achalasia
Pharyngeal pouch
Plummer–Vinson syndrome
Barretts' oesophagus
Carcinoma of the oesophagus

5.1   Chest Drainage and Thoracotomy

Chest drains

The indications for chest drainage are as follows.

1 A pneumothorax.

2 A pleural effusion — serous fluid or pus.

3 Haemothorax.

4 To prevent the collection of fluid or air, e.g. after thoracotomy.

The procedure of insertion is described in some detail as it is something most housesurgeons will have to do.

Operation: inserting a chest drain

Make sure that all the equipment you require is ready before you start. This includes the following.

1 Local anaesthetic (1 or 2% Xylocaine).

2 Skin preparation.

3 A suitable tube drain (e.g. 20−26 Ch gauge 'Argyle'), preferably with a radio-opaque line in it.

4 Stitches for:

    (a) holding the drain in;

    (b) later closure of the skin.

It is useful to use materials of different colours.

5 The underwater seal drain with water in it.

6 Straight artery forceps.

7 Available wall suction and a suitable connection for it.

8 A tube clamp.

The procedure should be done in the treatment room or theatre if possible.

The drain is usually inserted in the fourth or fifth inter-costal space in the mid-axillary line, or in the second space anteriorly.

Position of the patient. He should be sitting up, and can either lean forward over a suitably placed bed table with his arms folded in front of the body (for a posterior or lateral approach), or lie back on pillows (for an anterior approach).

If you are about to drain an effusion check the presence of fluid by inserting a 19-gauge needle on a syringe at your chosen site. It can be helpful to mark the skin before scrubbing up.

1 Clean the skin.

2 Inject local anaesthetic, infiltrating the underlying tissues

down to the parietal pleura. The presence of fluid can also be checked during this manoeuvre.

3 Incise the skin with a sharp, pointed scalpel and cut down on to the rib below the intercostal space chosen for the drain. Move upwards to the centre of that space and enlarge and deepen the hole by inserting closed artery forceps into the pleura, thus creating a track for the drain.

4 Put in two sutures:

(a) a 2/0 nylon across the incision. This is left loose for tying to close the wound when the drain is removed.

(b) a 0 silk purse string for securing the drain.

5 Push in the chest drain on its introducer until it touches the rib. Then 'walk' the tip up the rib until it slides over the top, following the preformed track, to penetrate the pleura. This avoids damaging the intercostal bundle (see Fig. 39). Use your middle finger as a depth marker to guard against too deep an initial insertion.

6 Angle the introducer to aim the drainage tube up to the apex. Then slide the tube over the introducer into the chest.

7 Withdraw the introducer. As a precaution, clamp the drain as the introducer is taken out to prevent further pulmonary collapse.

8 Connect the drain to the underwater seal as shown in Fig. 40 and, when the system is air-tight, unclamp the tube.

9 Tie it in securely and check that the meniscus is fluctuating.

10 Suction should be applied to the venting tube of the bottle whenever significant drainage of fluid or air is expected. For preference use wall suction providing a high volume at low pressure. A Roberts pump is often inadequate. Ten to twenty millimetres of mercury suction are applied and adjusted to obtain a gentle flow of bubbles or fluid.

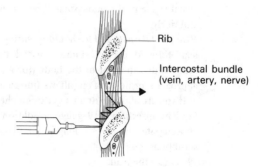

Rib

Intercostal bundle
(vein, artery, nerve)

Fig. 39. Avoiding damage to the intercostal bundle when entering the pleural cavity.

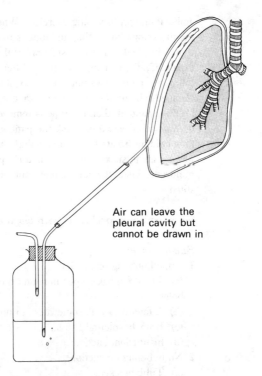

Air can leave the
pleural cavity but
cannot be drawn in

Fig. 40. Underwater seal drainage.

Postoperative care

1 Check the position of the tube and the expansion of the
lung by an early chest X-ray. This should be repeated daily.

2 *Position of the bottle.* The water seal must at all times be
kept below the patient, ideally on the floor. If it is lifted up
above the patient, the water may siphon into the patient's
chest. Everyone, including the patient, nurses, auxiliaries
and ward cleaners, must be told this.

3 *Moving the patient.* Have two clamps next to the patient to
double clamp the tube when a change of position is required.
One clamp may give way. Be certain these clamps are
removed again once the move is over. *Never clamp a bubbling
drain.*

4 *Checking patency.* The tube can be seen to be patent, and
therefore draining, by observing the meniscus fluctuate on
breathing or coughing. The swing reflects changes in pressure in the pleural sac and will remain high if the lung
compliance is high.

5 *Re-expansion of the lung.* This is encouraged by early

ambulation and breathing exercises. When the meniscus in the tube stops fluctuating, the lung is fully expanded or the tube is blocked. Take a chest X-ray. If the lung is seen to be expanded, then clamp the tube. After lung puncture or following spontaneous pneumothorax, it is usual to leave the clamped tube *in situ* for 24 hours, then re-X-ray. If the lung is still expanded, then the tube is removed.

6 *Removal of chest drain.* Ask the patient to breathe in and then hold his breath (i.e. to do a Valsalva manoeuvre). In this way no air is sucked into the pleural space as the tube is removed. When the tube comes out, tie the skin closure stitch.

Some common problems with chest drainage

Failure to drain
1 Tube bubbling on suction.
   (a) The drain has slipped out and exposed one of the side holes.
   (b) A fault or a leak somewhere in the circuit.
   (c) Broncho-pleural fistula.
   (d) Insufficient suction.
2 No bubbling on suction.
   (a) Tube blocked.
   (b) Tube in incorrect space.
   (c) Clamp still attached.
   (d) Tube kinked.

Breathlessness
1 Pneumothorax (? tension pneumothorax).
2 Pneumothorax on the opposite side of the chest.
3 Haemothorax.
4 Haemopericardium.

Thoracotomy

A thoracotomy is quite often performed on a general surgical unit and you should be familiar with the pre- and postoperative care that this entails.

Preoperative management
Explain to the patient that he will have one or two tubes draining the chest postoperatively and tell him why (see below). It will be important that he breathes fully and coughs adequately and to do this he must be given adequate analgesia.

   One of the three following major incisions may be used.

Operation: postero-lateral thoracotomy

This is used for access to the oesophagus or descending aorta. The patient is placed in a prone or lateral position. The fifth, sixth or seventh intercostal space is opened and part of a rib may be resected to enlarge the opening.

Operation: antero-lateral thoracotomy

This approach may be used for access to the heart, pericardium or lung. The patient lies obliquely with the side to be opened uppermost. Access is gained through the fifth space.

Operation: median sternotomy

This is the best approach for the heart, pericardium, great vessels and mediastinal structures. The patient lies supine and the sternum is split longitudinally with a special circular saw.

During closure, after the procedure has been completed, chest drains are inserted. There are usually two-one at the apex and one at the base. They are brought out through a separate incision below the main one, usually through the seventh or eighth space.

The chest drains are attached to an underwater seal drain.

Codes

Blood	4 or more units . . . .
GA/LA	GA . . . .
Opn time	Depends on indication for thoracotomy . . . .
Stay	7–10 days (except for oesophagectomy, see pp. 251–254) . . . .
Drains out	2–3 days (depending on drainage) . . .
Sutures out	7–10 days . . . .
Off work	6–8 weeks . . . .

Postoperative care

It is most important that the patient has sufficient analgesia to breathe adequately and cough. This may be achieved either by intercostal nerve blocks with long-acting anaesthetic (e.g. Marcain), a thoracic epidural (which requires intensive nursing care) or parenteral opiate drugs.

The management of the chest drain has already been described.

Tracheostomy

Tracheostomy is indicated in three situations.

1 Upper airways obstruction, e.g.

   (a) impacted foreign body;

(b) laryngeal oedema due to epiglottitis, angioneurotic oedema of the tongue or spreading infection of the floor of the mouth (Ludwig's angina);

(c) severe facial injury;

(d) facial burns;

(e) assault with direct laryngeal injury.

2 Conditions requiring prolonged ventilation.

3 In severe respiratory disease, to decrease the dead space and allow regular direct suction of the airways.

In an emergency situation the simplest and fastest method of establishing an airway is through the cricothyroid membrane (laryngotomy). Tracheostomy is, however, the method of choice when there is rather less urgency (Fig. 41).

Operation: laryngotomy

Hold the head still and make a transverse stab incision between the Adam's apple of the thyroid cartilage above and the cricoid cartilage below, using any available knife blade or, if necessary, a 14-gauge intravenous needle. Stay in the midline and continue backwards until air is heard hissing in and out. The cricothyroid membrane has now been pierced. Insert a sterile laryngotomy tube if available or else any tube which will help keep the hole open. Once breathing has been restored, the procedure can be completed tidily.

Operation: tracheostomy

The cricoid cartilage is palpated. A transverse skin incision is made over the trachea below this at the level of the second tracheal ring, usually two finger-breadths above the sternal notch. The strap muscles are separated and retracted sideways. The thyroid isthmus is either retracted or divided and

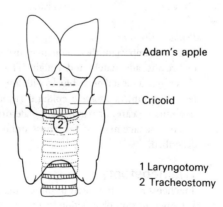

Adam's apple

Cricoid

1 Laryngotomy
2 Tracheostomy

Fig. 41. Sites for laryngotomy and tracheostomy.

sutured. When all bleeding has been controlled, a 1 cm disc is excised or an '∩' shaped flap is made in the trachea over the third or fourth ring and a tracheostomy tube is inserted and secured. The skin is loosely sutured around the tube.

Codes

Blood	0 . . . .
GA/LA	LA/GA . . . .
Opn time	30−45 minutes . . . .
Stay	Variable . . . .
Drains out	Nil . . . .
Sutures out	7 days . . . .
Off work	Variable . . . .

Postoperative care
A spare tube, introducer, retractor and sucker should be available by the patient's bed. The airways must be aspirated regularly to remove retained secretions. The inspired air must be humidified to prevent the secretions becoming too viscid.

5.2 Dysphagia

Assessment

Dysphagia is defined as difficulty in swallowing. A list of common causes of dysphagia is shown in Table 16.

Table 16. Common causes of dysphagia

Arising within the oesophagus
Chronic benign stricture
Carcinoma of the oesophagus
Foreign body
Achalasia
Oesophageal perforation
Acute caustic stricture
Pharyngeal pouch
Plummer–Vinson syndrome
Oesophageal candidiasis

Compressing the oesophagus from outside
Bronchial carcinoma
Thoracic aneurysm
Enlarged left atrium
Enlarged mediastinal lymph nodes
Large retrosternal goitre

Generalized conditions which are usually neurological
Bulbar palsy
Bulbar polio
Myasthenia
Hysteria
Anxiety state

Making the diagnosis

The characteristic clinical patterns of various conditions are given in the subsequent pages but certain points in the history and examination are helpful in reaching a diagnosis.

History
1 *Onset.* Dysphagia due to a foreign body is sudden in onset whereas that due to carcinoma comes on over a period of weeks. With achalasia and benign stricture, the symptoms develop over several years.
2 *Site.* Food sticking in the pharynx suggests a high lesion such as a pharyngeal pouch or carcinoma. Generally speaking, the level at which the patient feels the dysphagia is at or above the lesion, rarely below.

238

3 *Progression.* Carcinoma produces a rapidly progressive dysphagia. Other conditions such as benign stricture and achalasia progress very slowly.

4 *Severity.* Is the dysphagia for fluids or solids? This gives an indication of how tight the stricture is.

5 *Pain.* Benign stricture is usually associated with a history of heartburn, whereas achalasia is characteristically painless. Carcinoma of the oesophagus may progress to produce a constant central chest or epigastric pain. Oesophageal pain is commonly referred between the shoulder blades in the back.

6 *Regurgitation.* A long-standing history of reflux is characteristic of a hiatus hernia. Patients may begin to regurgitate oesophageal contents from any tight obstructive lesion once oesophageal stasis develops. This symptom is often associated with the onset of paroxysms of coughing at night due to tracheal aspirations.

7 *Systemic symptoms.* A history of weight loss suggests carcinoma, although it can follow long-standing obstruction due to other causes. Patients with a neurological cause may have a past history of stroke or symptoms from other neurological deficits. Non-steroidal anti-inflammatory drugs and potassium preparations may cause benign strictures when given for other conditions such as arthritis or heart failure.

On examination

Look carefully for cervical or other lymphadenopathy (spreading from a lesion in the chest), and for hepatomegaly or an abdominal mass. A neurological examination may give a clue to the presence of more generalized neurological disease.

Investigations

Every patient with mechanical dysphagia should have a barium swallow and oesophagoscopy.

The barium swallow may demonstrate the site and length of the oesophageal narrowing. It will show if it is extrinsic or intrinsic and reveal any features of malignancy. Oesophageal reflux can be demonstrated by tipping the patient head down.

Oesophagoscopy is carried out with either a flexible fibrescope or a rigid instrument and is described below.

Routine blood tests should look for anaemia, a raised ESR, and abnormal liver function tests (low plasma proteins and abnormal clotting). Any regurgitated fluid may be tested for acid. A plain chest X-ray may reveal a fluid level behind the heart, evidence of aspiration, or a mediastinal mass.

Operation: fibroscopy

A fibrescope is a flexible instrument with a tip that may be angled in four directions. The tip has a light beam, a suction channel and a channel for biopsy forceps or a brush. The patient is sedated and lignocaine spray used to anaesthetize the throat. The instrument is then passed down the oesophagus. The examination may be combined with examination of the stomach and duodenum (oesophagogastroduodenoscopy). An oesophageal stricture can be biopsied, and also dilated as described on p. 246.

Codes

Blood	0 . . . .
GA/LA	LA . . . .
Opn time	30 minutes . . . .
Stay	Day case . . . .
Drains out	0 . . . .
Sutures out	0 . . . .
Off work	1–2 days . . . .

Operation: rigid oesophagoscopy

This is performed with the patient anaesthetized, intubated and relaxed. A sandbag is placed underneath the shoulders. An assistant controls the position of the head and neck. Under direct vision with the head and neck flexed, the rigid oesophagoscope is introduced. The distance of the tip from the incisor teeth is measured by a scale on the instrument. As the tube is advanced the head and neck are gradually extended. The cardia of the stomach is seen at about 40 cm. A stricture can be dilated under direct vision (see p. 246).

Codes

Blood	0 . . . .
GA/LA	GA . . . .
Opn time	30 minutes . . . .
Stay	24–48 hours . . . .
Drains out	0 . . . .
Sutures out	0 . . . .
Off work	48 hours . . . .

Whichever method is used, the cause of the dysphagia can be directly visualized and if it is within the oesophagus a biopsy is taken. Any gastric reflux or oesophagitis may also be noted.

Postoperative care

Both these procedures carry the risk of oesophageal perforation. The patient requires close observation postoperatively.

1 Admit for 24 hours (day case).
2 Do not allow anything by mouth for 8–12 hours.
3 Regular observations (pulse, blood pressure, temperature).
4 Perform a chest X-ray after the procedure to look for mediastinal air or surgical emphysema in the neck.
5 If there is pain or pyrexia when the patient attempts to swallow or if surgical emphysema develops in the neck, an urgent barium swallow should be performed to look for a perforation.

Management

The further management of lesions in the oesophagus is discussed below. The treatment of an oesophageal perforation is dealt with on p. 242. Lesions causing dysphagia which are outside the oesophagus or which are neurological are not discussed further here but are listed in Table 16 (p. 238).

Impacted foreign body

The condition

This can occur either in a normal oesophagus or at the site of a carcinoma or a stricture. In a normal oesophagus there are three sites of narrowing.
1 At the level of the cricopharyngeus.
2 Where the oesophagus passes behind the left main bronchus with the arch of the aorta crossing its left side.
3 At the level of the diaphragm.
These three positions are respectively at about 15 cm, 25 cm and 40 cm from the incisor teeth.

Recognizing the pattern

The history
The patient notices that something has stuck in the back of the throat resulting in acute difficulty in swallowing. There is severe pain which is increased by any attempt to swallow.

On examination
The patient is distressed and retching. Occasionally there may be signs of perforation or mediastinitis (surgical emphysema, tachycardia and fever).

Proving the diagnosis

The foreign body may occasionally be seen on plain chest X-ray if it is radio-opaque. It may be demonstrated on a barium swallow. An oesophagoscopy should always be undertaken.

Management

The primary treatment is oesophagoscopy (see p. 240) with removal of the foreign body.

Postoperative care
The patient must be admitted for observation (see p. 240). A chest X-ray is performed to detect signs of perforation. If the foreign body was swallowed deliberately, then a psychiatric assessment may be advisable.

If the foreign body passes on into the stomach, the management is conservative. An X-ray is taken to establish its position and the patient is reassured that foreign bodies usually pass straight through the gastrointestinal tract. In the unlikely event of the gut being perforated lower down (causing abdominal pain and peritonism), a laparotomy will be necessary.

Oesophageal perforation

The condition

A common cause of oesophageal perforation is injury during oesophagoscopy or other oesophageal instrumentation. The site of the rupture is usually through Killian's dehiscence above the crico-pharyngeus or just above the stricture. Perforation may be due to a crushing injury against osteoarthritic cervical vertebrae or may follow biopsy, dilatation of a stricture, or removal of a sharp foreign body. Finally, it may occur spontaneously after violent vomiting or rarely after a penetrating injury. Perforation is followed by spreading mediastinitis and collapse due to septicaemic shock and hypovolaemia. The mortality is very high if the condition is not treated within 12 hours.

Recognizing the pattern

The history
The patient is distressed and experiences severe pain at a site related to the level of the perforation. The pain is worse on attempted swallowing even of saliva. There may also be dyspnoea if the pleural space is involved (pneumothorax and/or pleural effusion).

On examination
The patient is shocked and pyrexial and has a tachycardia. Palpation of the neck may reveal crepitation beneath the skin. This is due to air leaking from the oesophagus into the tissues of the neck (surgical emphysema). If the cervical oesophagus is perforated, there is localized tenderness.

Proving the diagnosis

1 A chest X-ray (normal and over-penetrated) will demonstrate surgical emphysema in the mediastinum. It may also show widening of the mediastinum. Look for a pleural effusion or pneumothorax.
2 An urgent barium swallow usually, but not always, demonstrates the perforation. A lateral decubitus film on the side

of the pleural effusion may reveal an otherwise undetected leak of barium.

Management   The management is exploration and suture or excision of the tear under antibiotic cover. This should be done urgently to minimize the degree of mediastinal contamination.

Preoperative management
The patient is started on intravenous broad spectrum antibiotics, e.g. gentamicin (80 mg 8-hourly), ampicillin (500 mg 6-hourly), metronidazole (500 mg 8-hourly).

Operation: repair of oesophageal perforation

A Cervical oesophagus
The upper oesophagus is approached through the neck. The incision is made anterior to the sternocleidomastoid on the side of the emphysema (if present) and the carotid sheath is retracted laterally. The tear is oversewn and the wound drained.

Codes

Blood	Group and save ....
GA/LA	GA ....
Opn time	1−2 hours ....
Stay	7−10 days ....
Drains out	6−7 days ....
Sutures out	5−7 days ....
Off work	6−8 weeks ....

B Perforation of the middle or lower oesophagus
A thoracotomy is performed (see p. 234). A tear in the middle third of the oesophagus is approached from the right side. One in the lower third is approached through a lower left thoracotomy. The tear is usually oversewn. Occasionally, if it is very ragged, that part of the oesophagus is excised and the stomach brought up to bridge the gap. If there is a distal stricture this should be excised.

Postoperative care
Leaks are not uncommon. The postoperative care is as for an oesophagectomy (see p. 254).

Acute caustic stricture

The condition   Ingestion of strong acid or alkali may be an accident or an attempted suicide. It causes a chemical burn of the oesophageal mucosa. The three sites mentioned above where foreign bodies commonly impact are also the sites commonly involved in caustic burns. The stomach may be involved. There is oedema, congestion and ulceration, which can lead to acute obstruction. This is followed by fibrosis with stricture formation.

Recognizing the pattern

The patient
The patient may be of any age or sex, although accidental ingestion of caustic fluids is common in children.

The history
This is one of severe pain which is continuous and increased by any attempt at swallowing. Find out the nature of the fluid swallowed and estimate the volume. The need for treatment is urgent and further enquiry as to motive can be carried out when the patient has recovered.

On examination
There may be signs of oropharyngeal inflammation. Look for evidence of circulatory collapse.

Management

Give immediate, strong, intravenous opiate analgesia. As soon as the patient has calmed down, wash away any remaining fluid with mouthwashes. The patient should swallow some water if possible. If the nature of the fluid is known, neutralize it (see Table 17).

Table 17. Agents causing stricture and their neutralizers

Common agents causing stricture	Neutralizing agent
Bleach	Sodium thiosulphate
Sodium hydroxide/sodium carbonate (lye)	Dilute acetic acid or citric acid
Other inorganic bases	Dilute acetic acid or citric acid
Mineral acids	Magnesium hydroxide or sodium bicarbonate
Paraquat	Fuller's earth
Phenol or organic solvents	Liquid paraffin, olive oil or castor oil

Do not attempt to wash out the stomach or provoke vomiting because the oesophagus is easily perforated. Check the airway. If the oropharynx has been badly burned, a tracheostomy may be required.

The oesophagus itself must be rested and the patient may be given fluid either intravenously or via a gastrostomy. Some centres initiate early treatment with steroids (hydrocortisone 200 mg, 4–6-hourly i.v.) and antibiotics and there is some evidence that this decreases the incidence of stricture formation. The patient must then be observed very carefully for evidence of oesophageal perforation. He or she will already be in pain but signs of fluid in the chest, a developing pyrexia and the development of surgical emphysema may indicate that this complication has occurred. Regular chest X-rays should also be carried out.

Following this, the patient is observed for evidence of stricture development. In some centres the patient is asked to swallow a fine tube or guide wire as any resulting stricture is often tortuous and a wire greatly assists the passing of oesophageal dilators. Fibroscopy may then be performed (see p. 239) with the help of the guide wire, to assess the extent of damage.

Should oesophageal dilatation be required, it is usually started 3–4 weeks after the incident. Long-term management may require resection of the stricture.

Remember to check for and manage any systemic manifestations of poisoning, e.g. renal failure (see relevant medical texts).

Chronic benign stricture

The condition

Recurrent episodes of oesophagitis scar the oesophagus and result in a circumferential stricture. This is commonly secondary to a hiatus hernia with reflux. Other causes include reflux in pregnancy, non-steroidal anti-inflammatory agents, and potassium preparations.

Recognizing the pattern

The patient
The patient is usually an elderly woman.

The history
There is a long history of reflux oesophagitis with a more recent onset of dysphagia, the food sticking at the lower sternal level. If the obstruction is severe there is usually regurgitation of food immediately after swallowing and there may be episodes of aspiration of gastric contents into the chest associated with paroxysms of coughing, especially at night.

On examination
The patient may look cachectic if the obstruction has been

severe and prolonged. Otherwise the examination is usually normal.

Proving the diagnosis

The stricture is demonstrated either by oesophagoscopy or by barium swallow. A barium swallow reveals a narrowing of the oesophagus with a ragged edge. If the patient is tipped upside-down, oesophageal reflux can be demonstrated.

On oesophagoscopy (see p. 239) the stricture is seen, together with surrounding oesophagitis. It is important to biopsy the lesion to exclude carcinoma. Malignant change can occur in a previously benign chronic stricture.

Management

Cimetidine and mucosal protectives help to reduce oedema and spasm and may relieve the symptoms in an early case. Otherwise the initial management is oesophagoscopy and dilatation of the stricture.

Operation: dilatation of oesophageal stricture

This may be carried out through either a fibrescope or a rigid oesophagoscope (p. 240). Using a fibrescope a guide wire is passed through the stricture and bougies are then threaded down over the guide wire and the stricture dilated. A rigid oesophagoscope is wide enough to allow gum-elastic bougies to be passed directly through the instrument to dilate the stricture.

Codes

Blood	0 ....
GA/LA	GA ....
Opn time	30 minutes ....
Stay	24 hours, variable ....
Drains out	0 ....
Sutures out	0 ....
Off work........	2−3 days, variable ....

Postoperative care

After this procedure the main complication is perforation of the oesophagus. The postoperative management is described on p. 240. Long-term management of a chronic benign stricture is to repair the underlying cause. Patients usually develop strictures secondary to hiatus hernia. They should have the hiatus hernia repaired as soon as they are fit enough (see p. 262).

Oesophageal achalasia

The condition

Oesophageal achalasia is a condition affecting the whole oesophagus in which the main feature is failure of relaxation of the circular muscles at the lower end of the oesophagus. The muscles hypertrophy and the oesophagus then dilates above the achalasia. The condition is thought to be due to neuromuscular incoordination and the histology shows a partial or complete loss of the myenteric plexus of nerves.

Recognizing the pattern

The patient
The patient is typically aged 30–40 years old and the condition is slightly more common in females.

The history
The history is one of gradual and slowly progressive dysphagia coming on over several years. Regurgitation of stagnant, undigested food occurs together with foul belching. Aspiration often takes place at night when the patient lies down, and it results in a fit of coughing. Recurrent chest infections due to aspiration pneumonia are common. There may be loss of weight.

On examination
There may be signs of chronic chest infection and possibly loss of weight.

Proving the diagnosis

1 *Chest X-ray.* The mediastinum is wide with a mass behind the heart appearing as a second shadow. This represents the dilated oesophagus. It usually contains a fluid level. There may also be evidence of pneumonitis.
2 *Barium swallow.* There is dilatation and tortuosity of the oesophagus down to a narrow lower segment of achalasia.
3 *Oesophagoscopy* (p. 239). This will show a grossly dilated oesophagus containing a pool of stagnant undigested food. Biopsy shows no evidence of malignant disease.

Management

Mild achalasia may be treated by amyl nitrite and anti-cholinergics. However, the definitive management is surgical.

Operation: Heller's operation
The lower oesophagus is exposed by either an abdominal or a thoracic approach. The muscle coats of the oesophagus are slit for at least 5 cm above the constriction, and no further than 1.5 cm on to the stomach below the gastro-oesophageal junction. This allows the mucosa to bulge through. The mucosa is not opened.

Codes
Blood . . . . 2 units . . . .
GA/LA . . . . GA . . . .

Opn time	60−90 minutes	
Stay	7−10 days	
Drains out	24 hours	
Sutures out	7 days	
Off work........	1 month	

Postoperative care

Oral fluids are reintroduced after about 48 hours and, providing there is no pain on swallowing, they may be gradually increased. Once free fluids are established, a light diet and then more solid food can be given providing swallowing is satisfactory. A normal diet can usually be established 5−7 days postoperatively.

The earliest complication that may occur after this procedure is oesophageal perforation (see p. 242). Incomplete myotomy may result in persistent dysphagia. This may respond to dilatation but, if not, re-operation is required. Late complications include reflux oesophagitis and stricture formation and, rarely, oesophageal diverticulum.

Pharyngeal pouch

This is a rare cause of dysphagia due to a pulsion diverticulum occurring in the base of the neck. It is described on p. 147.

Plummer−Vinson syndrome

The condition

This syndrome consists of:
1 iron deficiency anaemia;
2 dysphagia due to a post-cricoid web in the oesophagus.
It was described by Plummer and Vinson in 1921 and by Paterson and Kelly two years earlier.

There is hyperplasia of the squamous epithelium with hyperkeratosis in the mucosa of the upper oesophagus associated with patches of desquamation. This can lead to the formation of a web, which usually lies anteriorly.

Recognizing the pattern

The patient
The patient is typically a woman aged between 40 and 50.

The history
The history is one of high dysphagia, the patient complaining that food appears to stick in the back of the throat. This may be associated with retching and a choking sensation. There may be symptoms of anaemia.

On examination
The patient is usually anaemic with spoon-shaped nails (koilonychia), smooth tongue and angular stomatitis. He or she may also occasionally have a palpable spleen.

Proving the **diagnosis**	1 A barium meal shows a narrowing of the upper oesophagus due to a web-like fold in the anterior wall. 2 A full blood count shows anaemia with a hypochromic, microcytic picture. 3 Oesophagoscopy shows a friable web across the lumen of the oesophagus. 4 Biopsy of the bone marrow shows absent iron stores.
Management	The web is dilated at the time of oesophagoscopy. The condition is premalignant and so it must be biopsied.

Postoperative care
The patient is put on iron therapy and vitamin supplements. Provided the anaemia is corrected, the condition does not usually recur. Occasionally a blood transfusion is required.

If the biopsy shows malignant cells, then the lesion is treated as a post-cricoid carcinoma (see p. 251).

Barrett's oesophagus

This is a term which describes changes consisting of replacement of the normal squamous epithelial lining of the oesophagus proximal to the lower oesophageal sphincter by a mixture of columnar epithelial cell types. It appears deep red, as opposed to the pink colour of the normal squamous lining. There is a malignant predisposition (8−15%).

Carcinoma of the oesophagus

The condition The oesophagus is lined by stratified squamous epithelium down to the lowest 2−3 cm.

In the proximal third of the oesophagus almost all cancers are squamous cell in origin.

In the middle third squamous cell types are also the most common except where columnar epithelium extends up to this level.

In the lower third squamous cell tumours historically predominate in a ratio of 7:3. Adenocarcinomata are, however, increasingly reported, probably associated with chronic gastro-oesophageal reflux and the change to a columnar cell epithelium associated with this.

Predisposing factors include oesophageal achalasia, a long-standing benign stricture and the Plummer−Vinson syndrome mentioned above. It is more common in smokers. There is an environmental factor involved and the condition occurs more commonly in certain areas (e.g. Brittany, Normandy and Transkei).

The tumour typically spreads by submucosal invasion along the oesophagus. Lymphatic spread is either to the supraclavicular, subdiaphragmatic or mediastinal nodes. The oesophagus lies near other vital structures in the mediastinum, which may be involved by local invasion. For these reasons effective surgical removal is difficult to achieve in other than early lesions, and the prognosis is usually poor.

Recognizing the pattern

The patient
The patient is usually over the age of 60. Lower-third carcinomas are more common in males than females. The sex incidence for carcinomas of the middle and upper thirds is equal. Post-cricoid carcinoma is more common in females.

The history
The patient typically presents with a short history of progressive dysphagia. This initially affects solids only, but gradually increases until even swallowing liquids becomes a problem. Retrosternal pain may occur but is usually a late symptom. There may be regurgitation of food or fluids, or bloodstained vomiting. There is frequently a history of significant weight loss.

On examination
The patient is usually cachectic. Look for palpable nodes and an enlarged liver. Often, however, there are no abnormal signs. Sometimes it can be instructive to watch the patient attempting to swallow.

Proving the diagnosis

1 *Barium swallow.* A carcinoma of the oesophagus has a characteristic appearance on barium swallow consisting of a narrowing of the lumen, which has an irregular, craggy, pitted surface and raised, rolled edges. The length of the narrowed lumen is used in staging (see below).
2 *Oesophagoscopy and biopsy.* The carcinoma may be seen either as a malignant ulcer, a papillary growth or an irregular stricture. A biopsy must be taken to confirm the diagnosis.
3 *Oesophageal lavage and cytology.* A cytological diagnosis of carcinoma may be made from cells picked up from oesophageal washings.

Management

The first step is to assess the degree of spread and the patient's general condition. This can be done as follows.
1 Haemoglobin and ESR. The patient may be anaemic.
2 Liver function tests. These may suggest the presence of metastases (elevated bilirubin and alkaline phosphatase) or show evidence of malnutrition (hypoproteinaemia).
3 The length of narrowing demonstrated by barium swallow:

90% of tumours have involved regional lymph nodes when the narrowed segment is more than 5 cm long.

4 Chest X-ray with or without bronchoscopy. This will show involvement of the trachea and bronchi with resultant risk of tracheo-bronchial fistula.

5 Lymph node biopsy. Any enlarged cervical nodes should be biopsied before major surgery is contemplated.

6 Computerized axial tomography. This may give a picture of the degree of mediastinal involvement.

As a result of these investigations it should be possible to determine whether the tumour is potentially curable by local resection or not, and whether the patient is fit for major surgery.

Forms of therapy

This carcinoma may be treated by one of the following:
(a) surgical resection;
(b) radiotherapy;
(c) palliation — intubation or bypass.

Squamous cell carcinoma can be treated by either surgery or radiotherapy. Adenocarcinoma is not sensitive to radiotherapy.

Surgical resection

Curative resection is only attempted for growths confined to the oesophagus with no evidence of lymphatic or mediastinal spread. Of the patients considered operable, one-third will be found to have more extensive tumours at the time of operation. Because of the likely presence of submucosal invasion, curative resection requires wide excision of the oesophagus above and below the growth.

Operations for oesophageal carcinoma

The type of operation performed depends on the site of the growth (Fig. 42). Three types of curative procedure will be described (Fig. 43).

1 Pharyngo-laryngo-oesophagectomy.
2 Total oesophagectomy.
3 Oesophago-gastrectomy.

Preoperative management

The patient may require a supplemented diet or even intravenous nutrition to correct malnutrition. Oesophageal washouts are needed for lower-segment growths. The mouth should also be cleaned. Some centres give prophylactic antibiotics.

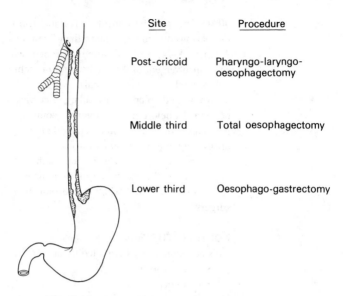

Site	Procedure
Post-cricoid	Pharyngo-laryngo-oesophagectomy
Middle third	Total oesophagectomy
Lower third	Oesophago-gastrectomy

Fig. 42. Carcinoma of the oesophagus: the sites of origin and the relevant surgical procedures.

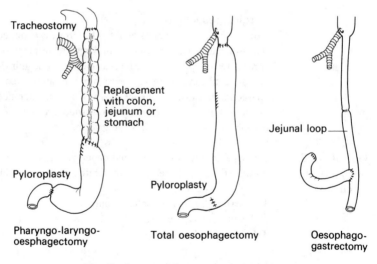

Fig. 43. Operations for carcinoma of oesophagus.

Operation: pharyngo-laryngo-oesophagectomy

In this operation it is necessary to resect the larynx as well as the oesophagus. A permanent tracheostomy is therefore inevitable. Continuity is restored by suturing the fundus of the stomach up to the lower pharynx in the neck, or by interposing a loop of colon or jejunum as a conduit. This conduit may be brought up inside the chest (retrosternally or prevertebrally) or subcutaneously in front of the sternum.

Codes

Blood	10 units ....
GA/LA	GA ....
Opn time	About 5 hours ....
Stay	3–4 weeks ....
Drains out	Pleura 48 hours, neck anastomosis 7 days, mediastinum 3–5 days ....
Sutures out	7 days ....
Off work........	2–3 months....................

Operation: total oesophagectomy

This operation is performed for carcinoma of the mid-oesophagus. Through an abdominal incision the stomach is mobilized and the degree of spread assessed. If the lesion is operable, the chest is opened through a right thoracotomy incision. The tumour is removed with a wide margin of normal oesophagus and either the stomach is brought up into the chest for anastomosis with the oesophageal stump (Ivor Lewis operation), or a piece of jejunum or large bowel is brought up on its vascular pedicle to act as a conduit.

Codes

Blood	6 units ....
GA/LA	GA ....
Opn time	3–4 hours ....
Stay	3–4 weeks ....
Drains out	Neck anastomosis 7 days, chest/pleura 48 hours, mediastinum 3–5 days ....
Sutures out	7 days ....
Off work........	3 months ....

Operation: oesophago-gastrectomy

This operation is performed for carcinomata of the oesophago-gastric junction and lower oesophagus. The stomach and lower oesophagus are mobilized and the liver palpated. If the tumour is considered resectable, the chest is then opened along the eighth rib (left thoraco-abdominal incision) and the lower oesophagus including the tumour, all or part of the stomach, the spleen and the omentum are removed. The continuity of the oesophagus is usually restored by anastomosis either to the stomach remnant or, if all the stomach is resected, to a loop of jejunum.

Codes

Blood . . . . 6 units . . . .
GA/LA . . . . GA . . . .
Opn time . . . . 3−4 hours . . . .
Stay . . . . 21−28 days . . . .
Drains out . . . . . . Chest 5 days, anastomosis 7 days . . . .
Sutures out . . . . . 7−10 days . . . .
Off work . . . . 2−3 months . . . .

Postoperative care

If the chest has been opened the routine care of a thoracotomy is appropriate (pp. 234−235). A chest X-ray should be performed daily for the first few days. Patients who have had a thoracotomy and resection are usually nursed in intensive care.

The major postoperative complication of all these procedures is pulmonary aspiration. Leakage of the anastomosis is also common. If this occurs an oesophageal fistula results. This is more debilitating if it drains via the pleural cavity. Hence anastomoses in the neck are safer. Because of the danger of leakage, the patient is usually kept 'nil by mouth' until the anastomoses are healed. Further management is then as follows.

1 Feeding. Some surgeons routinely perform a gastrostomy or enterostomy and use this to feed the patient once he has recovered from his abdominal ileus. Alternatively a nasogastric tube may be passed through the anastomosis into the jejunum and feeding instituted through this after 4 or 5 days.

2 A barium swallow is performed 6 or 7 days after the operation to look for signs of a leak.

3 If this shows a healed anastomosis, clear fluids are instituted and gradually increased up to a light diet.

4 If the barium swallow shows a leak, the patient continues to have nothing by mouth until the leak has healed. Nutrition is maintained either as above or intravenously. Occasionally re-exploration and resuture of the anastomosis are required or the ends may have to be exteriorized.

A second common complication is a chest infection associated with pulmonary collapse or pneumothorax. You must make sure that the chest drains remain patent and the patient should have good analgesia and physiotherapy.

Between 10 and 30% of these patients experience some recurrent dysphagia. Some may need oesophageal dilatation.

Radiotherapy

At present this is used for squamous cell carcinoma in

patients unfit for surgery or patients with a carcinoma involving the oesophagus above the arch of the aorta. Radiotherapy is also effective for palliative treatment of dysphagia in some cases. Fifty per cent of patients need follow-up oesophageal dilatation.

Complications include leucopenia, pulmonary fibrosis and spinal cord compression, all of which are rarer with modern techniques.

Palliation

Of any 100 patients with oesophageal carcinoma, 60 will be found to have inoperable tumours and many of these will require some form of symptomatic relief. The most significant symptom is dysphagia. This may be relieved by:

1 intubation of the tumour;
2 a bypass operation;
3 radiotherapy.

Operation: intubation of carcinoma of the oesophagus
This procedure involves implanting a tube in the stricture to maintain sufficient lumen for a liquid and semi-solid diet. Such tubes tend to block and they may become dislodged. There are different types of tube (see Fig. 44).

(a) Celestin tube
This has an olive-shaped head. A flexible pilot bougie is passed through the stricture under direct vision and into the

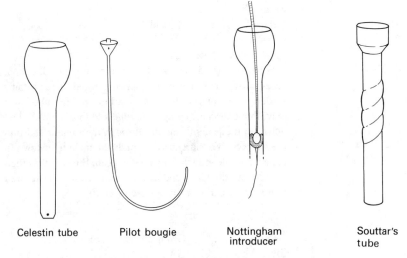

| Celestin tube | Pilot bougie | Nottingham introducer | Souttar's tube |

Fig. 44. The Celestin and Souttar tubes.

stomach and recovered through a high gastrotomy. The Celestin tube fits on the end of the bougie and can then be pulled down the oesophagus into position. The tube is cut to the required length and may be sutured to the stomach wall. Recently the development of a specifically adapted introducer has enabled this tube to be inserted from above and thus avoiding a gastrotomy (Nottingham introducer, Fig. 44).

Codes

Blood	Group and save serum ....
GA/LA	GA ....
Opn time	30−60 minutes ....
Stay	7−10 days ....
Drains out	0 ....
Sutures out	7 days ....
Off work	Variable ....

(b) Souttar's tube

A metal guide wire is first passed through the growth using an oesophagoscope. Bougies can be introduced to dilate the stricture. The tube is then pushed down over the guide wire or a bougie and impacted into the structure.

Codes

Blood	0 ....
GA/LA	GA ....
Opn time	30−60 minutes ....
Stay	3−5 days ....
Drains out	0 ....
Sutures out	0 ....
Off work	Variable ....

(c) Mousseau−Barbin tube

A bougie is passed through the stricture in either direction, access to the stomach being gained through a gastrotomy made in the stomach during a laparotomy. The tube has a long, thin end like a nasogastric tube and this is then pulled down via the patient's mouth, through the tumour and into the stomach. The surgeon then pulls the main tube down to impact it in the growth. The tube beneath the growth is then excised and the lower end of the prosthesis may be sutured to the lesser curve of the stomach (see Fig. 45).

Codes

Blood	Group and save serum ....
GA/LA	GA ....
Opn time	30−60 minutes ....

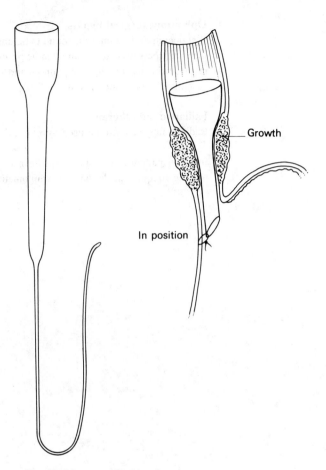

Fig. 45. Mousseau–Barbin tube.

Stay . . . . 7–10 days . . . .
Drains out . . . . . . 0 . . . .
Sutures out . . . . . 7 days . . . .
Off work . . . . Variable . . . .

Postoperative care
The patient must be instructed about diet and told to
swallow only well-masticated soft food with plenty of fluids.
Fizzy drinks are effective in flushing and cleaning the tube.
It is useful to show the patient an identical tube to the one
that has been inserted.

Operation: surgical bypass

If at operation the tumour is found to be unresectable, some form of bypass procedure can often be performed. This may involve bringing up a loop of jejunum and suturing it to the oesophagus above the growth.

Palliative radiotherapy

Radiotherapy can also be used to relieve dysphagia.

In some patients the appropriate form of treatment is to provide adequate analgesia and symptomatic relief only.

6   Abdominal Pain and Related Symptoms

6.1 Stomach and duodenum
Abdominal pain
Hiatus hernia
Peptic ulcers
Haematemesis and melaena
Carcinoma of the stomach
Post-gastrectomy syndromes

6.2 Liver, pancreas and spleen
Gall-stones
Surgical jaundice
Portal hypertension
Bleeding oesophageal varices
Hepatic tumours
Hepatic transplantation
Benign tumours of the pancreas
Carcinoma of the pancreas
Pancreatitis
Surgical conditions of the spleen

6.3 Adrenal glands
Adrenal tumours

6.4 Central abdominal pain
Acute appendicitis
Mesenteric adenitis
Intestinal obstruction
Meckel's diverticulum
Ischaemic bowel
Intussusception in adults
Crohn's disease
Small bowel tumours

6.5 Colorectal presentations and skeletal pain
Ulcerative colitis
Rectal bleeding in adults
Change in bowel habit
Colonic polyps
Carcinoma of the colon
Carcinoma of the rectum
Diverticular disease

Sigmoid volvulus
Rectal prolapse
Skeletal pain (referred pain)

Stomach and Duodenum

Abdominal pain

When a patient presents with abdominal pain the site of pain gives a primary clue as to the organ involved (see Fig. 46). In this book most abdominal conditions will be included according to the site where the pain typically presents. Disease states may of course present in other ways apart from pain (e.g. haematemesis, jaundice, change in bowel habit, etc.) and the more important of these are included as seems appropriate in relation to other conditions discussed.

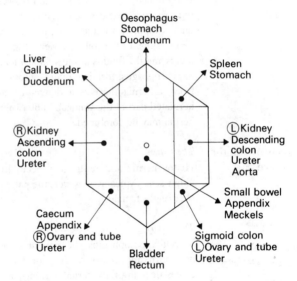

Fig. 46. Typical sites of presentation of visceral pain from different organs.

Upper abdominal pain

Important conditions presenting with upper abdominal pain, together with their complications and management, are dealt with on the following pages.

Hiatus hernia (p. 262)

Gastric ulcer (p. 265)

Duodenal ulcer, including perforated ulcers,
pyloric stenosis, and haematemesis and melaena (p. 268)

Gall-stones, including obstructive jaundice (p. 288)

Carcinoma of the stomach (p. 281)

Carcinoma of the pancreas (p. 314)

Pancreatitis (p. 318)

Less commonly, upper abdominal pain may arise from disease in the liver, spleen or diaphragm. Examples discussed in this book are as follows.

Hepatic abscess (p. 74)

Hepatic metastases, secondary to malignant disease from many sites

Subphrenic abscess (p. 72)

Ruptured spleen (p. 595)

Liver injury (p. 594)

Hiatus hernia — *sliding*

Two main types of hiatus hernia are recognized (Fig. 47). In the sliding variety (Fig. 47a) the gastro-oesophageal angle is straightened out and the junction between the oesophageal mucosa and gastric mucosa slides up into the chest. The main symptoms are due to reflux of gastric contents into the oesophagus. In the rolling variety (Fig. 47b) there is a large hiatus and the fundus of the stomach tends to roll up next to the oesophagus, forming a para-oesophageal hernia. In this type of hernia there is a danger of strangulation of the herniated part of the stomach. The two main types of hiatus hernia may be combined.

Recognizing the pattern

The patient

Hiatus hernia and reflux may occur in any age-group in either sex. Typically, however, the patient is a middle-aged, overweight female.

The history

In reflux oesophagitis the patient develops symptoms of heartburn and reflux of acid or food. Heartburn is an epigastric or low retrosternal burning pain, which may radiate to the back, to the neck or even down the arms. The symptoms are worse on bending forward or lying flat at night. Symptoms often come on when the patient has recently gained weight and are common in the last trimester of pregnancy.

With strangulation of a rolling hernia the patient complains of a sudden onset of very severe constricting lower chest and upper abdominal pain. The symptoms mimic those of a myocardial infarction.

Proving the diagnosis

The diagnosis of hiatus hernia is proved by performing a barium swallow and meal, or by fibroscopy. When requesting the barium swallow, you must ask for studies of reflux. The

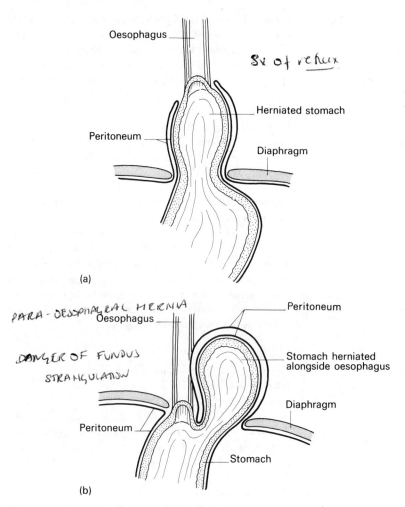

Oesophagus

S̶x̶ of reflux

Herniated stomach

Peritoneum

Diaphragm

(a)

PARA - OESOPHAGEAL HERNIA

Oesophagus

DANGER OF FUNDUS
STRANGULATION

Peritoneum

Stomach

Peritoneum

Stomach herniated
alongside oesophagus

Diaphragm

(b)

Fig. 47. (a) Sliding hiatus hernia. (b) Rolling hiatus hernia.

radiologist will then take films with the patient tilted head down. On fibroscopy the oesophagitis is visible and the endoscopist may see active reflux. A chest X-ray may also show signs of aspiration pneumonia.

Management
The initial management of a hiatus hernia is usually conservative. The most important thing is for the patient to lose weight. Symptoms will often abate when even a few pounds of weight have been shed. In addition to advice about this, the patient is given an H_2 (histamine receptor type II) blocker such as cimetidine and an oesophageal mucosal protective such as Gaviscon.

Operation is indicated when the medical treatment fails to control symptoms or when complications such as ulceration of the oesophagus, stricture formation or haemorrhage occur. Patients with a rolling hernia who have had a possible episode of strangulation should always have an operation.

Preoperative management
Patients should be advised to stop smoking and to lose as much weight as possible. The surgeon may elect to perform the operation either through the chest or through the abdomen and you should find out which approach is intended.

Operation: repair of hiatus hernia and Nissen's fundoplication
The oesophageal hiatus is approached either through an incision in the bed of the eighth rib or through a vertical incision in the epigastrium. Any rolling hernia is reduced into the abdomen and the oesophageal hiatus is narrowed by inserting sutures into the crura posterior to the oesophagus. An anti-reflux procedure is then undertaken. The most popular is Nissen's procedure (Fig. 48).

Codes

Blood	2 units . . . .
GA/LA	GA . . . .
Opn time	90–120 minutes . . . .
Stay	7–10 days . . . .
Drains out	Abdomen 0, chest 24 hours . . . .
Sutures out	7 days . . . .
Off work	6–8 weeks . . . .

Postoperative care
The patient usually has a nasogastric tube for about 48 hours after the operation and fluids are introduced as he recovers from the ileus. He often complains of dysphagia during the first few days and even weeks after the operation. He should keep to a fairly liquid diet and drink plenty of water with his meals until the symptoms settle. Occasionally the patient may also suffer from the 'gas bloat syndrome'. Air is trapped in the stomach and cannot be belched upwards because of the anti-reflux procedure. Symptoms are often associated with air swallowing and the patient should try and avoid this habit.

Peptic ulcers
Peptic ulcers are of two types — those in the stomach and those in the duodenum. Although both present with pain

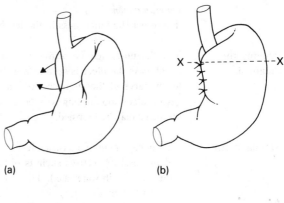

(a)   (b)

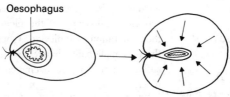

Oesophagus

Nissen's fundoplication

(c) T.S. at X---X   (d)

Fig. 48. (a) and (b) Nissen's fundoplication. A pouch from the anterior and posterior gastric fundus is pulled forwards (and to the patient's right) around the oesophagus. (c) and (d) Anti-reflux mechanism after Nissen's fundoplication. Raised intragastric pressure occludes the enclosed portion of the oesophagus.

after eating, they are two rather different conditions with different pathogeneses. They will be dealt with separately.

Gastric ulcer

Recognizing the pattern

The patient
He is typically middle-aged or elderly, debilitated and thin.

The history
The patient complains of poor appetite, loss of weight, and pain which comes on immediately after eating. The pain may be relieved by lying flat (when the gastric contents fall back into the fundus of the stomach and away from the ulcer on the lesser curve) and also by antacids. He may also present with haematemesis or melaena and there is a danger of malignant change (see Carcinoma of the stomach, p. 281).

On examination
There may be tenderness in the left hypochondrium.

**Proving the
diagnosis**

The diagnosis may be proved by doing a barium meal, in which case the ulcer is seen as a niche projecting from the lesser curve of the stomach. All patients with a suspected gastric ulcer should, however, be endoscoped in order that the ulcer may be biopsied.

Management

The management of a gastric ulcer is medical, with antacids and mucosal protectives such as bismuth chelate (De-Nol 5 ml 6-hourly in water a.c.). The main danger of treating a gastric ulcer medically is that a malignancy may be overlooked. It is, therefore, essential to monitor healing by repeated endoscopy. If the ulcer fails to heal completely, then operation is indicated. Operation is also indicated if there is malignant change in the biopsy or if the patient suffers from repeated haematemesis or perforation of the ulcer.

The surgeon will usually wish to resect a gastric ulcer and this may either be combined with a partial gastrectomy or a vagotomy and drainage procedure. A partial gastrectomy is probably the method of choice at the present time. Some surgeons also treat benign gastric ulcers by highly selective vagotomy together with excision of the ulcer. The vagotomy operations will be dealt with in more detail under Duodenal ulcer (p. 268).

Preoperative management
Patients with a gastric ulcer frequently have a severe gastritis and there may be gastric stasis. Attempts should be made to get the stomach as clean as possible before operation by instituting a liquid diet for at least 24 hours before surgery and possibly by washing out the stomach if stasis is severe. We also give prophylactic antibiotics when the stomach is being opened (e.g. flucloxacillin).

Operation: partial gastrectomy
In a partial gastrectomy the pylorus, the antrum and the lesser curve containing the gastric ulcer are resected. Two major types of reconstruction are then possible. In the Billroth I reconstruction the upper stomach is re-anastomosed to the cut end of the duodenum (see Fig. 49). In the Billroth II (Polya) type of anastomosis, the duodenal stump is closed and the proximal end of the stomach is anastomosed to a loop of jejunum. This loop may be brought up either in front of (antecolic) or behind the colon (retro-

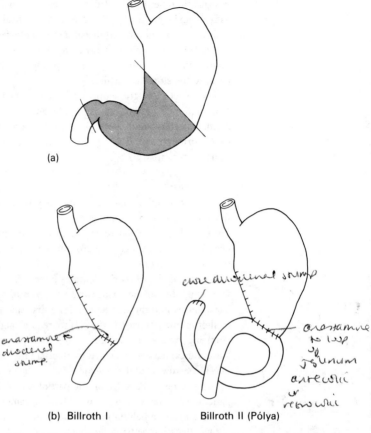

(a)

(b) Billroth I   Billroth II (Pólya)

Fig. 49. Two types of partial gastrectomy (the terms refer to the type of reconstruction). (a) Resection. (b) Reconstruction.

colic), the latter passing through an artificial hole in the mesocolon (as in a gastroenterostomy, see Fig. 51, p. 272).

Codes

Blood	4 units	
GA/LA	GA	
Opn time	2–3 hours	
Stay	7–10 days	
Drains out	3–6 days	
Sutures out	7 days	
Off work	6 weeks	

Postoperative care
The stomach must be kept empty until adequate gastric emptying occurs. This is achieved by hourly aspiration of the

nasogastric tube. Provided this is draining satisfactorily the patient can be given $15-30$ cm^3 of water to drink each hour. This keeps the mouth and throat more comfortable and has a beneficial 'washing' action on the stomach. A Billroth I gastrectomy takes longer to start emptying than a Billroth II because the stoma is smaller.

The onset of gastric emptying is noted when the gastric aspirate diminishes and the patient begins to pass flatus per rectum. At this point oral fluids can be increased and the nasogastric tube removed. The intravenous drip is removed shortly afterwards.

Complications

Postoperative anastomotic bleeding may occur in the first few hours after surgery or again at $7-10$ days. This usually settles. Adequate blood replacement must be available and occasionally it is necessary to take the patient back to theatre to stem the bleeding.

Persistently high gastric aspirates after a gastrectomy are frequently due to the nasogastric tube passing through the anastomosis into the duodenum. The first step is therefore to shorten the nasogastric tube. If there is no sign of gastric emptying by a week or more after the operation, then a barium meal may be indicated to ascertain the cause. There may be narrowing of the anastomosis, which will settle as the oedema resolves. Patience on the part of the doctor and the patient is usually rewarded. Metoclopramide (10 mg 8-hourly) can be helpful in assisting gastric emptying.

Once gastric emptying has been established, a light diet can be introduced and the patient's recovery thereafter is usually uncomplicated.

Late sequelae of gastrectomy include symptoms of bilious vomiting, dumping and diarrhoea. These are dealt with below (p. 283). Patients may also develop anaemia due to vitamin B$_{12}$ or iron deficiency. Patients who have had a gastrectomy should usually be put on iron and vitamin B$_{12}$ injections for the rest of their lives.

Duodenal ulcer

The condition

The condition is associated with gastric hyperacidity. The ulcer in the duodenum usually heals with treatment which lowers gastric acidity, such as antacids and H$_2$ (histamine receptor type II) blockers.

Recognizing the pattern

The patient

The patient is usually young and the condition is more common in males than in females. Unlike gastric ulcer patients, those with a duodenal ulcer tend to be overweight, as eating helps to ease the pain. Duodenal ulcers are more common in smokers.

The history
The pain is situated in the epigastrium and may radiate through to the small of the back. It comes on 1−2 hours after meals and also when the patient is hungry. It has a tendency to wake the patient up in the early hours of the morning when acidity is high and the stomach is empty.

Another feature of the typical history is 'periodicity'. That is to say there are periods (often weeks) when the ulcer is active and painful, followed by periods (often months) of inactivity and absent symptoms. Characteristically duodenal ulcers are worse in the autumn and spring and better in the summer months.

If the ulcer is chronic, the patient may develop the symptoms of perforation (see p. 273) or of fibrosis and gastric outlet obstruction (pyloric stenosis, p. 275) or the ulcer may erode a vessel and the patient present with haematemesis and melaena (p. 277).

On examination
There is tenderness to the right of, and above, the umbilicus, deep in the abdomen.

Proving the diagnosis

The diagnosis is proved either on a barium meal or on fibroscopy. The presence or absence of pyloric stenosis should also be noted on these investigations.

Gastric acid function studies will show that the stomach is producing acid at a high normal or above normal rate. Two major types of test are used:
(a) the pentagastrin test stimulates the parietal cell mass maximally and produces the greatest acid output;
(b) the insulin test induces hypoglycaemia and this in turn stimulates the vagus in the brain stem. This test is only positive if the vagal fibres are intact. The insulin-stimulated gastric output is about 75% of the peak acid output obtainable with pentagastrin.

Management

The initial management of an acute duodenal ulcer is medical. Treatment is with full dosage of H_2 blockers (e.g. cimetidine 200 mg t.d.s. after food and 400 mg nocte, or ranitidine 150 mg 12-hourly) for one month.

The indications for surgery are failed medical management or the onset of complications.

Medical management may fail due to the following factors.

1 The patient continues to have pain whilst on H_2 blockers (this is rare).

2 The symptoms recur as soon as the dosage is lowered or the drug stopped.

3 The symptoms recur after a period of weeks or months of treatment but are rapidly brought under control by further treatment. When this has been going on for more than 3 years, surgery should be considered.

Surgical management
Surgery is always indicated when the patient perforates a duodenal ulcer or if he has developed outlet stenosis. The management of haematemesis is described on p. 277.

Several procedures are available which satisfactorily lower the gastric acid output either by removing the antrum (gastrin mechanism) or part of the parietal cell mass, or by dividing the vagus nerves. These procedures are illustrated in Fig. 50 and include:

(a) partial gastrectomy;
(b) truncal vagotomy and drainage (either pyloroplasty or gastroenterostomy);
(c) truncal vagotomy and antrectomy;
(d) highly selective vagotomy (parietal cell vagotomy).

Preoperative management
Many duodenal ulcer patients are heavy smokers and they should be warned that continued smoking is liable to give them severe postoperative chest problems. They should be given chest physiotherapy before the operation.

Operation: truncal vagotomy and drainage
The trunks of the vagus nerve are cut as they enter the abdomen through the oesophageal hiatus. Total vagal denervation of the stomach results in gastric stasis and because of this a drainage procedure is necessary. Various types of pyloroplasty and gastrojejunostomy are shown in Fig. 51.

Codes

Blood	Group and save serum . . . .
GA/LA	GA . . . .
Opn time	60 – 90 minutes . . . .
Stay	7 days . . . .
Drains out	5 days (if used) . . . .
Sutures out	7 days . . . .
Off work	6 weeks . . . .

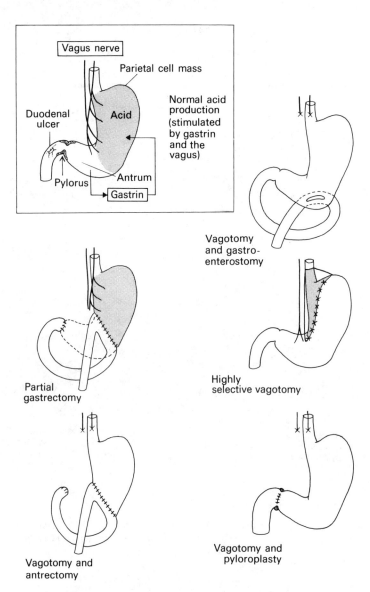

Fig. 50. Operations to lower gastric acidity.

Operation: truncal vagotomy and antrectomy
The distal part of the stomach which produces gastrin is
excised together with the pylorus. The stomach is usually
reconstituted using a Billroth I procedure (see Gastric
ulcer). The trunks of the vagal nerves are also divided.

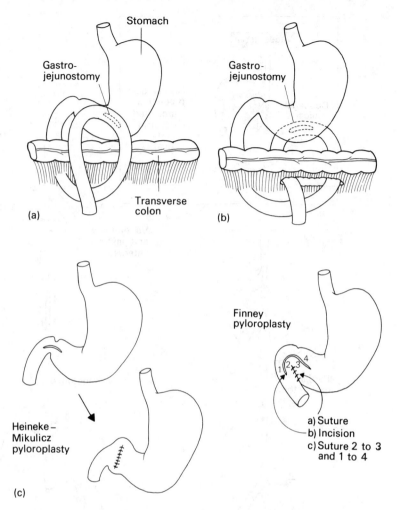

Fig. 51. (a) An antecolic anterior gastrojejunostomy. (b) A retrocolic posterior gastrojejunostomy. (c) Two types of pyloroplasty.

Codes

Blood	4 units	....
GA/LA	GA	....
Opn time	About 2 hours	....
Stay	7–10 days	....
Drains out	3–6 days	....
Sutures out	7 days	....
Off work........	6 weeks	....

Operation: highly selective vagotomy

Only the nerve fibres supplying the parietal cells in the body and fundus of the stomach are cut. The fibres supplying the antrum remain intact. In this operation, gastric emptying is almost normal and no drainage procedure is necessary. The procedure has the advantage of being free of the side-effects of diarrhoea, dumping and bilious vomiting.

Codes

Blood	Group and save serum . . . .
GA/LA	GA . . . .
Opn time	90–150 minutes . . . .
Stay	5–7 days . . . .
Drains out	0 . . . .
Sutures out	7 days . . . .
Off work	6 weeks . . . .

Postoperative care

The postoperative care of patients who have had a truncal vagotomy and antrectomy or truncal vagotomy and drainage is similar to that for patients who have had a partial gastrectomy (p. 266).

The postoperative care of highly selective vagotomy patients is usually very straightforward. The only major complication to be aware of is lesser-curve necrosis and this occurs in about 0.3% of patients. The patient suddenly deteriorates about 48 hours after the operation and shows signs of increasing peritonitis. It may be difficult to diagnose the perforation because there is already air under the diaphragm on a straight abdominal X-ray. A limited barium meal will show the defect, however, and if in doubt a laparotomy is advisable.

Many patients complain of dysphagia after vagotomy. This is always transient. The patient should be advised to stick to soft, semi-liquid foods until the dysphagia improves. The symptom has usually disappeared by about 6 weeks after the operation. It is worth while warning patients about this symptom before they leave hospital and explaining that it is due to the fact that the operation takes place around the lower oesophagus and that the difficulty in swallowing will settle as the operation site heals.

Perforated peptic ulcer

The condition

Either gastric or duodenal ulcers may perforate, although perforation of the latter is more common. As gastric ulcers are frequently posterior, they may perforate into the lesser sac. Anterior duodenal ulcers perforate direct into the main peritoneal cavity.

<table>
<tr><td>

Recognizing the pattern

</td><td>

The history

The typical pattern of symptoms suggesting gastric or duodenal ulcer has already been described. Not infrequently, however, patients present with a perforation without much in the way of past history of indigestion. When the ulcer perforates there is a sudden, defined onset of severe epigastric pain. The patient frequently remembers the precise time of onset (e.g. 'just as the nine o'clock news was beginning'). The pain rapidly spreads first to the right iliac fossa and later all over the abdomen. When a gastric ulcer perforates into the lesser sac, the symptoms are much more localized until gastric contents leak out of the foramen of Winslow, giving rise to a right-sided peritonitis. This picture can be confused with acute appendicitis.

</td></tr>
</table>

On examination
There is typically marked tenderness over the whole of the abdomen with 'board-like rigidity'. Percussion of the liver may reveal absent liver dullness. This sign is due to gas lying between the liver and the anterior abdominal wall.

Proving the diagnosis

The diagnosis is proved by doing an erect chest X-ray together with a supine and erect abdominal X-ray. Gas may be seen under the diaphragm.

Management

The management of an acute perforation is usually surgical. It is, however, possible on occasion to manage these lesions conservatively.
1 A nasogastric tube is positioned in the stomach and regularly aspirated. It is essential that the stomach is kept empty.
2 Adequate intravenous fluid replacement is given. These patients have usually lost a lot of fluid into the peritoneal cavity and are markedly dehydrated. A central venous line may be needed when large amounts of fluid have to be given. A fluid requirement in excess of two litres is not uncommon.
3 The patient is given broad-spectrum antibiotic cover.

Operation: for perforated peptic ulcer
The abdomen is opened through a vertical incision. Deep sutures are placed through the oedematous tissue around the perforation and a patch of omentum sewn over to close the defect (Fig. 52). If the perforation is less than 8 hours old, a definitive ulcer curing operation may be performed at

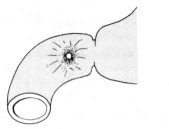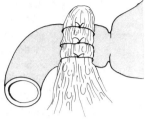

Fig. 52. Oversewing a perforated duodenal ulcer.

the same time. The peritoneum is carefully washed out and all food residue removed. Drains are placed at the site of the perforation and in the subphrenic spaces if there is extensive contamination.

Codes

Blood	Group and save serum . . . .
GA/LA	GA . . . .
Opn time	1 hour . . . .
Stay	If uncomplicated, 7 days . . . .
Drains out	3−5 days . . . .
Sutures out	7 days . . . .
Off work	Variable, 4−6 weeks . . . .

Postoperative care

The main problem is of persistent intra-abdominal sepsis either in the subphrenic regions or in the pelvis. This may delay recovery. The management of intra-abdominal abscesses is dealt with on pp. 72−75.

Pyloric stenosis

The condition

The condition known as 'pyloric stenosis' in adults is usually, in fact, a duodenal stenosis secondary to scarring from a chronic duodenal ulcer. (Pyloric stenosis in babies is dealt with on p. 545).

Recognizing the pattern

Pyloric stenosis can arise as a complication in any patient with a duodenal ulcer and the developing obstruction is usually heralded by the onset of vomiting. Characteristically the vomiting becomes copious and the patient recognizes food which has been digested a day or two previously. In severe long-standing pyloric stenosis the patient may become very ill and dehydrated with lassitude and loss of weight. In some elderly patients there is very little history of previous indigestion until the stenosis develops.

On examination

If the vomiting has been prolonged the patient is dehydrated and weak and may show signs of loss of weight. In the abdomen there may be tenderness over the duodenal region. The characteristic sign is a 'succussion splash'. A stethoscope is placed over the stomach and the patient gently shaken from side to side. Food can be heard splashing in the stomach several hours after the previous meal.

Proving the diagnosis

The diagnosis is proved either radiologically or by fibroscopy. The grossly distended stomach may be visible on a plain abdominal X-ray. If contrast studies are needed either very dilute barium or gastrografin should be used. Normal barium tends to solidify in the obstructed stomach and can cause problems. On fibroscopy the stenosed duodenum is usually clearly seen and the fibrescope cannot be made to pass through it. The food residue in the stomach is also noted in spite of the fact that the patient has starved.

Management

The development of pyloric stenosis is one of the absolute indications for surgery in duodenal ulcer. Before surgery is undertaken, however, electrolyte and nutritional disturbances must be corrected. Several days of conservative management may be needed to achieve this. Prolonged loss of gastric vomitus leads to a metabolic alkalosis with a low serum potassium. Adequate intravenous therapy including potassium and chloride ions must, therefore, be given. A nasogastric tube is passed and the stomach kept empty. Intravenous cimetidine can also be given. Not infrequently the stomach begins to empty again with this management. Nevertheless, once obstruction has developed it is likely to recur and surgical treatment should be undertaken.

Operation: for pyloric stenosis

The most common procedure performed is a truncal vagotomy and pyloroplasty or gastroenterostomy. Some surgeons prefer to perform a highly selective vagotomy and in this case the stenosis is dealt with either by a duodenoplasty or by dilatation. In a duodenoplasty the stenosis in the duodenum is incised longitudinally and sewn up vertically, thus widening the area. These manoeuvres allow the pylorus to be retained and thus obviate the development of problems related to abnormal gastric emptying after a drainage procedure (pp. 283–287).

Codes

Blood	2 units . . . .
GA/LA	GA . . . .
Opn time	1–2 hours . . . .
Stay	7–10 days . . . .
Drains out	3–5 days . . . .
Sutures out	7 days . . . .
Off work	4–6 weeks . . . .

Postoperative care
See p. 273.

Haematemesis and melaena

Haematemesis and melaena are due to bleeding from the upper gastrointestinal tract. Bleeding from the lower gastrointestinal tract is discussed under 'rectal' bleeding (p. 349). Upper gastrointestinal haemorrhage may be from the following sites.

1 The pharynx: e.g. vomiting of swallowed blood from a nasal haemorrhage.

2 The oesophagus: oesophagitis with ulceration secondary to hiatus hernia, oesophageal varices secondary to portal hypertension.

3 The stomach:
  (a) gastritis — biliary, drug-induced or alcoholic;
  (b) gastric ulcer;
  (c) benign tumours, e.g. leiomyoma;
  (d) carcinoma;
  (e) Mallory–Weiss tear.

4 The duodenum: duodenal ulcer.

The shocked patient vomiting blood is a common and dramatic surgical emergency. A houseman's training can be severely tested in these circumstances and the condition will ·be dealt with in some detail here.

A scheme of management

A suggested scheme is as follows.
1 Initial assessment.
2 Resuscitation.
3 Secondary assessment.
4 Further management.

A Initial assessment

An assessment must be made of the following.

1 Amount of blood lost by the patient

This is assessed by an estimate from the history, state of the patient's blood pressure, pulse, peripheral circulation and level of consciousness. After a sudden bleed a patient who is unconscious with a minimal blood pressure, a rapid, thin pulse and cold clammy extremities has probably lost 1½–2 litres of blood. A patient who is conscious but mildly shocked, with a low blood pressure and a tachycardia, may have lost about one litre. Signs of shock are not usually present when the patient has lost less than 500 cm^3.

2 Rate of bleeding

How rapidly are they bleeding? Is the history of a true massive single haematemesis or a more prolonged loss of blood? A patient who has had a massive haematemesis is likely to have another one which may prove fatal. Further assessment of the rate of blood loss is made after regular monitoring has been instituted.

3 General condition

The age and general fitness of the patient will give an indication as to how much blood loss he can stand.

At the end of this initial assessment you should have a good idea as to how serious the situation is and how immediate the following steps must be.

B Resuscitation

1 Intravenous infusion

Insert a large-bore intravenous needle (14-gauge if possible). Take blood for cross-matching using this needle. Six to eight units should be cross-matched and blood sent for haemoglobin and packed cell volume estimation. Set up an intravenous infusion.

Types of intravenous fluid

For the patient who is not suffering from shock, set up an infusion of 500 cm^3 of normal saline over 4 hours, thus maintaining intravenous access until blood arrives or in case the situation deteriorates rapidly.

For the shocked patient, any suitable intravenous infusion (e.g. normal saline) is better than nothing. Colloidal solutions (e.g. dextran or Haemaccel) are better than electrolyte solutions. Whole blood is better than colloid solutions, although it may not be available in the early stages.

Amount of intravenous fluid

Infuse sufficient to rapidly restore the blood pressure to

an acceptable level (e.g. systolic blood pressure up to 100–120). In elderly or decrepit patients a CVP line may be essential during this process, to avoid overloading the patient and precipitating heart failure.

2 Install a urinary catheter
The urinary output per hour is a good indication of the perfusion of the central organs during shock.

3 Institute regular monitoring
For example, quarter-hourly pulse and blood pressure, CVP levels, and hourly urine output.

After the initial assessment and resuscitation the situation should be coming under control. You must then push on rapidly with the next phase.

C Secondary assessment
A full history should be taken either from the patient or from relatives, looking for symptoms suggestive of the causative pathology. Note particularly any indigestion, heartburn or reflux, abdominal pain, alcohol intake, or recent use of drugs.

A general assessment of the patient's health must also be undertaken. Unless this is done, there are likely to be large gaps in the patient's record and these may become important as management continues. You should also review the parameters measured so far and revise your assessment of the rate of bleeding.

Investigations
Investigations should now be undertaken to confirm your provisional diagnosis. These will include urgent fibroscopy and/or a barium meal.

D Further management
Most patients with upper gastrointestinal haemorrhage are controlled by conservative means, including the following.
1 Blood replacement.
2 Sedation and bed rest.
3 Antacid or other relevant medical therapy.
The patient should, therefore, be admitted and kept under close observation.

If bleeding continues or recurs, then further management is usually surgical and depends on the causative lesion as below.

Bleeding peptic ulcer

The surgeon should be informed of any patient with gastro-intestinal bleeding and called upon to see anyone who has:
(a) lost in excess of 6 units of blood;
(b) had a massive haematemesis;
(c) re-bled during adequate medical management.

Elderly patients are more likely to continue bleeding than younger ones because their arteries tend to be arterio-sclerotic and less able to contract down.

Operation: for bleeding peptic ulcer

A bleeding gastric ulcer is usually treated by emergency partial gastrectomy. The ulcer may be adherent posteriorly to the pancreas and may have eroded the splenic artery. In that case massive blood loss may be encountered. At least 10 units should be cross-matched for a posterior bleeding gastric ulcer.

A bleeding duodenal ulcer is usually treated by a vagotomy and pyloroplasty with under-running of the ulcer. Some surgeons prefer partial gastrectomy with excision of the duodenal ulcer. Surgeons who favour highly selective vagotomy may perform this procedure as an emergency and open the duodenum by a longitudinal incision to under-run the ulcer.

Postoperative care

In general, this is as described in the previous sections (pp. 267–273). However, there is an increased risk of recurrent haemorrhage and the patient must be carefully monitored for this.

Mallory–Weiss tear

This lesion is a tear of the gastro-oesophageal junction occurring during an episode of vomiting. The patient often gives a history of vomiting at the end of which blood is noted. The condition is diagnosed on endoscopy and usually settles with conservative management. If laparotomy is required, the stomach is emptied and the bleeding point oversewn.

Acute gastritis

This is a frequent source of gastric haemorrhage. There may be a history of drug ingestion, particularly of drugs used in the management of arthritis, such as phenylbutazone, indomethacin, steroids and aspirin compounds. Acute gastritis can also occur in septicaemia.

In most cases the condition settles with adequate medical therapy and withdrawal of the offending drug. In some cases, however, bleeding continues unabated and in that case operation becomes mandatory. There is no agreed surgical policy for dealing with this diffuse gastric condition. The majority of surgeons would probably perform a partial gastrectomy of the Polya type.

Oesophagitis

The management of oesophagitis and hiatus hernia is dealt with on p. 262. Bleeding from these lesions usually settles with conservative management.

Oesophageal varices

These are dealt with in detail on p. 303.

Carcinoma of the stomach

The condition

Adenocarcinoma of the stomach is thought occasionally to arise on the basis of a previous gastritis or benign gastric ulcer. The macroscopic appearance varies from an ulcer to a cauliflower growth or the more diffuse 'leather-bottle stomach'. The latter is due to diffuse spread of malignant cells along the submucosal layer of the stomach. Carcinoma of the stomach is more common in those of blood group A.

Sixty-four per cent of growths are situated in the prepyloric region. Spread is by direct invasion into neighbouring organs, through the lymphatics, and in the blood. Transcoelomic spread may give rise to peritoneal secondaries and secondaries in the ovary (Krukenberg's tumour).

Recognizing the pattern

The patient

The patient is typically aged between 40 and 60 and the condition is more common in males.

The history

There may or may not be a preceding history of indigestion due to a gastric ulcer. The patient begins to suffer from symptoms of nausea, anorexia and epigastric pain. The pain is initially worse after meals but later becomes continuous and starts to keep him awake at night. He also begins to lose weight.

On examination

There may be a mass palpable in the left hypochondrium. Signs of spread of the disease should be looked for, including enlarged supraclavicular nodes in the neck (Troisier's sign) and enlargement of the liver. The patient is usually cachectic and may be jaundiced.

Carcinoma of the stomach may also present with haematemesis and melaena.

Proving the diagnosis

The diagnosis is demonstrated on a barium meal which shows an irregular craggy filling defect in the stomach. A fibroscopy is mandatory and a biopsy will confirm the diagnosis. Very small gastric carcinomas may be picked up on fibroscopy and these are the lesions which are most amenable to treatment.

Management

Patients with carcinoma of the stomach are frequently debilitated and both the haemoglobin and serum albumin must be checked before surgery is contemplated. Carcinoma of the stomach carries a poor prognosis and the only method of management that has any success is surgical removal of the lesion. Where surgical cure is impossible (e.g. where there are already distant metastases), operation is only indicated to relieve local symptoms such as persistent pain or obstruction with vomiting. 5-Fluorouracil occasionally provides effective palliation for carcinoma of the stomach.

The surgical management is to excise the tumour and the local lymph nodes if a cure is to be attempted. Either a subtotal or total gastrectomy may be required. The latter may be carried out through the abdomen alone, or through a thoraco-abdominal incision.

Preoperative management
As with all cases of malignant disease, both the patient and his relatives will need careful counselling. The patient may require transfusion of blood or intravenous feeding for several days before the operation. If he is able to take oral fluids satisfactorily, then a high nutrition oral diet should be instituted. Adequate vitamins should be given including vitamin C.

If there is gastric outlet obstruction and stasis, the patient should be put on clear fluids for 48 hours and the stomach washed out preoperatively.

Operation: partial gastrectomy (see under Gastric ulcer, p. 266)
In the case of cancer of the stomach, a more radical procedure is undertaken, removing the omentum and the spleen, but the postoperative management is similar to the usual partial gastrectomy.

Operation: total gastrectomy

In this operation the whole of the stomach is removed, usually for a cancer on the lesser curve or the body. The oesophagus is anastomosed either to a loop of jejunum (with closure of the duodenal stump) or, rarely, directly to the duodenal stump. The oesophago-jejunal anastomosis is vulnerable and leaks are common. Because of this, the surgeon may pass a nasogastric tube down through the anastomosis into the proximal jejunum.

Codes

Blood	4−6 units . . . .
GA/LA	GA . . . .
Opn time	3−5 hours . . . .
Stay	2−3 weeks . . . .
Drains out	7 days . . . .
Sutures out	7−10 days . . . .
Off work	6−9 weeks . . . .

Operation: thoraco-abdominal gastrectomy

This operation is undertaken where the carcinoma of the stomach involves the lower oesophagus. In this case an oblique incision is extended up along the bed of the eighth rib and the chest opened. The anastomosis to the oesophagus is then carried out inside the chest.

Codes

Blood	4−6 units . . . .
GA/LA	GA . . . .
Opn time	3−5 hours . . . .
Stay	2−4 weeks . . . .
Drains out	Pleural 2 days, anastomotic 5−7 days, abdominal drain 7 days . . . .
Sutures out	7−10 days . . . .
Off work	8−12 weeks . . . .

Postoperative care

The patient is given no fluids at all by mouth for 7 days, at the end of which a limited barium swallow is performed. If the anastomosis is intact, oral feeding can recommence. If it is not, then the patient can be fed either down the nasogastric tube or intravenously. Intravenous feeding may in any case be continued throughout the early postoperative period.

Post-gastrectomy syndromes

These include the following:
Bilious vomiting.

Dumping.

Diarrhoea (e.g. post-vagotomy diarrhoea).

A fourth problem is recurrent pain, which may be due to the dumping syndrome, recurrent peptic ulcer disease, intestinal obstruction due to adhesions, gastritis due to helicobacter infection or other new pathology.

Bilious vomiting

The condition

This is vomiting of pure bile and occurs in up to 10% of patients following a gastrectomy. The cause is not clearly understood but it can follow any operation in which the pylorus has been removed or bypassed. It is more common after a Polya II type of reconstruction or after a gastro-enterostomy. The symptom is associated with a marked 'biliary gastritis' visible on endoscopy. It may be associated with symptoms of abdominal pain and dumping.

Recognizing the pattern

The history

This is of intermittent sudden attacks of vomiting 15−30 minutes after a meal. The vomit typically consists of pure bile with no food. This may be preceded by epigastric cramping pain which is relieved by the vomiting.

Management

Bilious vomiting is more common immediately after a gastric operation and tends to settle as time passes. It is therefore worth while exhibiting patience providing the vomiting is not too severe. The patient should be reassured that the symptoms usually settle.

Medical management includes substances which help to bind bile salts such as hydrotalcite (Altacite). Meto-clopramide (Maxolon) may also be of value.

If the symptoms persist some form of bile diversion or gastric reconstruction procedure is required.

Operation: gastric reconstruction for bilious vomiting

If the original procedure was a truncal vagotomy and gastro-enterostomy (see p. 270), the gastroenterostomy can be closed, providing a year has elapsed since the vagotomy was performed. Similarly, a pyloroplasty can be taken down and reconstructed.

Bile diversion is best achieved by converting the standard enterostomy loop to a Roux-en-Y procedure (see Fig. 53). This results in the bile entering the intestine well away from the stomach.

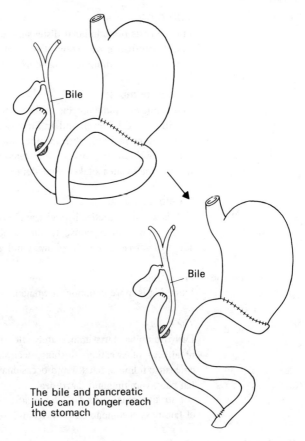

Fig. 53. Roux-en-Y conversion for biliary gastritis.

The bile and pancreatic juice can no longer reach the stomach

Codes

Blood	2 units	
GA/LA	GA	
Opn time	About 2 hours	
Stay	7 days	
Drains out	2–5 days	
Sutures out	7 days	
Off work........	4–6 weeks	

Postoperative care

There are no special problems after these procedures. Oral fluids can be reintroduced as soon as the stomach is seen to be emptying (as evidenced by diminished gastric aspirate and passage of flatus).

Dumping

This consists of abdominal distension and colic, and vaso-motor disturbance occurring after meals. It is seen after a gastrectomy or a drainage procedure. There are two types.

1 Early dumping

This is due to rapid emptying of the stomach, a high osmotic load in the small bowel, and an increased splanchnic blood flow resulting in a fluid shift from the vascular compartment to the bowel lumen. This is precipitated particularly by hot, sweet or bulky meals taken with fluid.

2 Late dumping

This is due to a reactive hypoglycaemia caused by increased insulin output in response to the earlier hyperglycaemia. The hyperglycaemia itself follows rapid gastric emptying.

Recognizing the pattern

The patient
Dumping is more common in women.

The history
Early dumping starts immediately after a meal and consists of attacks of sweating, flushing, tachycardia, palpitations, epigastric fullness, nausea and occasionally colicky abdominal pain, vomiting and diarrhoea.

Late dumping starts 1−2 hours after meals and consists of faintness accompanied by sweating, tremor and nausea.

Proving the diagnosis

The diagnosis of dumping is made on the history. Hypoglycaemia may be confirmed by measuring the blood sugar during an attack.

Management

The symptoms are difficult to treat and are best managed by persuading the patient to modify his intake of food so as to minimize the rapid gastric emptying of foodstuffs. Patients with dumping must have the causes explained to them and should be reassured that the condition usually settles with time. After 6 months only 1−2% of patients are still affected.

Early dumping can be prevented by small, dry meals, with a diet consisting of fat and protein and restricted carbohydrate. Drinks should be taken between and not during meals. Late dumping is made worse by exercise after a meal so susceptible patients should rest for an hour after eating.

Severe persistent dumping can be treated by closing a gastroenterostomy or pyloroplasty as above, or by inserting a short reversed segment of jejunum just beyond the pylorus.

Diarrhoea

The condition

Truncal vagotomy not only decreases gastric secretion and motility, thereby delaying stomach emptying, but also affects the rest of the bowel to a variable extent. Up to 50% of patients after a truncal vagotomy suffer some increase in bowel habit and 5% need treatment for this. The diarrhoea is typically 'episodic'. That is to say, the patient has normal bowel actions most of the time but is then suddenly struck with episodes of urgency and looseness. The mechanism is uncertain and several factors may be responsible. The rapid emptying of the stomach which follows the accompanying gastric drainage procedure results in hyperosmolar contents arriving in the small bowel lumen. As the bowel rapidly dilutes this, vigorous peristalsis ensues, producing some of the symptoms of early dumping and also diarrhoea. There may also be a direct effect of loss of vagal influence on the small bowel and on the biliary tract. Diarrhoea is not seen following a highly selective vagotomy.

Recognizing the pattern

The patient complains of an increase in bowel habit which in severe cases may consist of attacks of uncontrollable, watery diarrhoea. These attacks are episodic and unpredictable.

Management

The diarrhoea sometimes responds to codeine phosphate (45−120 mg daily in 3−6 divided doses), diphenoxylate (Lomotil) or loperamide (Imodium). A short course of neomycin or phthalyl sulphathiazole occasionally provides long-lasting relief. For severe cases re-operation and insertion of a 10 cm reversed segment of jejunum at the gastric outlet or 100 cm down the jejunum can relieve the symptoms.

6.2　　　Liver, Pancreas and Spleen

Gall-stones

The condition

Gall-stones precipitate from bile concentrated in the gall bladder. They may be either basically formed from cholesterol or from bile pigment though most stones are mixed. Ten per cent of gall-stones are radio-opaque due to the presence of calcium salts. Stones cause symptoms either by obstructing the neck of the gall bladder and causing pain and cholecystitis or by moving into the common bile duct and causing obstructive jaundice or pancreatitis.

Rarely a large gall-stone may ulcerate through the gall bladder wall and enter the gut. The stone may then cause intestinal obstruction (gall-stone ileus).

Recognizing the pattern

The patient

Gall-stones are particularly common in the typical fat, fertile female in her forties. However, they do also occur in other age-groups and in men.

The history

The typical symptoms are of two types. First there is flatulent dyspepsia. This consists of a feeling of epigastric fullness and distension coming on about an hour or two after meals and particularly after fatty foods. Often the patient has already subconsciously decided to keep off fats and does not therefore give a positive history of fat intolerance. The dyspepsia commonly occurs in the evenings.

The second type of symptom is gall-bladder 'colic' and is probably due to obstruction of the outlet of the gall bladder by a stone. It is a much more severe pain coming on an hour or two after meals, often after eating fats or pastry. The pain is situated in the epigastrium or the right hypochondrium and radiates around the costal margin to the right shoulder blade. The severe pain lasts a few hours and usually results in the patient seeking medical advice. It settles with an injection of pethidine but the patient still feels sore under the right hypochondrium for several days afterwards. This soreness is worse on coughing or moving.

If the contents of the gall bladder become secondarily infected (acute cholecystitis), the patient can become very unwell with rigors, anorexia, nausea and vomiting.

On examination

The patient may have a fever. Palpation of the abdomen reveals upper abdominal tenderness maximal beneath the right, ninth costal cartilage over the gall bladder. If the examining hand is placed 2–3 finger-breadths below the costal margin and the patient is asked to inspire deeply, he feels a sharp pain as the gall bladder descends on to the palpating hand (Murphy's sign).

Proving the diagnosis

During an acute attack there may be mild derangement of the liver function tests. The presence of gall-stones is confirmed by an ultrasound scan of the gall bladder and once the acute attack is over they may also be demonstrated on an oral cholecystogram. A Hida scan may show non-filling of the gall bladder during an acute attack.

Management

Gall-stones can sometimes be dissolved by medical treatment, shattered by lithotripsy, or removed percutaneously. All these methods share the disadvantage of stone recurrence due to disease in the gall bladder wall. This disease also carries a small but definite long-term risk of malignancy.

The definitive management of gall stones is therefore removal of the gall bladder. This may either be carried out by open operation or through a laparoscope.

Acute cholecystitis

A patient with acute cholecystitis is usually managed conservatively with bed rest and antibiotics (e.g. a parenteral cephalosporin). Some surgeons prefer to perform cholecystectomy as an emergency during the acute attack. The gall bladder is usually easy to remove in the early stages (48 hours) as it is surrounded by oedema.

Obstructive jaundice due to gall-stones

The management of obstructive jaundice will be dealt with on p. 291. If the jaundice is known to be associated with gall-stones, it is allowed to settle and a cholecystectomy is performed later. The patient should be given an antibiotic which is effective in bile (e.g. ampicillin or a cephalosporin) to treat associated cholangitis. It is also important to maintain adequate hydration as there is a danger of associated renal failure.

Operation: cholecystectomy and exploration of common bile duct

The operation is usually carried out through a vertical or an oblique (Kocher's) incision. An operative cholangiogram may be performed and the X-ray department must be warned of this. The cholangiogram demonstrates the presence or absence of stones in the common bile duct. Before the operation starts the patient must be positioned carefully on the table so that the X-ray plate is beneath the patient's biliary tree. If there are no stones in the duct, the cystic artery and duct are ligated and the gall bladder is removed. A drain may be placed down to the gall bladder bed.

If stones are demonstrated in the common bile duct, the duct is explored and the stones removed. The surgeon may wish to inspect the duct using a choledochoscope. Occasionally a stone impacted in the ampulla of Vater cannot be removed through an incision in the common bile duct and in this case the duodenum has to be opened and a sphincterotomy performed. The stone can then be removed through the widened ampulla of Vater. The common bile duct (CBD) is closed over a T-tube which is brought out to the surface (see p. 120).

Codes

Blood	Group and save serum . . . .
GA/LA	GA . . . .
Opn time	1 hour (+ CBD exploration 90–120 minutes) . . . .
Stay	7–10 days . . . .
Drains out	Drain 2–5 days, T-tube 7–10 days (see below) . . . .
Sutures out	7 days . . . .
Off work	4–6 weeks . . . .

Postoperative care

Oral fluids are given after 36 hours or so when the patient's ileus recovers. If the common bile duct has been explored, a T-tube cholangiogram is performed after a week. This is to exclude the presence of further retained stones before the T-tube is removed. If the X-ray is clear, the T-tube can be taken out. Some surgeons prefer to clamp the tube intermittently before it is removed.

The drain to the gall bladder bed can usually be removed at 48 hours, although some surgeons prefer to leave it longer, particularly if they use catgut to tie off the cystic duct stump.

If the patient is not jaundiced, bile-stained drainage after a gall bladder operation is of ominous significance, and indicates a biliary fistula. If the patient is jaundiced, however, all serous collections in the peritoneum will be bile-stained and this is nothing to worry about.

A biliary fistula can be demonstrated by doing a T-tube cholangiogram, or a sinogram if there is no T-tube. An intravenous cholangiogram or Hida scan may also be helpful. The drain should not be removed until the surgeon in charge has decided on the further course of action. Fistulae will often heal if there is adequate drainage of the biliary tree, but there is a danger of stricture formation later. The surgeon may decide to re-explore the patient and repair the bile duct using a loop of jejunum.

After a cholecystectomy the patient is gradually returned to a normal diet and there is no need for him to keep off fatty foods in the convalescent period. He may need reassurance that his digestion should be normal after he has lost his gall bladder.

Operation: laparoscopic cholecystectomy
The gall-bladder area is visualized on a video screen connected to a camera on a laparoscope. Operative manoeuvres are carried out through secondary laparoscopic ports. A cholangiogram can also be performed. The main abdominal incision is therefore avoided in favour of four or more stab wounds for the laparoscopic cannulae.

Codes

Blood	Group and save serum . . . .
GA/LA	GA . . . .
Opn time	1–4 hours . . . .
Stay	24–48 hours . . . .
Drains out	12 hours . . . .
Sutures out	24–48 hours . . . .
Off work	1–2 weeks . . . .

Postoperative care
The patient suffers very little pain and can usually resume drinking within a few hours after operation and oral feeding after 24–36 hours. Apart from excessive tiredness for a week, recovery is remarkably rapid and the patient can return to full activity 1–2 weeks after surgery.

Surgical jaundice
Patients with jaundice are referred to surgeons because it is believed the cause may be obstructive and hence possibly amenable to operative treatment. Faced with such patients the first task is to establish that the jaundice is indeed obstructive and then to determine the cause of the obstruction. An understanding of the physiology of bile metabolism is necessary.

Jaundice is due to excessive accumulation of bile pigment (bilirubin and its derivatives). The normal metabolism of bile is shown in Fig. 54. An excess of bilirubin may be due to any of the following.

1 Excessive production — prehepatic jaundice, e.g. haemolytic anaemia.

2 Defective processing of bilirubin in the liver — hepatic jaundice, e.g. hepatitis.

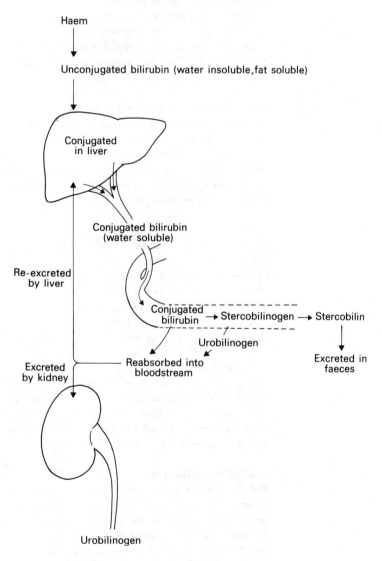

Fig. 54. Normal bilirubin metabolism: Bilirubin is conjugated in the liver and excreted into the gut.

3 A blocked excretion of bile from the liver — post-hepatic or obstructive jaundice, e.g. stone in the common bile duct or carcinoma of the pancreas.

The main features of these three types of jaundice are given below.

1 Prehepatic jaundice

This occurs in a younger age-group and is common in children. There is an excessive production of bilirubin due to an increased red cell turnover. This may be due to a haemolytic disorder such as spherocytosis, drug-induced haemolysis, or an incompatible blood transfusion. Laboratory tests show an increased unconjugated bilirubin in the peripheral blood and a low haemoglobin. Other liver function tests including the serum alkaline phosphatase, alanine transaminase (ALT) and the serum albumin are all normal. Blood clotting studies are also normal. The absence of liver damage makes this type of jaundice easy to separate from the other two. Because of the satisfactory liver function the jaundice is always mild and the patient is usually a lemon-yellow colour.

2 Hepatic jaundice

In this condition there is liver damage from one of a variety of causes including viral hepatitis, leptospirosis, alcoholic cirrhosis, and drug- or chemical-induced liver damage. The patient is usually markedly jaundiced and ill from the effects of the liver disease. Laboratory tests show a raised serum ALT and a less marked rise in the serum alkaline phosphatase. Some bile is usually still being processed in the liver and the stools may remain a normal colour.

On examination the liver is enlarged and tender.

3 Post-hepatic obstructive jaundice (Fig. 55)

In this condition the liver function is initially normal but the liver may become secondarily damaged due to back pressure or ascending infection. Characteristically the alkaline phosphatase is very high and the ALT less elevated. The serum albumin should be normal. The jaundice is usually deep but it may be intermittent if the obstruction is intermittent (e.g. gall-stones).

Investigation of obstructive jaundice

1 Test the urine for urobilinogen and urobilin. Urobilinogen is raised in prehepatic jaundice and bilirubin is present in post-hepatic jaundice. Urobilinogen is absent from the urine if the obstruction is complete.

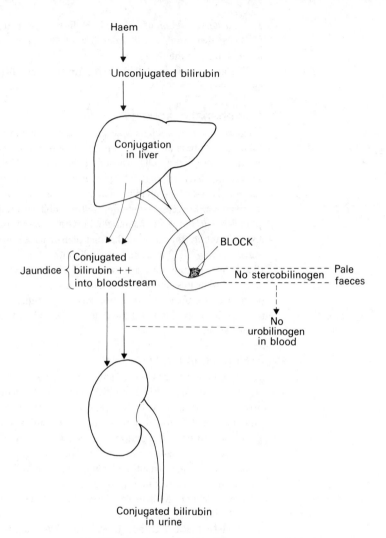

Haem

↓

Unconjugated bilirubin

↓

Conjugation
in liver

BLOCK

Jaundice { Conjugated
bilirubin ++
into bloodstream

No stercobilinogen — Pale faeces

No
urobilinogen
in blood

Conjugated bilirubin
in urine

Fig. 55. Obstructive jaundice. When conjugated bilirubin cannot get into the gut it appears in the bloodstream and is excreted in the urine.

2 Liver function tests. The pattern of results in various types of jaundice is shown in Table 18. In addition, the prothrombin time gives a useful indicator of liver function and may be important in the future management of the patient.

If these tests indicate an obstructive picture or are indecisive, an ultrasound examination is carried out to determine the size of the intrahepatic bile ducts.

3 Ultrasound. If the intra-hepatic bile ducts are dilated, the

Table 18. Laboratory results in jaundice

	Prehepatic (haemolytic)	Hepatic* (hepatitic)	Post-hepatic (obstructive)
Bilirubin			
Unconjugated	Raised	Raised	May be raised
Conjugated	Normal	Raised	Raised
Alanine			
transaminase (ALT)	Normal	Raised	May be raised
Alkaline		Slightly	
phosphatase	Normal	raised*	Raised
Plasma proteins	Normal	May be low	Normal

* There is often an element of obstruction in hepatic jaundice due to intra-hepatic cholestasis.

cause is obstructive. The investigation may also detect the presence of gall-stones in the gall bladder or other masses within the liver parenchyma.

4 If dilated ducts are found, a percutaneous transhepatic cholangiogram is performed. This should show the level of the obstruction and possibly its cause. The lower end of the common bile duct may also be cannulated using a fibroscope (endoscopic retrograde cholangio-pancreatography, ERCP). The ampulla of Vater can be inspected during this procedure.

5 If the ducts in the liver are not dilated, a liver biopsy may be performed and may give a diagnosis of the cause of hepatic damage.

6 In cases where a carcinoma of the head of the pancreas is suspected a CAT scan may be helpful.

At any stage of this process the surgeon may decide that enough investigation has been done to warrant proceeding with a laparotomy. This may also be indicated if the above work-up has failed to settle the question of whether the jaundice is obstructive or not. Such a laparotomy will be combined with intraoperative cholangiography and a liver biopsy.

Preoperative management

Patients with liver damage may have abnormal clotting factors and should be given vitamin K preoperatively. Where the jaundice is severe, there is a danger of induction of renal failure at the time of surgery (hepato-renal syndrome). This can be avoided by adequately hydrating the patient and by giving him a peroperative infusion of mannitol (dose 0.5 g/kg, e.g. 200 cm^3 of 20%) intravenously. Before the operation is started, a urinary catheter should be inserted so that the urinary output can be monitored.

Operations

The operations to deal with obstructive jaundice are dealt with under the individual conditions.

Exploration of the common bile duct, p. 289.

Whipple's operation, p. 316.

Bypass operation for carcinoma of the pancreas, p. 318.

In some cases an obstruction of the common bile duct due to stricture or carcinoma may be relieved by an intraluminal tube. This can be inserted percutaneously through the liver by a radiologist.

Portal hypertension

The condition   The portal venous pressure is raised when there is an obstruction in the portal system. This can be situated before, in or after the liver. The causes of such an obstruction are shown in Fig. 56. The commonest aetiology in Western countries is cirrhosis. Schistosomiasis is the main cause world-wide. The normal portal venous pressure is 5–10 mmHg and the pressure may reach 30–40 mmHg in portal hypertension. Elevated portal pressure leads to the development of venous collaterals between the portal and systemic venous circulation. The most important of these are in the oesophagus, where varices may develop. Collaterals also develop at the umbilicus and in the rectum and anal canal (see Fig. 57). The patient also develops ascites if there

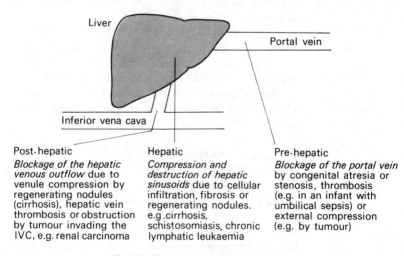

Liver

Portal vein

Inferior vena cava

Post-hepatic

Blockage of the hepatic venous outflow due to venule compression by regenerating nodules (cirrhosis), hepatic vein thrombosis or obstruction by tumour invading the IVC, e.g. renal carcinoma

Hepatic

Compression and destruction of hepatic sinusoids due to cellular infiltration, fibrosis or regenerating nodules. e.g.cirrhosis, schistosomiasis, chronic lymphatic leukaemia

Pre-hepatic

Blockage of the portal vein by congenital atresia or stenosis, thrombosis (e.g. in an infant with umbilical sepsis) or external compression (e.g. by tumour)

Fig. 56. The causes of portal hypertension.

is coexistent liver failure with hypoproteinaemia and hyper-aldosteronism. Splenomegaly is common and there may be a degree of hypersplenism with leucopenia and thrombo-cytopenia. Portal systemic encephalopathy may occur due to the fact that blood from the gut bypasses the liver and its filtering and detoxifying mechanisms.

Recognizing the pattern

The history
The usual presentation of portal hypertension is haema-temesis and melaena. This is described on p. 277. There may also be symptoms of anaemia. There is usually a past history suggestive of liver disease or alcoholism. The patient may have noticed easy bruising or a purpuric rash.

On examination
The signs of portal hypertension include splenomegaly

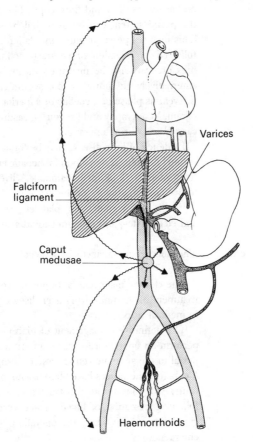

Fig. 57. Portal hypertension results in the enlargement of veins at the sites of porta-systemic venous anastomoses.

(80−90%), ascites and occasionally dilated veins around the umbilicus (caput medusae) over which there may be a venous hum on auscultation. Look for purpura and stigmata of chronic liver disease. These include jaundice, skin pigmentation, clubbing, spider naevi, palmar erythema, gynaecomastia, testicular atrophy and a female distribution of pubic hair.

The liver is a variable size in cirrhosis.

Hepatosplenomegaly and ascites with no history of alcohol abuse suggest hepatic vein obstruction.

Signs of encephalopathy include confusion, drowsiness and tremor, increased tendon reflexes, up-going plantar responses and constructional apraxia (e.g. inability to copy a star).

Proving the diagnosis

The presence of oesophageal varices can be demonstrated on barium swallow and fibroscopy. The precise anatomy of the portal system can be displayed by splenoportography. This involves percutaneous cannulation of a splenic venule followed by injection of contrast medium. Portal venous pressure can also be measured during such a procedure. Alternatively, the portal venous system can be visualized in the venous phase of a coeliac or superior mesenteric arteriogram. Venography and pressure measurements can also be carried out during operation.

Evidence of liver disease may be found by measuring the serum bilirubin, serum albumin, hepatic enzymes and alphafetoprotein (to look for hepatoma). A liver biopsy may help to diagnose the nature of the disease.

Finally the haemoglobin, platelets, clotting screen, urea and electrolytes, and calcium should also be measured.

Management

The emergency management of bleeding oesophageal varices is described on p. 303.

The elective management of portal hypertension includes treatment of the underlying liver disease. This is described in medical texts.

The definitive management of high portal pressure is to perform an operation to create an artificial shunt from the portal to the systemic venous system. Prophylactic shunting (i.e. before the varices have bled) has not been found to be of value. A shunt is usually constructed as an elective procedure following cessation of bleeding and restabilization of the circulation. Occasionally the operation is performed as an emergency.

Alternative procedures for dealing with varices involve interrupting them locally either by direct ligation or by transection and re-anastomosis of the oesophagus or upper stomach. Such procedures are effective but recurrence is common. They are described on pp. 305−6.

Finally, varices can also be treated by injection sclerotherapy.

Operation: sclerotherapy of oesophageal varices

This may be performed through a rigid or flexible oesophagoscope (see p. 240), and as an emergency or elective procedure. Sclerosant (4−6 ml) (e.g. ethanolamine oleate) is injected into each varix. These are then compressed with a balloon for 24 hours. The injections can then be repeated later. The patient can sometimes be maintained for a long time by regular re-injection. Alternatively, following control of the varices, he may be considered for surgery.

Shunt procedures

These are carried out in the following circumstances.

1 The patient is under 50 years old.
2 The serum albumin is more than 30 g/litre.
3 The bilirubin is not significantly raised (>35 mmol/litre).
4 There is no medical history of encephalopathy.
5 Portal and systemic venography has shown that the planned anastomosis is possible. Venograms may be done during operation.

Preoperative management

Before an elective shunt the patient should be put on a low protein, high carbohydrate diet if not on one already. The bowels should be cleared of all protein by careful bowel preparation (see p. 110). Neomycin (1 g 4−6-hourly) may also be given.

Additional preoperative measures include blood transfusion, platelet transfusion, correction of clotting defects and a mannitol infusion to prevent the hepato-renal syndrome.

Operation: portacaval anastomosis

An end-to-side or side-to-side anastomosis of the portal vein to the inferior vena cava is performed where the vessels lie around the foramen of Winslow (see Fig. 58).

Codes

Blood . . . . 8−10 units . . . .
GA/LA . . . . GA . . . .
Opn time . . . . 3−4 hours . . . .

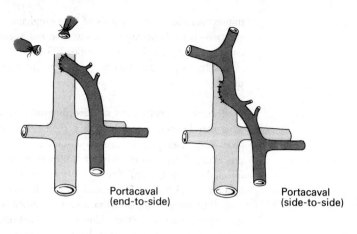

Portacaval
(end-to-side)

Portacaval
(side-to-side)

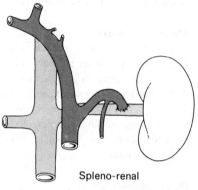

Spleno-renal

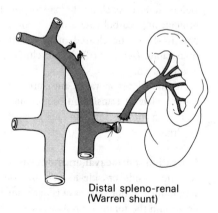

Distal spleno-renal
(Warren shunt)

Fig. 58. Portacaval shunt operations.

Stay .... 10—14 days depending on preop.
                condition ....
Drains out ...... Subhepatic space 48 hours ....

| Sutures out | 7–10 days | .... |
| Off work | Variable | .... |

Postoperative care

There is usually no further bleeding and the spleen decreases in size. However, there is a 20–30% incidence of post-operative encephalopathy, and fluid retention may occur due to further impairment of liver function.

Operation: spleno-renal anastomosis

This is indicated if the portal vein is thrombosed. A splenectomy is performed, leaving as long a length of splenic vein as possible. This is anastomosed end-to-side to the left renal vein (see Fig. 58).

Codes

Blood	8–10 units	....
GA/LA	GA	....
Opn time	3–4 hours	....
Stay	10–14 days	....
Drains out	48 hours	....
Sutures out	7–10 days	....
Off work	Variable	....

Operation: distal spleno-renal shunt (Warren shunt)

Here the spleen is preserved. The splenic vein is ligated behind the neck of the pancreas and the free end is anastomosed to the left renal vein. The right and left gastric veins are divided. This causes selective decompression of the lower end of the oesophagus, which now drains via the short gastric veins into the shunt. The hepatic portal blood flow is preserved and there is therefore a low incidence of encephalopathy (see Fig. 58).

Codes

Blood	8–10 units	....
GA/LA	GA	....
Opn time	3–4 hours	....
Stay	Variable	....
Drains out	48 hours	....
Sutures out	7–10 days	....
Off work	Variable	....

Operation: mesenterico-caval shunt

An anastomosis is made either end-to-side between the inferior vena cava and the superior mesenteric vein, or by a Dacron graft placed between these two vessels ('H' graft).

The latter is technically easier. This shunt is suitable for cases of portal venous thrombosis (see Fig. 59).

Codes

Blood	6−8 units . . . .
GA/LA	GA . . . .
Opn time	2−3 hours . . . .
Stay	Variables . . . .
Drains out	0 or 48 hours . . . .
Sutures out	7 days . . . .
Off work	Variable . . . .

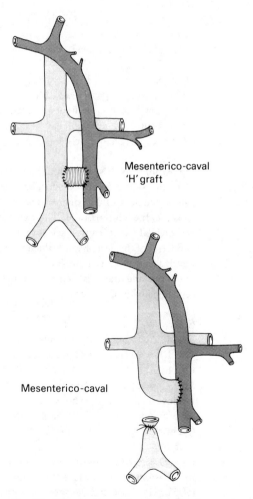

Mesenterico-caval
'H' graft

Mesenterico-caval

Fig. 59. Other portacaval shunts: mesenterico-caval anastomoses.

Postoperative care
The general management of liver failure ascites and porta-systemic encephalopathy is described in medical texts.

Bleeding oesophageal varices

These occur as part of the syndrome of portal hypertension and can bleed massively. The hospital mortality is high and 60% of those who recover re-bleed within one year. Blood in the bowel may precipitate encephalopathy.

Patients with portal hypertension may bleed from other sites, usually a gastric or duodenal ulcer or haemorrhagic gastritis.

Recognizing the pattern

The history
The haematemesis is usually profuse. There may be a history of similar episodes, and also of previous liver disease (e.g. cirrhosis, jaundice, hepatitis). The patient may be an alcoholic.

On examination
The patient is usually shocked. Stigmata of portal hypertension, liver disease and alcoholism are usually present to a varying degree. Look for the signs of encephalopathy (p. 298).

Proving the diagnosis

The bleeding site must be confirmed by a fibroscopy as soon as the patient is stabilized. Other emergency investigations include the following.
1 Haemoglobin and cross-match.
2 Clotting screen.
3 Platelet count.
4 Urea, electrolytes and calcium.
5 Liver function tests.

Management

Resuscitation is carried out as on pp. 277–279. A CVP line is usually needed. Use fresh blood if possible as this contains more clotting factors and platelets than stored blood. Fresh frozen plasma and platelet transfusion may be required. Vitamin K (10 mg i.v.) is given. Neomycin (1 g 6-hourly) and lactulose (30–50 ml 8-hourly) are given to decrease the urea-splitting organisms in the bowel and to clear the bowel of blood. This is done to try and prevent encephalopathy. Gastric and colonic washouts are also helpful.

If bleeding continues, vasopressin can be given. This causes splanchnic vasoconstriction. It may be given either as an intravenous bolus (20 units in 100 ml 5% dextrose over

20 minutes and repeated after 2 hours if necessary) or as an intravenous infusion (0.4 units per minute over 24 hours).

The further management depends on the patient's overall condition. Patients in severe liver failure with gross oedema and encephalopathy are poor operative risks. In these patients the varices may be controlled by sclerotherapy (see p. 299), or transhepatic embolization of the left gastric vein can be attempted.

If the patient is considered fit for surgery and still bleeding, then a Sengstaken tube is inserted (see Fig. 60).

Sengstaken tube

This compresses the varices and fundal veins. The tube is passed into the stomach and the gastric balloon inflated. This balloon is impacted on the lower end of the gastro-oesophageal junction by traction on the tube. The upper oesophageal balloon is then inflated. Regular aspiration of the stomach is carried out through the tube to ensure that bleeding is not continuing. The oesophagus is aspirated to prevent inhalation of nasopharyngeal secretions. The tube is unpleasant for the patient and can be dangerous. Complications of its use include aspiration, pressure necrosis of the oesophageal and gastric mucosa, rupture of the oesophagus and respiratory obstruction.

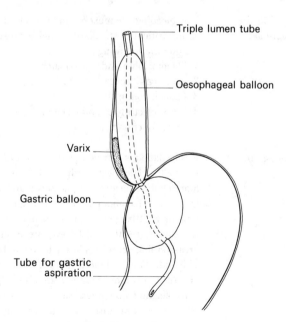

Fig. 60. The Sengstaken tube: the oesophageal balloon compresses the varices.

If the bleeding is controlled after a few hours the tube is deflated and left *in situ* for up to 24 hours before removal. Should bleeding recur during this time, the tube must be reflated and emergency operation will be required.

Sclerotherapy can be used as an emergency measure to try and control bleeding.

Surgical management

The operations described below are aimed at obliterating the varices. Operations for the general management of portal hypertension have already been described. In the emergency situation the varices may be either under-run or transected, or an emergency portacaval shunt may be performed. The choice depends on the rate of bleeding, the overall condition of the patient and the experience of the surgeon. The indications for portacaval shunting are listed on p. 299. Three other operations will be described here.

1 Oversewing of varices.
2 Oesophageal transection.
3 Gastric transection.

Preoperative management

Before operation the patient's haemoglobin, coagulation screen and platelet numbers must be as normal as possible. A mannitol infusion may be required to prevent the hepato-renal syndrome.

Operation: oversewing of oesophageal varices

A left thoracotomy is performed and the oesophagus opened just above the diaphragm to expose the varices.

The varices (usually in three columns) are then oversewn using continuous chromic catgut sutures.

Codes

Blood	6–10 units . . . .
GA/LA	GA . . . .
Opn time	90–120 minutes . . . .
Stay	Variable . . . .
Drains out	Pleura 24 hours, mediastinum 5–7 days . . . .
Sutures out	7–10 days . . . .
Off work	Variable . . . .

Postoperative care

A barium swallow can be performed on the fifth or sixth day and, if this is normal, fluids are reintroduced slowly.

Operation: oesophageal transection

The oesophagus is exposed through a lower, left thoracotomy, the vagal trunks are dissected clear and the oesophagus is transected. It is then resutured with continuous sutures to obliterate the vessel. Alternatively, the procedure can be performed through the abdomen with a stapling gun introduced through the stomach. This is technically easier and has the advantage that the chest is not opened.

Codes

Blood	6–10 units ....
GA/LA	GA ....
Opn time	2–3 hours ....
Stay	Variable ....
Drains out	Pleura 24 hours, mediastinum 5–7 days ....
Sutures out	7–10 days ....
Off work........	Variable ....

Postoperative care

Fluids are reintroduced slowly as above.

Operation: gastric transection

The stomach is exposed through a left thoraco-abdominal incision and the stomach transected and resutured just below the gastro-oesophageal junction.

Codes

Blood	10 units ....
GA/LA	GA ....
Opn time	3–4 hours ....
Stay	Variable ....
Drains out	Subphrenic space 7 days ....
Sutures out	7–10 days ....
Off work........	Variable ....

Postoperative care

This is similar to that described for gastrectomy on p. 268.

Hepatic tumours

These may be benign or malignant.

Benign hepatic tumours

The condition

Benign hepatic tumours include the following.

1 Haemangioma.
2 Focal nodular hyperplasia.
3 Liver cell adenoma.

Benign tumours of the liver are uncommon and frequently asymptomatic, being found incidentally at laparotomy. The cavernous haemangioma is the most common benign tumour of the liver. It presents in adults most commonly between 30 and 70 years of age and may grow to a very large size. Focal nodular hyperplasia and liver cell adenoma are most commonly found in women of child-bearing age and are associated with the use of the oral contraceptive pill. Stopping this medication may result in regression of the tumour.

Recognizing the pattern

A cavernous haemangioma is usually asymptomatic but may present with vague abdominal symptoms (swelling, pain, nausea). The diagnosis is confirmed by ultrasound, CAT scan and angiography. Biopsy is usually contraindicated in this condition.

Focal nodular hyperplasia tumours are usually small and found incidentally. Liver cell adenoma tumours are often larger and more likely to present with symptoms, particularly bleeding into the peritoneal cavity. The diagnosis is made by ultrasound, CAT scan and biopsy. The latter may involve total excision depending on the location and size.

Management

The risk of spontaneous haemorrhage from a haemangioma is very small. However, resection may be indicated in the symptomatic case, the technique depending on the size and location of the lesion.

Patients with focal nodular hyperplasia or liver cell adenoma should be advised to stop the oral contraceptive pill. Distinguishing these tumours from malignant hepatoma may be difficult and justify excision. Having made the diagnosis, large tumours may require resection and small tumours may be managed conservatively.

There is no evidence that these lesions are pre-malignant.

Malignant hepatic tumours

The condition

Malignant hepatic tumours are of the following kinds.
1 Primary:
   (a) primary hepatocellular carcinoma (hepatoma);
   (b) cholangiocarcinoma.
2 Secondary.

The incidence of primary hepatocellular carcinoma shows considerable geographic variation, being common in the Far East and Africa and relatively uncommon in Europe and North America. Its incidence is strongly associated both with chronic hepatitis B infection and with cirrhosis of other aetiologies. It is commoner in males (3:1). Other, less significant, aetiological agents include the ground-nut fungal toxin, aflatoxin, and the oral contraceptive pill.

Cholangiocarcinoma (primary carcinoma of bile duct) occurs most commonly after 60 years of age and more frequently in males (2:1). It may develop at an earlier age, particularly in association with sclerosing cholangitis (10%) or (rarely) Caroli's disease (cystic disease of the biliary tract).

The majority of malignant tumours of the liver are secondary to primary tumours in the gastrointestinal tract (stomach, pancreas, colon) or elsewhere.

Proving the diagnosis

The diagnosis of a malignant neoplasm of the liver includes ultrasound and CAT scan (this may also detect extrahepatic spread of disease, particularly to portal or para-aortic lymph nodes). Coeliac arteriography may demonstrate an abnormal 'tumour' circulation. Histological confirmation is obtained by percutaneous CAT-guided biopsy. Even after a needle biopsy, it is important to exclude the presence of a gastro-intestinal primary tumour by endoscopy (stomach), CAT scan (pancreas) and barium enema (colon). A cholangio-carcinoma may be very small and present with biliary ob-struction; this may be difficult to biopsy and the diagnosis may be made by cholangiography (endoscopic or transhepatic).

Management

1 Resection.
2 Palliation.

If it appears that complete removal of the tumour is possible, the patient should undergo hepatic resection. The risks of hepatic resection in patients with chronic liver disease must be carefully considered. In some cases where a primary liver tumour is too extensive for resection but appears confined to the liver, patients are considered for hepatic transplantation. Hepatic resection for secondary liver tumours (usually colonic) is considered only if there is good evidence that the recurrence is solitary and after some months have elapsed following excision of the primary tumour.

In tumours unsuitable for resection and causing unac-ceptable symptoms, palliation is attempted. Most commonly this involves relief of jaundice either by transhepatic or endoscopic stenting of the biliary system or by surgical bypass.

Operation: hepatic resection
1 Left hemihepatectomy (removal of the anatomical left lobe).

2 Right hemihepatectomy (removal of the anatomical right lobe).

3 Right trisegmentectomy (removal of the right lobe and medial segment of the left lobe).

The porta hepatis is explored and the appropriate branches of the portal vein, hepatic artery and hepatic duct ligated and divided. The liver parenchyma is then divided, carefully ligating or clipping all vessels which cross the line of section. The appropriate hepatic vein is identified, clamped and oversewn. A large silicone drain is placed in the region of the cut surface of the liver.

Codes

Blood	8 units	
GA/LA	GA	
Opn time	2–4 hours	
Stay	10–21 days	
Drains out	7–10 days	
Sutures out	10 days	
Off work........	2–3 months....................	

Postoperative care

After hepatic resection, a patient requires monitoring on the intensive care unit for at least 24 hours or until cardiovascular parameters are stable. The nasogastric tube should remain in place until the patient passes flatus. The patient should be observed for postoperative haemorrhage and, later, for signs of bile leakage or of hepatocellular insufficiency, particularly coagulopathy and/or hypoglycaemia. (Full blood count, coagulation studies and liver function tests should be performed daily.)

Hepatic transplantation

Indications

The indications for liver transplantation include the following.

1 Chronic liver disease.

2 Acute liver failure.

3 Metabolic defects.

4 Liver tumours.

1 Chronic liver disease

The common causes of chronic liver disease leading to transplantation are the following.

Primary biliary cirrhosis.

Post-hepatic cirrhosis (chronic active) hepatitis.

Auto-immune chronic active hepatitis.

Sclerosing cholangitis.

Cryptogenic cirrhosis.
Alcoholic cirrhosis (carefully selected cases).

Liver transplantation should be considered in patients with these diseases who develop life-threatening complications, particularly gastro-oesophageal variceal haemorrhage, encephalopathy, spontaneous bacterial peritonitis or intractable ascites and malnutrition. In some patients without such complications, symptoms of fatigue and itching may be so severe as to warrant transplantation.

2 Acute liver failure

Patients suffering from fulminant hepatic failure (liver failure within 8 weeks of the onset of symptoms) or subacute hepatic failure (liver failure between 8 and 26 weeks of the onset of symptoms) may require urgent liver transplantation. The most common aetiological agents are viral hepatitis (hepatitis B, non-A non-B), drug reactions and toxins.

3 Metabolic diseases

A number of life-threatening metabolic diseases are characterized by the deficiency of a hepatic enzyme. Examples of this include α-1-antitrypsin deficiency, primary hyperoxaluria and Wilson's disease. Successful replacement of the diseased liver results in permanent cure of the condition.

4 Liver tumours

Patients with primary liver tumours may be suitable candidates for liver transplantation if the growth is too extensive to allow conventional hepatic resection and if there is no evidence of extrahepatic disease. Secondary liver tumours are not an indication for transplantation.

Preoperative management

The extent of liver disease is assessed by liver function tests, coagulation screen, and the presence or absence of complications of liver disease. The size of the portal vein can be assessed by Doppler ultrasound. The patients undergo a microbiological screen, including looking for cytomegalovirus. Blood grouping and antibody studies are undertaken. A full general medical and anaesthetic assessment is also carried out.

Operation: hepatic transplantation

The donor

Brain-dead, heart-beating donors are used. The liver is fully mobilized until it is attached only by its vascular connections (inferior vena cava (IVC), portal vein, hepatic artery). Cannulae are placed in the aorta and portal vein and, when the circulation stops (when the heart is excised for transplantation), *in situ* cooling is carried out. The liver, perfused and stored in suitable preservation solution, can remain ischaemic, at ice temperature, for up to 24 hours.

The recipient
The recipient operation often has the following complications.
1 Portal hypertension.
2 Coagulopathy.
3 Adhesions due to previous upper abdominal surgery.
   The liver is mobilized with careful attention to haemostasis. The bile duct is divided, the blood vessels clamped and the liver excised. The donor liver is then transplanted, anastomosing the suprahepatic IVC, infrahepatic IVC, portal vein, hepatic artery and bile duct. Some patients tolerate the clamping of the IVC and portal vein poorly and require bypass from the infrahepatic IVC and portal vein, back to the right side of the heart.

Codes

Blood	30 units	
GA/LA	GA	
Opn time	5−8 hours	
Stay	3−6 weeks	
Drains out	2−7 days	
Sutures out	2 weeks	
Off work	3 months	

Postoperative management
All liver transplant recipients require a period of ventilation and intensive monitoring of cardiopulmonary, renal and liver function. Immunosuppressive medication is started at the time of operation. Particular problems include bleeding, graft infarction, infection, rejection and biliary complications.

Benign tumours of the pancreas

The condition
The most important benign tumours of the pancreas are those derived from the islet cells. These are part of the APUD system (see p. 177). An insulinoma is a tumour derived from the beta cells of the islets. It produces an excess of insulin. A gastrinoma is derived from non-beta cells and produces an excess of gastrin. The latter results in gastric hyperacidity and severe duodenal ulceration (Zollinger−Ellison syndrome).

Other tumours may secrete vasoactive intestinal peptide (VIP), causing diarrhoea and hypocalcaemia (the Verner−Morrison syndrome), or glucagon, causing mild diabetes.

Most of these tumours are benign and for convenience both benign and malignant forms are described here. They may be associated with other lesions in the APUD system.

Insulinoma

The condition

Ten per cent of beta cell tumours are multiple and 10% are malignant. Over 90% are situated in the pancreas, the remaining few being found in ectopic pancreatic tissue. The tumour is frequently less than 2 cm in diameter.

Recognizing the pattern

The patient is usually between the ages of 20 and 40. The excessive insulin production results in marked hypoglycaemia and the patient suffers from attacks of unconsciousness or strange behaviour and may become intensely hungry. He may gain a lot of weight.

Proving the diagnosis

This may be difficult. Patients are frequently misdiagnosed as having epilepsy or psychiatric disease. Whipple's triad is helpful when trying to make the diagnosis and states the following:

1 The attacks are induced by starvation or exercise.
2 Hypoglycaemia is present during an attack (blood glucose less than 2 mmol/litre).
3 The episode is relieved by giving sugar orally or intravenously.

Once the possibility of this condition has been recognized the diagnosis can be confirmed by the following:

1 Measuring the plasma insulin levels by radio-immunoassay. The levels are elevated even in the presence of hypoglycaemia.
2 Fish insulin test. The patient is given an injection of fish insulin. This produces hypoglycaemia which would normally suppress the patient's own insulin production. In the presence of an insulinoma this suppression does not occur.
3 The actual tumour may occasionally be identified by the following:
(a) abdominal CAT scan or ultrasound;
(b) selective coeliac axis arteriography. An abnormal tumour 'blush' is seen in 60−70% of cases;
(c) venous sampling. The portal vein is cannulated transhepatically and blood is sampled from various sites around the pancreas. The level of insulin is measured and can give an indication of the site of a tumour.

Management   The tumour is excised. Medical treatment can be used when the tumour is not found at operation or if there is a malignant tumour with metastases. Diazoxide (5 mg/kg daily in divided doses) suppresses insulin release and is effective in 50% of patients. Streptozotocin (1 g/m² body surface) can be used for malignant insulinomas. It is selectively toxic to malignant islet cells.

Preoperative management
Set up an intravenous infusion of 5−10% dextrose 12 hours before the operation to maintain the blood sugar during the preoperative fast.

Operation: excision of an insulinoma
A laparotomy is performed and the pancreas and surrounding tissues explored to search for the tumour. When it is found, it is excised. If no tumour is found, the surgeon may elect to remove the body and tail of the pancreas in the hope that an impalpable tumour will be found on microscopy. Alternatively, the patient can be treated with diazoxide and re-explored after a period, when the tumour may be larger and easier to find. If a tumour is found, the rest of the pancreas must be palpated to exclude multiple adenomas. A blood sugar may be measured after enucleation. Persistent hypoglycaemia suggests that a second tumour is present.

Codes

Blood	2−4 units	
GA/LA	GA	
Opn time	2−3 hours	
Stay	7−14 days	
Drains out	5−7 days	
Sutures out	7 days	
Off work........	6 weeks........................	

Postoperative care
The remaining beta cells may be suppressed by the chronic hypoglycaemia. When the tumour is removed, rebound hyperglycaemia may develop in the first 4−5 days and insulin therapy may be needed for a short period. There is also a danger of postoperative pancreatitis, and pancreatic sepsis and fistula formation are not uncommon. If a pancreatic fistula develops, the skin must be protected from autodigestion, using a barrier cream. The fistula will usually heal spontaneously in 2−3 weeks.

Zollinger–Ellison syndrome

The condition

In this condition there is excessive production of gastrin by a non-beta cell adenoma often situated in the pancreas. The patient develops severe duodenal and gastric ulceration and his life may be threatened by recurrent haemorrhage or perforation. Fifty per cent of such tumours are malignant and 30% are multiple.

Recognizing the pattern

The usual age at presentation is around 40 and the condition is slightly more common in males. The symptoms and signs are those of an aggressive duodenal ulcer which is difficult to control (see p. 268). The condition should always be considered in patients who develop recurrent ulcers after adequate surgical treatment.

Proving the diagnosis

The diagnosis is proved by finding high serum gastrin levels in spite of a low gastric pH (which normally inhibits gastrin secretion).

The gastric function tests show a raised basal acid output (e.g. over 15 mmol/hour). A barium meal and endoscopy show extensive ulceration and scarring.

Secretin or calcium administration produces an abnormal rise in serum gastrin. This rise is not seen with simple hyperplasia of the antral cells.

Methods of localizing the tumour are the same as those already described for insulinoma.

Management

This may be medical or surgical, and is still controversial. Symptoms may be relieved by cimetidine or ranitidine (cimetidine 1–3 g daily). This may be used either for short-term treatment before operation or in the long term.

Operative treatment is by total gastrectomy. If a tumour is found, it may also be excised at the same time. There is a high incidence of multiple tumours, however, and simple excision of one tumour may not cure the condition. Total gastrectomy is described on p. 282.

Carcinoma of the pancreas

The condition

Carcinoma of the pancreas is an adenocarcinoma arising from the ductal epithelium. Histologically it is usually solid and fibrous (scirrhous) but may be medullary or rarely a cystadenocarcinoma. The incidence is increasing in the UK and the USA. Two-thirds of pancreatic carcinomata occur in the head of the gland and these tend to compress the common bile duct, causing jaundice. A carcinoma in the body and tail may remain undetected until it is quite large. Further spread occurs to the liver, lung and peritoneal cavity.

Recognizing the pattern

The patient
The patient with this disease is typically middle-aged or elderly (aged 50–70).

The history
The presentation is often non-specific with a gradual onset of ill-health and weight loss. If pain is present, it is usually dull and situated deep in the epigastrium. It radiates through to the back. The pain is characteristically relieved by sitting forwards. The disease is sometimes associated with episodes of spontaneous venous thrombosis, 'thrombo-phlebitis migrans'.

On examination
The patient with a carcinoma of the head of the pancreas may be jaundiced and show signs of weight loss. In the presence of jaundice the gall bladder may be palpable as a smooth, rounded mass below the liver. Courvoisier's law states that if the gall bladder is palpable in a case of obstructive jaundice then the cause is unlikely to be gall-stones. (Gall bladders containing stones are usually fibrotic and shrunken.)

Carcinomas of the tail of the pancreas present late and by then a mass is often palpable in the left upper quadrant.

Proving the diagnosis

Ba enema
ERCP
✓ x-ray
CT
USS / arteriogram

LFT

faecal occult blood

This may be very difficult. A barium meal may show fixity and indentation of the posterior wall of the stomach, or indicate a mass enlarging and indenting the duodenal loop. An endoscopic retrograde cholangio-pancreatogram (ERCP) may show visible distortion of the duodenum and narrowing or kinking of the pancreatic duct. An ampullary carcinoma can be visualized and a biopsy taken. Once the diagnosis is suspected, a CAT scan may demonstrate the presence of the mass in the body of the pancreas. Ultrasound and arteriography are also useful. Liver function tests may confirm the obstructive nature of the jaundice (see p. 294). Faecal occult blood tests may be positive if the duodenum is involved. Carcinomas of the body and tail are often only diagnosed with certainty at exploratory laparotomy.

Management

Patients with carcinoma of the pancreas will usually require a laparotomy to confirm the diagnosis and assess curability. Carcinomas of the tail can be resected by distal pancreatectomy. Carcinomas of the head of the pancreas may be resected if they are small and in this case a Whipple's procedure is indicated. Larger growths are incurable by surgery. However, in these cases a bypass operation is undertaken to relieve the obstructive jaundice and potential obstruction of the duodenum. Chemotherapy, especially 5-fluorouracil, can be useful for prolonging life and palliating symptoms.

Preoperative management
A mannitol infusion may be required if the patient is jaundiced (see p. 295). We give prophylactic antibiotics (gentamicin and flucloxacillin). The patient's clotting factors should be checked and vitamin K_1 given if he is jaundiced.

Operation: distal pancreatectomy (Fig. 61)
The splenic vessels are ligated and the spleen removed *en bloc* with the specimen. The cut end of the pancreas is closed and drained.

Codes
Blood	4 units	
GA/LA	GA	
Opn time	2−3 hours	
Stay	2−3 weeks	
Drains out	7−10 days	
Sutures out	7 days	
Off work	About 2 months	

Operation: Whipple's operation (Fig. 61)
In this operation the neck of the pancreas is transected as it runs over the portal vein. The head of the pancreas is removed together with the distal part of the stomach, pylorus and complete duodenal loop up to the duodeno-jejunal flexure. The common bile duct is also divided. The gall bladder may or may not be removed. In the reconstructive phase of the operation the jejunal loop is brought up and anastomosed first to the common bile duct, then to the cut end of the body of the pancreas and finally to the stomach remnant. Drains are inserted through this loop to splint the anastomoses to the common bile duct and pancreatic duct. These stents are usually brought out through the jejunal loop and thence to the surface. A larger drain is put up to the outer surface of the pancreatic anastomosis. A truncal vagotomy may be added in order to reduce gastric acidity and prevent stomal ulceration of the gastro-jejunal anastomosis.

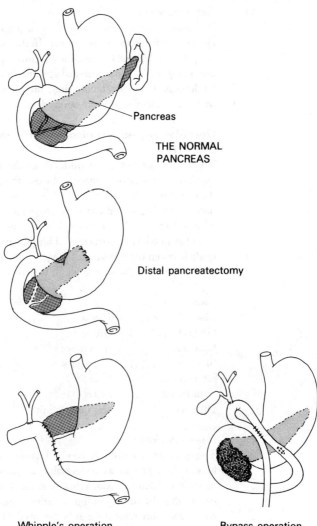

THE NORMAL
PANCREAS

Distal pancreatectomy

Whipple's operation

Bypass operation

Fig. 61. Pancreatic operations.

Codes

Blood	6 units ....
GA/LA	GA ....
Opn time	3−5 hours ....
Stay	3 weeks........................
Drains out	7−10 days ....
Sutures out	7 days ....
Off work........	2−3 months....................

317 SECTION 6.2

Postoperative care

Individual surgeons vary widely in their postoperative management of this complex procedure. In the author's practice the patient is kept nil by mouth until flatus is passed. If there are no signs of anastomotic leakage (increased drainage or tenderness at the operation site), the various stents and drains are removed at about seven days.

Operation: bypass operation for carcinoma of pancreas (Fig. 61)

Three anastomoses are performed. In the first a loop of jejunum is anastomosed either to the common bile duct or to the distended gall bladder, thus relieving the biliary obstruction. Secondly, the stomach is anastomosed to the side of this loop forming a gastro-jejunostomy. This relieves potential duodenal obstruction. Thirdly, an anastomosis is made between the two sides of the jejunal loop in order that food may bypass the loop going to the common bile duct.

Codes

Blood	2 units . . . .
GA/LA	GA . . . .
Opn time	90 minutes . . . .
Stay	7–10 days . . . .
Drains out	0 . . . .
Sutures out	7 days . . . .
Off work	May be indefinite . . . .

Postoperative care

The objective is to produce good palliation and it is essential to keep the patient as comfortable as possible after the operation. Adequate pain relief is given. Care is taken to ensure that the urinary output remains adequate postoperatively and more mannitol may be required. Once the patient has recovered from the operation, a decision is made about whether he or she should also be given chemotherapy.

Pancreatitis

Pancreatitis is inflammation of the pancreas and may be acute, relapsing or chronic.

Acute pancreatitis

The condition

Acute pancreatitis is the term applied to a vicious circle of events which follows damage to the pancreas from a variety of causes. Pancreatic enzyme precursors are released and activated by substances in the inflammatory exudate. The activated enzymes further damage the pancreas and subsequent inflammation and oedema tend to obstruct the pancreatic duct, aggravating the situation.

The disease progresses through well-recognized stages. Resolution may occur at any stage without progression to the next. It is important to understand these stages in order to monitor the patient's progress.

1 *Oedema*. In the first few days the pancreas is markedly oedematous and there is exudation of pancreatic enzymes into the peritoneal cavity resulting in autodigestion of fat and patchy fat necrosis throughout the peritoneum. During this stage the serum amylase will be high and if the process is severe there may be a fall in the serum calcium. The latter may be due to calcium being mopped up by the digested fats to form soaps.

2 *Haemorrhage*. In this next stage the digestion affects blood vessels and there is retroperitoneal bleeding. This phase also occurs early in severe disease, usually during the first week from the onset.

3 *Necrosis*. Once blood vessels have become damaged, there may be infarction of large areas of the pancreatic gland, leading to slough formation.

4 *Abscess and pseudocyst formation*. This occurs in the second to third week. Pseudocyst formation probably occurs as the residual pancreas recovers. Secretions and transudate accumulate in a damaged pancreatic bed and in the lesser sac. If the subsequent collection and residual slough become infected, a pancreatic abscess results.

Recognized causes of pancreatic damage are shown in Table 19.

Table 19. Aetiological factors in acute pancreatitis

1 Biliary disease (55–60% of cases in England)
2 Idiopathic (35–40%)
3 Alcoholic (1–5%)
4 Trauma
  Crush injury
  Abdominal surgery
5 Carcinoma of the pancreas
6 Mumps
7 Hypothermia
8 Drugs, e.g. steroids/thiazides
9 Polyarteritis nodosa
10 Hyperparathyroidism
11 Hyperlipidaemia

Recognizing the pattern

upper abdo pain ↓ *back*
P severe *vomiting usual*
↑ 24h.

Dehydration
shock
fever
jaundice

Grey Turner
Cullen

ΔΔ perf PU
mesenteric Disease
obstruction
MI

The patient

The disease is more common in the middle-aged and elderly. In this country it is usually seen in the type of patient who suffers from gall-stones (see p. 288).

The history

The patient presents with a sudden onset of upper abdominal pain which gradually becomes very severe. It tends to radiate through to the back and is usually associated with vomiting. Over the next 24 hours the patient becomes gradually more and more ill.

On examination

There is generalized abdominal tenderness, maximal in the upper abdomen. The patient also shows signs of dehydration and shock and is generally toxic with a fever. He may also be slightly jaundiced due to obstruction of the common bile duct by oedema or by the stone causing the pancreatitis.

Later careful examination may disclose bruising in the subcutaneous tissue of the flanks (Grey Turner's sign) or even around the umbilicus (Cullen's sign). These signs are due to bleeding from a severe haemorrhagic pancreatitis. Both the history and the signs are rather non-specific and the differential diagnosis includes perforated peptic ulcer, mesenteric infarction, intestinal obstruction and myocardial infarction.

Proving the diagnosis

Amylase >1-2000
ΔΔ PPU MI
acute cholecystitis
↓Hb ↓Ca = BAD
met Hbaemia
haemorrhagic pancreatitis
pseudo of later

The diagnosis is proved by measuring the serum amylase (normal range 80−150 Somogyi units). If this is above 1000−2000 units, acute pancreatitis is extremely likely. Other causes for a moderately raised amylase include a perforated duodenal ulcer, myocardial infarction and acute cholecystitis. The severity of the condition is not related to the amylase level. A falling haemoglobin or a falling calcium in the first few days after the onset or positive faecal occult bloods are of grave prognostic significance and imply the onset of haemorrhagic pancreatitis. Methaemalbuminaemia is also ominous. It is these patients who are likely to progress to pseudocyst or abscess formation in the second and third weeks (see below).

Apart from the amylase, other base-line investigations should include the following:
1 haemoglobin and white cell count;
2 liver function tests and serum calcium;
3 urine test for sugar and bilirubin;
4 a chest X-ray and an abdominal X-ray. These help to exclude a perforated ulcer or intestinal obstruction. They

may show a solitary dilated loop of jejunum which is suffering from localized ileus ('sentinel loop');

5 ECG;

6 blood gases.

After admission the daily progress of the disease is assessed by daily measurement of the following:

(a) urea and electrolytes,

(b) white cell count,

(c) calcium,

(d) urine for sugar content.

These detect any developing renal failure, hyperglycaemia (transient diabetes) or hypocalcaemia, which can then be treated accordingly.

Management
Medical treatment

1 *Bed rest.*

2 *Analgesia.* The pain is often severe and the patient should be written up for pethidine (50–100 mg intramuscularly 4-hourly). Some clinicians also give atropine (0.6 mg 6-hourly) or propantheline (15–30 mg 6-hourly) intravenously. These are to counteract spasm of the sphincter of Oddi.

3 *Blood and fluid replacement.* The oedematous process is associated with a huge loss of fluid into the retroperitoneal tissues, accompanied by a loss of protein and blood if the pancreatitis is severe. This results in oligaemia, which aggravates the tendency to renal failure. It is essential, therefore, to give the patient adequate fluid replacement early on. This should be sufficient to maintain a good urinary output. In the first 24 hours this is mainly fluid and electrolyte replacement. Later plasma and blood should be given. In a severe case of pancreatitis a CVP line should be set up and a urinary catheter inserted to monitor the fluid replacement.

4 *Resting the pancreas.* Every effort is made to minimize the degree of pancreatic stimulation during the disease. The stomach is kept empty by aspiration through a nasogastric tube and no food is given.

5 *Antibiotics.* The use antibiotics in acute pancreatitis is controversial. Some physicians believe it may delay or prevent the onset of late pancreatic sepsis but the evidence for this is not strong.

6 *Trasylol.* This substance acts as a pancreatic enzyme inhibitor but there is no clear evidence to show that it has any value in established pancreatitis.

7 *Glucagon.* Glucagon increases the blood flow to the pancreatic bed and is, therefore, used to try to decrease the amount of pancreatic necrosis. It also diminishes pancreatic

secretion. Again, its value in acute pancreatitis is theoretical rather than proved.

Surgical treatment

Although a few centres practice emergency total pancreatectomy for fulminant acute pancreatitis, operation is not generally required for the type of cases seen in the UK. There are, however, a few indications for operative intervention short of total pancreatectomy.

1 In the acute attack a laparotomy may be indicated to exclude other diseases and to prove the diagnosis of acute pancreatitis. This is, of course, best avoided as a laparotomy adds a further injury to the patient's problems. Where the diagnosis is in doubt, it can be justified. It is safe provided adequate fluid replacement is given preoperatively and postoperatively.

2 Late in the disease there may be a need to operate to drain a pancreatic pseudocyst or abscess. Occasionally patients also require operation because of persistent duodenal ileus (gastroenterostomy).

Management of complications

1 *Renal failure.* Renal failure occurs as a complication of the early stage of acute pancreatitis. Treatment is by peritoneal dialysis or in severe cases by haemodialysis.

2 *Diabetes.* A transient episode of hyperglycaemia is not uncommon in severe pancreatitis and insulin therapy may be needed. However, the diabetes usually recovers later.

3 *Hypocalcaemia.* Ten per cent calcium gluconate (10 ml) may be required once or twice a day.

4 *Pseudocyst formation* — see below.

5 *Duodenal ileus.* This is a rare complication. Although the patient's general health improves, he continues to show signs of duodenal obstruction with vomiting. The condition is due to persistent inflammation on the inner aspect of the duodenal loop. Occasionally a gastroenterostomy is required in order to start the patient feeding again (see p. 271).

6 *Haematemesis and melaena.* This is due to concurrent peptic ulceration.

After recovery

After recovery from the acute attack, identification and treatment of any underlying cause must be carried out so as to prevent recurrence. This may include cholecystectomy and exploration of the common bile duct, parathyroidectomy for hypercalcaemia or treatment of alcoholism. Whatever the cause of the pancreatitis, alcohol should be avoided for 3 months.

Pancreatic pseudocyst

Recognizing the pattern

The patient continues to run a swinging fever and a white count either remains elevated or begins to climb again. The abdomen should be examined regularly and a mass may become palpable in the epigastrium.

Proving the diagnosis

The diagnosis is proved by performing an ultrasound scan. The mass may also be seen displacing the stomach anteriorly on a barium meal.

Most pseudocysts settle spontaneously and a policy of patient observation should be adopted. Indications for operation are failure to resolve after 2−3 weeks, the presence of unremitting distressing pain, or a climbing fever. In the latter case the pseudocyst may have become infected and this is an indication for drainage. This may either be done percutaneously under ultrasound control by a radiologist, or by open operation.

Operation: drainage of a pseudocyst

The pseudocyst is drained by a transgastric approach. A routine laparotomy is performed and the anterior wall of the stomach opened. The posterior wall of the stomach is then incised and the pseudocyst, which is adherent to it, is drained into the stomach. The walls of the cyst are sutured to the gastric mucosa. A tube drain is then placed in the pseudocyst and brought out across the lumen of the stomach through the anterior abdominal wall and skin to the exterior.

Codes

Blood	4 units ....
GA/LA	GA ....
Opn time	1−2 hours ....
Stay	Variable−1 week minimum ....
Drains out	14−21 days (see below) ....
Sutures out	7−10 days ....
Off work........	Variable ....

Postoperative care

Oral fluids can be introduced once the ileus recovers. The transgastric tube is left in place until there is evidence that the cavity has shrunk down (usually about 2 weeks). The size of the cavity can be seen by injecting contrast down the drain and taking X-rays. The first of these is done on the tenth day. Once the tube has been removed, the gastrostomy is sealed with a pad of paraffin gauze and rapidly heals.

Chronic pancreatitis

The condition

In chronic pancreatitis there is gradual destruction and fibrosis of the gland. The pancreatic duct is narrowed and distorted and calculi or diffuse pancreatic calcification may occur.

This condition is associated with diabetes and malabsorption due to the failure of endocrine and exocrine function.

Recognizing the pattern

The patient is in poor health and may have chronic pain. Relapsing chronic pancreatitis is characterized by episodes of epigastric pain and vomiting with associated weakness. Obstructive jaundice may develop. Steatorrhoea, weight loss and diabetes indicate severe disease with failure of pancreatic function.

Proving the diagnosis

A plain abdominal X-ray may show calcification. The amylase is moderately elevated during a relapse. Stool analysis may show steatorrhoea (more than 6 g of fat lost per day). Pancreatic function can be measured by performing a glucose tolerance test and analysing pancreatic secretions (including bicarbonate and enzymes). These are obtained from a tube placed in the duodenum and the pancreas is stimulated with secretin/pancreozymin.

Management

Functional failure is treated medically with a high-protein, high-calorie diet, exogenous enzyme preparations and vitamin replacement. Insulin may be needed.

Surgery is required for pancreatic duct stricture, and a bypass procedure may be needed for obstructive jaundice. In some cases of unremitting pain greater splanchnic nerve resection may be performed.

Operation: for pancreatic duct stricture (Fig. 62)
If the stricture is in the head of the pancreas, a Whipple's operation may be performed. The distended distal duct is anastomosed to a Roux loop of jejunum. Where the stricture is in the neck or body of the gland, the distal distended pancreatic duct may be laid open and a loop of jejunum anastomosed to it side-by-side (pancreatico-jejunostomy). Occasionally there are multiple strictures in the pancreatic duct and such a procedure is not then possible. In these circumstances the whole pancreatic duct may be laid open and anastomosed along the length of the gland to a loop of jejunum (Puestow's operation).

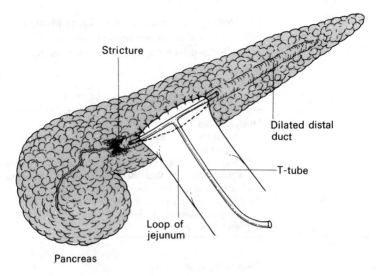

Stricture

Dilated distal duct

T-tube

Loop of jejunum

Pancreas

Fig. 62. Pancreatico-jejunostomy for stricture. A loop of jejunum is anastomosed end-to-side to the dilated pancreatic duct.

Codes

Blood	4 units ....
GA/LA	GA ....
Opn time	2−3 hours ....
Stay	About 2 weeks ....
Drains out	Pancreatic T-tube 10−14 days, after pancreatogram, main drainage tube about 7 days ....
Sutures out	7 days ....
Off work........	6−12 weeks ....

Surgical conditions of the spleen

The spleen is situated in the left upper quadrant of the abdomen protected by the ribcage. It receives blood from the splenic artery, which is a branch of the coeliac plexus. It also receives some blood from the short gastric and left gastroepiploic arteries. Blood returns to the portal system via the splenic vein. The spleen has important immunological functions, clearing antigens from the circulation and producing immunoglobulin M (IgM) and various factors which are important in the phagocytosis of encapsulated bacteria. It also produces lymphocytes and plays a role in red cell maturation.

The spleen can become enlarged as a result of a response to infection, connective tissue disorders, myelo- or lymphoproliferative disorders, infiltration by neoplastic cells from other sites, and in various types of anaemia. The indications for splenectomy can be grouped together as in Table 20.

Table 20. Indications for splenectomy

Hypersplenism
    Myeloproliferative disorders, e.g. myelofibrosis, chronic myeloid
      leukaemia
    Haemolytic anaemia: spherocytosis, elliptocytosis, pyruvate-
      kinase deficiency, thalassaemia, immune haemolytic anaemia
    Platelet disorders: thrombocytopenic purpura
Trauma (see p. 595)
Portal hypertension (see p. 301)
Lymphoma (see p. 154)

Preoperative management
The patient should be immunized against *Pneumococcus* by giving 1 vial of Pneumovax 2 weeks before an elective splenectomy. He or she should also be given pre- and postoperative penicillin (or erythromycin if allergic to penicillin).

Operation: splenectomy
A left subcostal or paramedian incision is performed. The short gastric vessels are divided. The peritoneum lateral to and above the spleen is opened and the spleen and tail of pancreas mobilized to the midline. The splenic flexure of the colon is freed, the splenic vessels divided between the pancreas and the spleen, and the spleen removed.

Codes
Blood	2 units	
GA/LA	GA	
Opn time	60–90 minutes	
Stay	7–10 days	
Drains out	3–7 days	
Sutures out	7 days	
Off work	4 weeks	

Postoperative care
Following splenectomy a number of complications can arise.
1 *Acute dilatation of the stomach.* This is quite common after a splenectomy and can be avoided by adequate aspiration of the stomach until the gastric ileus has fully recovered.
2 *Left basal pulmonary collapse and pneumonia.* Movements of the left base are diminished and it is important to give

adequate analgesia and physiotherapy to protect against this complication.

3 *Subphrenic abscess.* This may follow infection of a haematoma or damage to one of the organs in the neighbourhood of the spleen (see above). The abscess should drain spontaneously through the track provided.

4 *Thrombotic complications.* When the spleen is removed the platelet level rises and if the platelet count goes over 1000×10^9/litre there is a risk of thrombotic complications. Some surgeons use routine anticoagulant prophylaxis after this procedure or give dipyrimadole (50–100 mg 8-hourly) or aspirin (75 mg daily or 150 mg on alternate days) to decrease platelet stickiness until the platelet count falls to less than 1000×10^9/litre.

5 In the long term, patients, especially children, have an increased risk of dying from pneumococcal pneumonia and other infections, such as *Haemophilus influenzae*. They should be immunized after the operation if they have not been preoperatively. It is also reasonable to give penicillin V (250 mg b.d.) to patients for a year postoperatively or to children until the age of 21. Patients remain at a low risk of infection with penicillin-resistant organisms. Erythromycin can be substituted if the patient is allergic to penicillin.

6.3   Adrenal Glands

Adrenal tumours

The adrenal gland consists of an inner medulla and an outer cortex. The medulla originates from neuroectoderm and secretes catecholamines. The cortex develops from mesoderm and produces glucocorticoids, mineralocorticoids and some androgens and oestrogens.

Primary tumours may arise in both parts of the gland and can be benign or malignant. The adrenal gland is also occasionally a site for metastases, particularly from carcinoma of the breast or bronchus or from melanoma.

If the tumour is actively secreting hormones, specific treatment may be required before surgery can safely be undertaken. This section outlines the management of four conditions.

1 Phaeochromocytoma.

2 Cushing's syndrome due to adrenal adenoma or carcinoma.

3 Conn's syndrome due to adrenal adenoma or carcinoma.

4 Adrenal carcinoma.

The initial diagnosis is usually made by the physicians, who then refer the patient for surgery. A detailed account of the presentation and investigation is therefore not included, the emphasis in this section being placed on surgical management.

Phaeochromocytoma

The condition   This is a tumour of chromaffin cells which secretes noradrenaline and adrenaline. There is a familial incidence and an association with medullary carcinoma of the thyroid, parathyroid adenomas and neurofibromatosis (multiple endocrine adenomatosis). It usually occurs as a single benign tumour in the adrenal gland. It is useful to remember that 10% are bilateral, 10% are malignant and 10% arise outside the adrenal gland. Tumours arising from chromaffin cells outside the adrenal gland only secrete noradrenaline.

The tumour causes hypertension and sometimes hyperglycaemia. The hypertension may be persistent or paroxysmal.

Recognizing the pattern	The patient may present with attacks of sweating, pallor, palpitations, angina, nausea and vomiting, abdominal pain, headache and nervousness.
Proving the diagnosis	The diagnosis is proved by finding high concentrations of catecholamine metabolites in the urine (metanephrine, normetanephrine and vanilylmandelic acid (VMA)).

The tumour must be localized. An abdominal mass may be palpable or the blood pressure may rise during deep palpation in a particular site. If metanephrine (from adrenaline) is found in the urine then the tumour lies in the adrenal gland.

Various methods of localization have been used, including arteriography, intravenous pyelogram (IVP) and retroperitoneal air insufflation. The advent of CAT scanning has rendered all the others almost obsolete.

Management The tumour is treated by surgical removal.

Preoperative management
There is usually a degree of hypovolaemia in these patients due to prolonged vasoconstriction. A sudden drop in catecholamine levels as the tumour is removed may cause severe hypotension. The patient should be admitted 5 days before operation and given alpha- and beta-blockers in an attempt to reverse this vasoconstriction and restore blood volume. The drugs used are the following:
(a) Phentolamine (1 mg/kg orally or intravenously). One regime is to start with 10 mg 8-hourly and increase this dose until the blood pressure is controlled. Postural hypotension may occur.
(b) Propranolol (40 mg 8-hourly orally).
An alternative is to use phenoxybenzamine and α-methyl paratyrosine.

The preoperative management must be discussed with the anaesthetist.

Operation: excision of an adrenal phaeochromocytoma
During operation there are two potential problems.
1 Alpha- and beta-blockade inhibits the sympathetic response to hypovolaemia and so a CVP line is needed. A cardiac monitor and arterial line are also used.
2 Handling the tumour may cause a sudden surge in catecholamine levels which, despite the preoperative blockade, may cause a hypertensive crisis. A short-acting alpha-blocker, phentolamine (5 mg intravenously), must be available to treat this. Propranolol (0.5 – 1 mg intravenously) or sodium

nitroprusside (0.5−1.5 µg/kg/minute intravenously) may be used.

The tumour is usually approached trans-abdominally and the whole adrenal gland removed. This can be a difficult procedure, particularly in an obese patient. The contralateral adrenal and the para-aortic area should be examined to exclude other tumours.

Codes

Blood	4−6 units . . . .
GA/LA	GA . . . .
Opn time	2−3 hours . . . .
Stay	About 2 weeks . . . .
Drains out	48 hours . . . .
Sutures out	7 days . . . .
Off work	6 weeks . . . .

Postoperative care
A close watch must be kept on the central venous pressure to detect any hypovolaemia. A blood transfusion may be required. Occasionally an infusion of noradrenaline is needed.

Cushing's syndrome due to adrenal tumour

The condition
Cushing's syndrome is due to excess production of glucocorticoids. This is most commonly secondary to an abnormally high ACTH level, itself produced either by a pituitary adenoma or from an ectopic site (e.g. carcinoma of the bronchus). In 20% of patients with Cushing's syndrome there is a primary lesion in the adrenal gland, either an adenoma or a carcinoma. Adenomas may be bilateral.

Recognizing the pattern
The patient characteristically gains weight and develops a bloated appearance. The syndrome also consists of hypertension, hyperglycaemia and glycosuria, increased protein catabolism and a predisposition to infection.

Proving the diagnosis
The diagnosis is proved by finding an elevated serum cortisol with loss of the normal diurnal variation. There are increased levels of cortisol metabolites in the urine. An adrenal primary lesion is characterized by markedly depressed serum ACTH levels. The tumour can sometimes be localized by plain abdominal X-ray or IVP (showing displacement of the kidney), arteriography or a CAT scan.

Management
The tumour is removed surgically.

Preoperative management

The production of adrenal hormones by tissue other than the tumour will be suppressed and the patient will be unable to respond to the stress of operation by increasing steroid secretion. Supplemental therapy must therefore be prescribed starting at the time of premedication. The usual dose is hydrocortisone 100 mg intravenously or intramuscularly.

Operation: adrenalectomy for Cushing's syndrome

The tumour may either be approached anteriorly or posterolaterally. A postero-lateral approach is used when the tumour site has been positively identified, particularly if it is large and on the right side and the other adrenal has been shown to be normal. This approach may involve opening the pleura, so it is necessary to warn the patient and the anaesthetist of this. A chest drain may be required postoperatively.

During the operation 100–300 mg of hydrocortisone is given intravenously.

Codes

Blood	4–6 units	
GA/LA	GA	
Opn time	2–3 hours	
Stay	2–3 weeks	
Drains out	Chest 2 days, abdominal 2 days	
Sutures out	10–14 days	
Off work	2 months	

Postoperative care

Steroid supplements must be continued. The usual regime is as follows.

1st postop. day:	100 mg hydrocortisone i.m. 8-hourly.
2nd postop. day:	50 mg hydrocortisone i.m. or orally 8-hourly.
3rd postop. day:	50 mg hydrocortisone i.m. or orally 12-hourly.
4th postop. day:	25 mg hydrocortisone i.m. or orally 12-hourly.

After this the steroids may gradually be stopped in the hope that the other adrenal will start working. Occasionally a small dose of ACTH may be required. If, despite this, the other gland does not function, or if both glands have been removed at operation, replacement therapy will be required long term. This is as follows.

Hydrocortisone	20–30 mg/day
Fludrocortisone	0.1–0.2 mg/day

— in twice daily dosage, two-thirds given in the morning and one-third in the evening.

During the first 24—48 hours the blood pressure should be measured half-hourly to detect evidence of steroid insufficiency. A close watch must be kept on the electrolytes and blood sugar. If any complications arise, the steroid supplements must be increased.

Cushingoid patients are more susceptible to postoperative complications such as poor wound healing, wound infection or haemorrhage.

Conn's syndrome

The condition

This is due to excessive production of aldosterone by an adenoma of the glomerulosa cells of the adrenal gland. Occasionally it is due to bilateral hyperplasia. Carcinoma is a rare cause.

The syndrome is characterized by hypertension, renal damage, hypokalaemic alkalosis and muscle weakness.

Proving the diagnosis

Investigations show a high urinary potassium content despite a low serum potassium and a high serum bicarbonate. The serum aldosterone level is elevated.

Localization of the tumour is difficult as it is often small and may be multiple and bilateral. However, it may sometimes be identified by an intravenous urogram, venogram, arteriogram, CAT scan or differential venous sampling studies.

Management

The tumour must be removed.

Preoperative management
The body is potassium-depleted and this should be corrected before operation by a high-potassium, low-sodium diet. Spironolactone (200—400 mg/day) also helps. Steroid supplements as above should start with the premedication.

Operation: adrenalectomy for Conn's syndrome
An anterior approach is used. The tumour is removed and the other adrenal palpated. If no tumour is found, the left gland is resected and sliced up (the left gland is more commonly affected than the right). If this gland is normal, then the right may be partially or completely removed.

Hydrocortisone may be required during operation as described above.

Codes

Blood	4–6 units ....
GA/LA	GA ....
Opn time	2–3 hours ....
Stay	2–3 weeks ....
Drains out	Chest 2 days, abdominal 2 days .....
Sutures out	7 days ....
Off work	6 weeks ....

Postoperative care

Replacement therapy may be required as above.

Adrenal carcinoma

The condition

Carcinoma may occasionally present with no evidence of endocrine disturbance. It is usually fast-growing with rapid invasion and early metastases. It presents with loin discomfort, weight loss and possibly a palpable mass. It is localized with the aid of an abdominal X-ray, intravenous urogram, venogram, arteriogram or CAT scan.

Management

Removal must be accompanied by steroid supplements as outlined above.

For the operation note, codes and postoperative management, see under Adrenalectomy for Cushing's syndrome, p. 331.

Central Abdominal Pain

The condition

Acute appendicitis

This is the commonest surgical emergency in this country. The appendix has a narrow lumen and there is a rich collection of lymphatic tissue in the submucosa. Obstruction of the lumen can follow impaction of a faecalith or swelling of the submucosal lymphatic tissue. Once this occurs, a vicious circle ensues with further swelling and obstruction, blockage of blood supply, infection and ischaemia of the distal appendix.

Recognizing the pattern

The patient

Acute appendicitis can occur at any age, although it is particularly common between the ages of 10 and 30.

The history

The typical history is of central abdominal colic associated with nausea and vomiting. After a few hours the colic subsides and the pain settles in the right iliac fossa. At this stage the pain is worse on movement (walking, coughing).

On examination

The patient looks unwell and is flushed. There is often a fetor. The tongue is furred and the patient has a low-grade pyrexia, typically of 37.5°C (99.5°F). The fever is very rarely above 38.0°C (100.4°F) in the early stages of the disease. There is also a tachycardia.

Examination of the abdomen discloses marked tenderness in the right iliac fossa with guarding and rebound. By careful palpation it is usually possible to delineate a constant line of tenderness over the site of the appendix.

This localized tenderness is the single most important factor in making the diagnosis. Rectal examination may also disclose tenderness high up on the right side, especially if the appendix is in a pelvic position.

The clinical picture of appendicitis does, of course, vary widely and the presentation may be particularly confusing in the very young and the very old. A localized line of tenderness, together with signs of peritonitis, will indicate the need for operative exploration.

Proving the	Surprisingly there are no absolute tests to prove or disprove
diagnosis	the diagnosis of acute appendicitis. If the suspicion is strong

enough, a laparotomy must be performed in order to exclude
the disease.

Management   *Preoperative management*

The patient must be adequately rehydrated before operation
and the value of giving preoperative antibiotics with the
premedication has been demonstrated. A metronidazole
suppository is effective.

Operation: appendicectomy

The abdomen is opened through a grid-iron incision situated
in the right iliac fossa. The appendix lies under McBurney's
point, which is on a line between the anterior superior iliac
spine and the umbilicus, two-thirds of the way from the
umbilicus. The incision is best made almost horizontally in
Langer's lines (see Fig. 63). The muscles of the abdominal
wall are split in the line of their fibres (grid-iron incision)
and the peritoneum opened. The presence or absence of
peritoneal fluid is noted and a swab taken. The upper part of
the caecum is grasped and pulled out of the wound towards
the patient's feet. After completing this manoeuvre, the
caecum is then pulled upwards towards the patient's head
and the appendix is thus delivered. It may be necessary to
free adhesions in order to achieve this. With a retrocaecal
appendix it is necessary to mobilize the lower pole of the
caecum by dividing the peritoneum laterally. The appendix
stump is crushed and tied with catgut. The appendicular

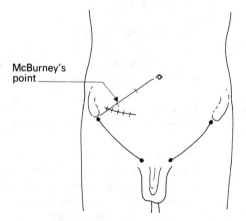

Fig. 63. Appendicectomy: the incision is made just below
McBurney's point, horizontally parallel to Langer's skin lines.

vessels are tied and the appendix is removed. The terminal 100 cm of small bowel is gently examined to see if there is a coincident Meckel's diverticulum. A drain is inserted into the peritoneum if there is pus at the appendix site. The wound may also be drained.

Codes

Blood	0 ....
GA/LA	GA ....
Opn time	15−30 minutes ....
Stay	5−7 days ....
Drains out	3−5 days ....
Sutures out	7 days ....
Off work	4 weeks ....

Postoperative care
The postoperative ileus is usually short-lived and fluids can be reintroduced orally after about 24 hours. Thereafter the postoperative recovery is usually uneventful. A careful watch must be kept for developing sepsis in the wound or in the pelvis. The temperature chart is the best guide to this (see p. 69).

The wound must be inspected before the patient leaves hospital and a rectal examination should also be done. Surgeons vary widely in their use of antibiotics in and around the time of an appendicectomy. If antibiotics are given post-operatively, it has to be remembered that abscess formation may be delayed and the patient and his doctor should be warned of this.

For the management of wound abscess and pelvic abscess, see pp. 68 and 75.

Mesenteric adenitis

The condition

The mesenteric lymph nodes may become inflamed as part of a general infection or a gastroenteritis. The importance of the condition lies in differentiating it from acute appendicitis.

Recognizing the pattern

The patient
The patient is usually under the age of 30.

The history
The complaint is of abdominal pain. This may be generalized or localized, possibly in the right iliac fossa. There may be symptoms of diarrhoea and/or vomiting, or of a recent upper respiratory tract infection.

On examination
The tenderness tends to be moderate with little guarding or rebound, and poorly localized. The patient may be pyrexial, often with a fever above 37.5°C.

Proving the diagnosis

A laparotomy may be indicated to exclude acute appendicitis. In that case the appendix is normal and large inflamed fleshy lymph nodes are seen in the mesentery. Otherwise the diagnosis is clinical and there are no specific confirmatory tests.

Management

If appendicitis can be excluded, the management is conservative and the patient can be allowed home.

Intestinal obstruction

The condition

The bowel may become obstructed from a variety of causes anywhere along its length. The obstruction may be mechanical or adynamic (localized or generalized paralytic ileus). Mechanical causes are usefully divided into those which compress the bowel from the outside, those which arise within the wall of the bowel and obstruct the lumen, and those which arise within the lumen (see Table 21). Paralytic ileus is described on p. 45.

Recognizing the pattern

The patient
The patient can be of any age from a newborn baby onwards.

The history
The patient complains of colicky central abdominal pains.

Table 21. Mechanical causes of intestinal obstruction

Outside the bowel	Adhesions or bands	p. 339
	Volvulus	p. 367
	Invasion by neighbouring malignant growths	
	Strangulated hernia, etc.	p. 395
In the bowel wall	Tumours	p. 344
	Infarction	p. 340
	Congenital atresia	pp. 555–565
	Hirschsprung's disease	p. 564
	Inflammatory bowel disease	pp. 342, 346
	Diverticulitis	p. 363
In the lumen	Impacted faeces	p. 40
	Bolus obstruction	
	Gall-stone ileus	p. 288
	Intussusception	pp. 344, 546
	Large polyps	pp. 344, 352

Some time after the onset of the colic, the patient begins to vomit and there is total constipation. The intervals between the waves of colic give some idea of the site of the obstruction. Higher obstruction is associated with a short interval between bouts of pain whereas obstruction of the ileum has longer intervals. Vomiting also occurs earlier in high intestinal obstruction. The three symptoms of abdominal pain, vomiting, and absolute constipation are almost diagnostic of intestinal obstruction.

On examination
The patient may be dehydrated due to fluid losses into the intestine and vomiting, and there may be visible peristalsis under the abdominal wall. The degree and site of abdominal distension varies with the level of obstruction. The distended loops of obstructed small bowel are often tender on palpation. On auscultation there are hyperactive high-pitched bowel sounds.

Proving the diagnosis

The diagnosis is proved by performing a supine and erect abdominal X-ray, which shows the presence of distended loops of small bowel together with fluid levels (see Fig. 64). If the colon is obstructed the caecum will also be distended.

Management

The initial management of small bowel obstruction is to replenish the fluid loss and keep the bowel empty by nasogastric suction. In many cases this will relieve the condition. Indications for operation are failure of conservative treatment after 48−72 hours, or a general deterioration in the patient's condition and the onset of abdominal tenderness and a

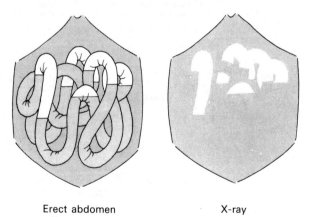

Erect abdomen   X-ray

Fig. 64. Fluid levels in obstructed small bowel.

tachycardia. These latter signs may indicate that part of the bowel is becoming ischaemic.

Operation: for intestinal obstruction
The procedure undertaken depends on the underlying cause.

(a) Intestinal adhesions
The adhesions are divided and loops of bowel mobilized so as to free the obstruction. Occasionally it is necessary to resect a damaged segment of small bowel.

(b) Volvulus
The volvulus is untwisted and the viability of the bowel checked. The surgeon may wait to see whether a dubious segment of bowel regains its colour satisfactorily after a period.

(c) Strangulated hernia
The hernia is repaired and the bowel dealt with as above.

Codes

Blood	2 units . . . .
GA/LA	GA . . . .
Opn time	Variable, depends on cause . . . .
Stay	Variable 1–2 weeks . . . .
Drains out	Nasogastric tube out when flatus passed; other drains according to general principles (see p. 120) . . . . .
Sutures out	7–10 days . . . .
Off work	Variable . . . .

Other causes of intestinal obstruction are dealt with in other sections (see Table 21, p. 337).

Meckel's diverticulum

The condition
This lesion is a remnant of the attachment of the small bowel to the embryological yolk sac. It arises from the antemesenteric border somewhere along the distal 100 cm of small bowel. The diverticulum may contain remnants of all types of intestinal mucosa (including acid-secreting gastric mucosa).

Recognizing the pattern
The patient may be of any age, although problems from a Meckel's diverticulum are more common in children.

The history
The lesion may remain asymptomatic for the whole of the

patient's life. If it does cause trouble, however, the presentation is in one of three ways.

1 *The picture of acute appendicitis.* This is due to obstruction of the lumen of the diverticulum in exactly the same way as the appendix becomes obstructed. This presentation is not common as the diverticulum usually has a wide neck.

2 *The picture of intestinal obstruction.* This is often due to the fact that the Meckel's diverticulum is associated with a band running up to the umbilicus and this may obstruct other loops of bowel.

3 *Intestinal bleeding.* If the diverticulum contains gastric mucosa a peptic ulcer may arise in the adjacent ileum. This bleeds and the patient passes fresh blood per rectum. This is perhaps the most common presentation of a Meckel's diverticulum in children.

Proving the diagnosis

This is difficult and frequently a laparotomy is necessary. An attempt should be made to define the diverticulum using radio-active technetium scanning, but this is not always reliable. The lesion may be demonstrated on a barium meal and 'follow-through', or even a barium enema, but again the investigation is unreliable. For this reason, if there is a strong suspicion that a Meckel's diverticulum might be present, a laparotomy is undertaken.

Management

Operation: for Meckel's diverticulum
The diverticulum is resected and the small bowel closed. If there is an ulcer in the ileum, this segment of ileum is resected together with the diverticulum. The appendix may be taken out in the same operation to avoid diagnostic confusion later.

Codes
Blood . . . .   0 (babies may require one unit) . . . . . .
GA/LA . . . .   GA . . . .
Opn time . . . .   1 hour . . . .
Stay . . . .   5−7 days . . . .
Drains out . . . . . .   0 . . . .
Sutures out . . . . .   7 days . . . .
Off work . . . .   3−4 weeks . . . .

Ischaemic bowel

The condition

Ischaemic bowel may arise either secondary to some of the causes of intestinal obstruction, or as a primary condition from interruption of the arterial or venous blood supply. This is usually due to an embolus from the heart or great vessels or due to thrombosis. Bowel infarction is a life-threatening condition and early laparotomy is mandatory. In this section primary ischaemia of the bowel will be considered. A more recent cause of intestinal necrosis is gas gangrene of the small intestine occurring in neutropenic patients while under treatment for leukaemia.

Recognizing the pattern

The patient
The patient is usually elderly and may have other signs of cardiac or vascular disease.

The history
The patient complains of a sudden onset of abdominal pain which rapidly becomes very severe. The patient becomes very distressed and shocked. There may be a history of recent myocardial infarction or arrhythmia.

On examination
The signs may not seem to coincide with the severity of the patient's pain. There is usually some localized tenderness but not a lot in the way of guarding or rebound tenderness in the early stages. Rectal examination may reveal blood. The patient may be in atrial fibrillation.

Proving the diagnosis

The most important point to remember is the possibility of bowel ischaemia in undiagnosed severe abdominal pain. Straight abdominal X-ray may show a slightly dilated loop of bowel with thickened walls. The serum amylase should be measured to exclude pancreatitis. Remember that mesenteric infarction can cause a slightly elevated level (600–900 Somogyi units).

Management

Preoperative management
Before laparotomy, resuscitation may be required to treat shock. Broad-spectrum parenteral antibiotics must be given.

Operation: laparotomy for ischaemic bowel
At operation the ischaemic loop of bowel is identified. Various causes may be found. The ischaemia may be secondary to a volvulus or band causing obstruction of the mesenteric vessels. In this case treatment of the cause may result in adequate perfusion of the ischaemic segment.

Another possible cause is embolism or thrombosis of one of the major arteries supplying the bowel. If the bowel is still potentially viable, an embolectomy or bypass operation may be performed to restore the blood supply. Any bowel which fails to recover must be resected. Occasionally where there is a long loop of ischaemic bowel and viability is dubious, it may be permissible to close the abdomen and take a second look after 24−36 hours to determine the viability of the bowel.

Codes

Blood	2 units . . . .
GA/LA	GA . . . .
Opn time	1−2 hours . . . .
Stay	7−10 days . . . .
Drains out	0 . . . .
Sutures out	7 days . . . .
Off work	Variable; at least 4 weeks but usually affected by the patient's general condition . . . .

Postoperative care

The patient is given intravenous fluids and nasogastric suction until flatus is passed and bowel function restored.

Intussusception in adults

Intussusceptions are much commoner in children and are dealt with on p. 546. The management in the adult is very similar, although open operation through a vertical incision, and not reduction by barium enema, is the method of choice. This is because there is almost always a causative lesion in an adult, such as a polyp or a leiomyoma, which forms the head of the intussusception. This will need to be resected.

Crohn's disease

The condition

Crohn's disease is a chronic inflammatory condition affecting the small or large bowel (or even the stomach). It is of unknown aetiology. It produces characteristic granulomas through the full thickness of the bowel wall (unlike ulcerative colitis, which only involves the mucosa). These progress to fissure formation and sepsis around the bowel, and eventually to fistulae and strictures.

Recognizing the pattern

The patient

He is usually between the ages of 15 and 55, and loss of weight is common in long-standing disease.

The history

1 Small bowel Crohn's disease presents either with chronic diarrhoea or with episodes of colicky abdominal pain due to obstruction. In acute terminal ileitis the picture is similar to appendicitis. In chronic disease there is often severe constitutional disturbance, e.g. lassitude, anaemia and weight loss.

2 Large bowel Crohn's disease presents with diarrhoea and frequently with perianal sepsis. Crohn's perianal fistulae are difficult to treat, tend to heal very slowly, and cause the patient a great deal of distress.

On examination
The patient may be pyrexial. In acute Crohn's disease a tubular mass may be palpable in the right iliac fossa. Otherwise there may be tenderness anywhere in the abdomen. Look carefully for signs of perianal sepsis.

Proving the diagnosis

The diagnosis is confirmed by a barium 'follow-through' study. The affected gut is seen with a thick wall and a narrow lumen ('string sign'). There are ulcers and fissures in the bowel, which are seen as spicules of barium or cobblestoning. The affected areas of the bowel are intermingled with normal bowel ('skip lesions'). Fistulae may be present. A biopsy shows the characteristic non-caseating granulomas.

The patient may have abnormal liver function tests (hypoalbuminaemia), and anaemia and an elevated sedimentation rate. The affected area of the bowel shows up on an indium scan.

Management

The main treatment of Crohn's disease is medical. Drugs used are sulphasalazine and steroids. Immunosuppression with azathioprine can also be effective.

Surgery should be avoided in an acute exacerbation because of the risk of fistula and abscess formation. If the disease presents as an episode of intestinal obstruction, this is managed conservatively for as long as possible. If Crohn's disease is found at laparotomy for suspected appendicitis, the bowel should not be opened.

Operative treatment is eventually required in 70−80% of cases to resect or bypass diseased bowel. As several areas of the bowel are affected, a long length may need to be resected in small bowel Crohn's disease. In large bowel Crohn's disease a panproctocolectomy may be required.

Preoperative management
Check that the serum proteins are satisfactory. If they are not, a period of intravenous feeding may be indicated. With large bowel Crohn's disease a bowel preparation is undertaken (p. 110). The operation will usually be covered by antibiotics. If the patient is already on steroids, the steroids must be increased preoperatively (pp. 27−28).

Operation: small bowel resection for Crohn's disease
The affected bowel is resected with an adequate margin and an end-to-end anastomosis is performed.

Codes

Blood	2 units	....
GA/LA	GA	....
Opn time	90–150 minutes	....
Stay	7–14 days	....
Drains out	7 days	....
Sutures out	7 days	....
Off work	6–8 weeks	....

Postoperative care
Nasogastric suction and intravenous fluids are continued until the patient has passed flatus. The care of patients on steroids postoperatively is dealt with on p. 27. The patient with severe Crohn's disease is often debilitated, and intravenous feeding may be continued postoperatively. Whenever an area of Crohn's disease has been resected, there is a danger of fistula formation. The patient should be kept in hospital long enough to make sure that this danger has passed (7–14 days).

Long-term follow-up will be needed as there is a tendency for the disease to recur. Recurrent disease can be monitored by performing an indium scan and measuring acute-phase proteins.

Operation: panproctocolectomy
See p. 348.

Small bowel tumours

The condition Small bowel tumours are rare. Benign tumours include adenomas, lipomas and leiomyomas. They may bleed, causing melaena and anaemia, and they can cause intussusception. Multiple hamartomatous polyps of the small bowel occur in association with melanin pigmentation of the lips and oral mucosa as part of the Peutz–Jeghers syndrome. Malignant change is rare.

Primary malignant tumours include the lymphosarcoma, spindle cell sarcoma and carcinoma. Again they present with symptoms of bleeding (melaena and anaemia), intestinal obstruction or general carcinomatosis. The bowel wall may perforate, causing acute peritonitis.

Carcinoid tumour is a malignant growth of the Kulchitsky cells (argentaffin cells, APUD system). Sixty-five per cent arise in the appendix and 25% in the ileum. Other primary sites include the rest of the gut and, very rarely, the bronchus, testis and ovary. The tumour may excrete serotonin and kinins (and possibly prostaglandins and histamine), resulting in the carcinoid syndrome. The main features of this are flushing attacks (precipitated by alcohol), diarrhoea, episodic bronchospasm and pulmonary stenosis. This only occurs once there are metastases in the liver, because hormones from the primary in the gut are detoxified in the hepatic circulation.

Proving the diagnosis

Small bowel tumours are often only found at laparotomy (e.g. for intussusception or bleeding). Occasionally, a barium meal may reveal a lesion in the duodenum or upper jejunum. Carcinoid syndrome is proved by demonstrating elevated levels of 5-hydroxyindole acetic acid (5-HIAA, the breakdown product of serotonin) in the urine (normal range is 2–20 mg in 24 hours). In this case a liver scan or CAT scan will show evidence of secondaries in the liver.

Management

Benign tumours are resected if they are causing symptoms of bleeding or obstruction. Malignant tumours are treated by wide excision including the local mesenteric nodes. Metastases in the liver are often found at operation. Partial hepatectomy may be considered for metastases although the tumour is very slow-growing and the patient may be managed conservatively for many years. Drugs used to control the carcinoid syndrome include methysergide, antihistamines and α-methyldopa. Another alternative is selective embolization or infusion of 5-fluorouracil in the hepatic artery.

Operations
1 See Intussusception, p. 342.
2 See Small bowel resection, p. 343.
3 See Right hemicolectomy, p. 354.

Colorectal Presentations and Skeletal Pain

Ulcerative colitis

The condition

Ulcerative colitis is a condition of unknown aetiology affecting the colon and rectum. It starts distally and may spread any distance proximally up the large bowel. Twenty per cent of cases involve the rectum only, 45% involve the rectum and part of the colon, while 35% involve the whole of the large bowel. The mucosa of the colon becomes ulcerated and tends to bleed. In severe acute disease the colonic wall may become very thin and lose its strength. There is a danger of perforation. This condition is called toxic megacolon and is an acute surgical emergency.

In long-standing disease there is a risk of carcinomatous change occurring in the large bowel.

Recognizing the pattern

The patient

The disease may affect patients of any age, although they are usually between the ages of 15 and 55. The sufferer is often thin. Many patients with ulcerative colitis are diagnosed as having mental illness, although it is probable that their mental condition is secondary to the diarrhoea rather than the other way round.

The history

The patient suffers from a marked increase in frequency of defaecation. This occurs in episodes, with periods of remission. The bowel frequency may go up to 8−12 times a day during an attack. The motion is liquid and there is blood and mucus in the stool. The patient also suffers with abdominal pain.

On examination

There may be tenderness over the colon in acute extensive disease, and the abdomen may be distended. On rectal examination there is a spongy feel to the mucosa and blood and mucus are noted on the examining glove.

Proving the diagnosis

The diagnosis is proved on sigmoidoscopy when the inflamed, haemorrhagic mucosa can be clearly seen. During this examination it may be possible to determine the upper extent of the disease. A biopsy should always be taken, as this is diagnostic and may help to differentiate the disorder from Crohn's disease. A barium enema or colonoscopy will also demonstrate the extent of the ulceration and in long-standing disease should be used to exclude secondary neo-plastic change.

Management

An acute attack is treated with bed rest, intravenous infusion and replacement therapy, together with steroids (e.g. pred-nisolone 60 mg/day). Sulphasalazine and antibiotics may also be used.

EXCLUDE TOXIC MEGACOLON (handwritten margin note)

The management of a severe case of acute colitis is dominated by the need to exclude and manage toxic mega-colon. In this condition the mucosa is lost and the colonic wall becomes very thin and distended. After a certain point the bowel wall is so badly damaged that there is no hope of recovery. Left untreated the colon will perforate and the subsequent peritonitis is frequently fatal. If the case is to be managed successfully, the colon must be removed before perforation occurs.

A case of acute colitis should therefore be managed jointly by the physicians and surgeons. The patient is given an increased dose of steroids and kept on bed rest in hospital. Daily abdominal X-rays are performed and the colonic diameter measured. If the pulse rate is steadily rising and the colonic diameter increases to over 8 cm, surgery should be considered.

Other investigations which help in assessing the severity of the disease, and are usually monitored daily, include:
1 haemoglobin and white cell count;
2 ESR;
3 urea and electrolytes (especially the potassium);
4 liver function tests (especially to monitor the serum albumin).

The indications for emergency surgery are as follows:
1 toxic megacolon (see above);
2 haemorrhage;
3 perforation;
4 failed medical treatment: this can be said to occur if the patient, despite adequate treatment, has:
   (a) persistent diarrhoea;
   (b) pyrexia more than 38°C;
   (c) tachycardia or increasing abdominal tenderness; or
   (d) a falling haemoglobin or serum albumin.

The indications for elective surgery include the following:
1 failed medical treatment, with chronic poor general health;
2 prolonged history (over 10 years);
3 malignant change.

Preoperative management

The patient must be made as fit as possible. Dehydration, anaemia and hypoproteinaemia are corrected. Bowel preparation is not usually indicated.

The necessity for operation must be explained to the patient, including the dangers inherent in leaving the diseased colon *in situ*. They must be told what the operation will entail, and that a permanent ileostomy may be required. This usually comes as a shock to the patients, although those who have had intermittent diarrhoea for many years may welcome the decision. The site of the ileostomy should be marked with the patient standing. It may be useful to introduce the patient to others who have had an ileostomy, as this can markedly diminish the fear of the unknown. The Ileostomy Association is particularly valuable in this regard. The hospital's stoma therapist should also be involved.

Operations

Three possible operations will be described here.
1 Panproctocolectomy and terminal ileostomy.
2 Total colectomy and ileo-rectal anastomosis.
3 Loop ileostomy.

Operation: panproctocolectomy and terminal ileostomy

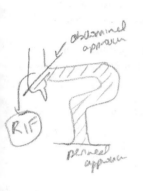

The whole colon is removed from the caecum to the anus using two incisions, one abdominal and the other perineal. The operation is frequently performed by two teams working at once, as in an abdomino-perineal resection of the rectum. A terminal ileostomy is brought out in the right iliac fossa and this is formed by eversion of the last part of the ileum. The empty pelvis is drained via the perineal wound (or occasionally via the vagina). Abdominal drains may also be inserted.

Codes

Blood	6 units ....
GA/LA	GA ....
Opn time	3−5 hours ....
Stay	10−14 days ....
Drains out	Perineum 5 days, abdominal 3−7 days, nasogastric tube until ileostomy is working properly ....
Sutures out	7−10 days ....
Off work........	2−3 months...................

Postoperative care
This is the same as for an abdomino-perineal resection of the rectum and is described on p. 363.

Operation: total colectomy and ileo-rectal anastomosis
The colon is removed but the rectal stump is left *in situ*. This leaves an option to re-anastomose the terminal ileum to it, either at the initial operation or as a secondary procedure. There is a risk of recurrent disease in the rectal stump. The terminal ileum may be fashioned into a pouch (Park's pouch) to form a reservoir above the rectal stump. In this operation the rectal mucosa is excised and the pouch anastomosed to the dentate line.

Codes

Blood	4 units
GA/LA	GA
Opn time	2–4 hours
Stay	10–14 days
Drains out	Pelvic 7 days, nasogastric tube 3–4 days
Sutures out	7–10 days
Off work	2–3 months

Operation: loop ileostomy
In certain circumstances the bowel contents can be diverted from the colon by bringing out a loop of ileum in much the same way as a loop colostomy is performed. This may allow the colonic disease to settle but recurrence is common if the ileostomy is closed.

Codes

Blood	2 units
GA/LA	GA
Opn time	1 hour
Stay	7–10 days
Drains out	0
Sutures out	7–10 days
Off work	Variable

Rectal bleeding in adults
Common causes of fresh rectal bleeding in adults include:
Haemorrhoids (p. 382).
Anal fissure (p. 387).
Inflammatory bowel disease (pp. 342, 346).
Neoplasms – benign or malignant (pp. 353–363).
Diverticular disease (p. 363).

Meckel's diverticulum (p. 339).
Rectal bleeding in children is dealt with on p. 553.
If the blood is old and black, a bleeding lesion higher up in the bowel must obviously be considered. Blood from the upper colon and above will be mixed in with the motion. In lower rectal bleeding the blood is coated on the outside of the motion and is noted in the pan and on the toilet paper.

Investigation

A full history and examination should be taken and particular attention paid to the presence of abdominal masses and tenderness. On rectal examination, note whether the examination is painful or not and whether the anal sphincter is tight or not. A painful examination may indicate a fissure. A tight sphincter is often associated with other perianal pathology such as piles or fissures. Also on rectal examination, feel high up to note whether there is a palpable neoplasm in the rectum or even in the sigmoid colon. The latter is felt outside the rectum lying in the pelvis. An area of diverticulitis may be felt as a tender mass high up on the left side.

All adults presenting with rectal bleeding should have a proctoscopy and sigmoidoscopy.

On proctoscopy the surgeon can note the presence of piles and whether the surface is haemorrhagic or not. An anal fissure can be seen or excluded. If the examination is impossible due to pain, then a fissure is likely.

On sigmoidoscopy the presence of blood and mucus in the bowel can be seen and a tumour within the rectum looked for. The character of the rectal mucosa and any evidence of proctitis can be noted. Any tumour or suspicious area of mucosa can be biopsied.

A barium enema should also be performed looking for polyps or carcinomas of the colon, and noting the presence or absence of diverticular disease.

The management of the condition found is dealt with under the appropriate section.

Change in bowel habit

A change in bowel habit is a serious symptom and must always be investigated if it persists for more than 3 weeks, especially if the patient is over 30. It is most commonly due to colonic disease and possible causes include the following.
Inflammation: ulcerative colitis, Crohn's disease, diverticular disease.
Neoplasia: polyps, carcinoma of the colon.
Other less common causes of a change in bowel habit are pancreatic disease, chronic mesenteric ischaemia, and gastric

and small bowel obstruction. These will not be considered further here.

Making a diagnosis

A full history is taken in order to determine the patient's normal bowel habit and the nature of the change. The changes in consistency and character of the motion and the presence of blood and mucus must be determined. With inflammatory large bowel disease (ulcerative colitis or Crohn's) there is a marked increase in frequency of defaecation and blood and mucus in the stool. This often lasts several weeks at a time with periods of normality between. The stools are watery.

With obstruction of the left side of the colon or rectum the patient suffers from continued alternating constipation and diarrhoea, usually occurring in cycles of a few days (see p. 355). This picture is seen in carcinoma of the left side of the colon or rectum or in diverticular disease with stricture formation.

With a sigmoid volvulus the patient has intermittent attacks of total constipation associated with abdominal pain and marked distension. In diverticular disease uncomplicated by stricture formation, there is an acute episode of severe, left-sided abdominal pain and diarrhoea which usually resolves completely. The motions are loose during the attack and may be pellet-like at other times.

A full examination is indicated and obviously a rectal examination must be included.

Sigmoidoscopy

This is done to look for a rectal lesion and the presence of blood and mucus coming down from a lesion higher up. Inflammatory disease of the mucosa is visible and can be biopsied. The nature of the stool in the rectum can provide valuable confirmatory evidence of the patient's history. Hard, rabbit pellet motions may be seen in the presence of diverticular disease.

Proctoscopy

This should be undertaken to look for the presence of piles. Patients sometimes complain of frequency of defaecation when they have piles as they believe they are not emptying their rectum fully due to the discomfort produced by the piles.

A barium enema

This is always indicated where there is a change in bowel habit in order to look for colonic polyps or a carcinoma.

The further management of a change in bowel habit is dealt with under the individual conditions as below.
Carcinoma of the colon (p. 353).
Carcinoma of the rectum (p. 359).
Diverticular disease (p. 363).
Sigmoid volvulus (p. 367).
Crohn's disease (p. 342).
Ulcerative colitis (p. 346).

Colonic polyps

The condition

Polyps of the colon may be either single or multiple. Familial polyposis coli is a condition of extensive polyposis of the large bowel, inherited as an autosomal dominant.

Benign adenomas may be either sessile or pedunculated. A villous adenoma is well differentiated and sessile, with a frond-like surface. Malignant change is common, particularly in familial polyposis. The polyps may bleed, or secrete mucus rich in potassium.

Other rare polyps include juvenile polyps, hamartomatous polyps of the Peutz–Jeghers syndrome, haemangiomas and lipomas. Metaplastic polyps are very common and are due to dysplasia rather than a neoplasm.

Recognizing the pattern

The patient
He is usually adult. The polyps of familial polyposis appear after puberty in the late teens, and affect men more commonly than women. Solitary polyps are rare before the age of 40.

The history
The patient may present with anaemia, or increased bowel frequency with mucous diarrhoea. Polyps may cause intussusception and intestinal obstruction. Familial polyposis coli may produce a picture resembling ulcerative colitis, with episodes of abdominal pain, loss of weight, diarrhoea and the passage of blood and mucus. Symptoms suggesting malignant change include weight loss, anorexia and a further change in bowel habit.

On examination
There is often nothing abnormal to find. A polyp in the rectum may be palpable or seen on sigmoidoscopy. It is usually a soft tumour protruding into the lumen. A hard area within it suggests malignant change.

Proving the diagnosis

The diagnosis is proved by sigmoidoscopic biopsy and barium enema. The faeces may be positive for occult blood. Other relevant investigations include a full blood count to look for anaemia, and serum electrolytes to check the potassium level. Profuse haemorrhage from a haemangioma can sometimes be localized by arteriography.

Management

Adenomatous polyps over 1 cm in diameter must be removed because of the risk of malignant change. If the polyp is solitary, it can be removed by local excision either through a colonoscope or by laparotomy. Familial polyposis coli may have to be treated by total colectomy. If the rectum is not seriously involved, a low ileo-rectal anastomosis is fashioned. Otherwise ileostomy is required.

The operation of total colectomy is described on p. 348.

Postoperative care
In familial polyposis coli, if there is a rectal stump, regular follow-up with sigmoidoscopy is required and any polyps found are treated by diathermy. Other members of the family must also be examined regularly until the age of 50. Anyone who has a colonic polyp removed should also be followed up regularly.

Carcinoma of the colon

The condition

The clinical features of carcinoma of the colon depend on the site of the growth. They can be divided into those affecting the right side and those affecting the left. Because the contents of the right side of the colon are fluid and those of the left side semi-solid, right-sided lesions tend to obstruct late and left-sided lesions obstruct early. Both lesions tend to bleed quietly into the bowel and iron deficiency anaemia is therefore common.

Right-sided colonic carcinoma

Recognizing the pattern

The patient
The patient is usually over 40 and the condition is common in 70–80 year olds. Women are more commonly affected than men.

The history
The patient may present with unexplained pain in the right iliac fossa or symptoms due to anaemia such as general malaise and weakness. He may notice a lump in the right iliac fossa and/or blood in the motions. Occasionally he presents with colicky abdominal pain when the lesion begins to obstruct the terminal ileum.

On examination
There may be a mass in the right iliac fossa and localized tenderness over the growth. Also look for hepatomegaly.

Proving the diagnosis

The stools may be positive for occult blood and the iron-deficiency anaemia can be detected on a blood film. The ESR is often raised. The diagnosis is confirmed by performing a barium enema. The radiologist must be asked to give particular attention to the caecum. False negative barium enemas are not uncommon and, if the condition is suspected and the barium enema negative, the investigation should be repeated after a few weeks. A colonoscopy may also help.

Management

In the general work-up of the patient, care is taken to look for metastases. Preoperative investigations include liver function tests, a liver scan and a chest X-ray. A barium enema is essential in order to exclude a second colonic lesion. Before operation is undertaken, the anaemia may have to be corrected by blood transfusion.

Preparation for surgery
The bowel must be adequately prepared so that hard faeces, which will cause obstruction below the anastomosis, are not present postoperatively (see p. 110).

Most surgeons give antibiotics when a colonic operation is planned. Antibiotics may be given orally in an attempt to sterilize the lumen of the bowel or they may be given intramuscularly with the premedication. Some surgeons continue giving antibiotics for 3−5 days postoperatively. The antibiotic combination used should be of broad spectrum and effective against bowel organisms, e.g. metronidazole, gentamicin and penicillin or ampicillin.

Operation: right hemicolectomy
The abdomen is opened and the terminal ileum, ascending colon and hepatic flexure of the colon are mobilized. The mesentery is divided and the growth and surrounding bowel removed. An anastomosis is made between the ileum and the transverse colon. It is not always possible to put an adequate drain to this anastomosis as it remains mobile within the peritoneal cavity.

Codes
Blood . . . . 2 units . . . .
GA/LA . . . . GA . . . .
Opn time . . . . 1−2 hours . . . .
Stay . . . . 7−10 days . . . .

Drains out	5−7 days ....
Sutures out	7 days ....
Off work	6 weeks ....

Postoperative care

The patient will require analgesics but the dose of opiates should not be excessive as these cause colonic spasm and have been implicated in an increased anastomotic disruption rate. The patient usually has an ileus for 3−4 days and oral fluids can be increased once flatus has been passed. The patient commonly gets diarrhoea in the first few days after the bowel recovers and he should be reassured that this will gradually settle down. Anti-diarrhoeal agents such as loperamide (Imodium) or diphenoxylate hydrochloride (Lomotil) may be helpful.

Left-sided colonic carcinoma

The condition

With left-sided lesions the main feature is the early onset of obstruction.

Recognizing the pattern

The patient

The patient is usually over the age of 40 and the disease is common in the over-70s. Men are slightly more commonly affected.

The history

The patient presents with a change in bowel habit. There is constipation due to the hold-up of faeces at the site of the growth. The faeces then liquefy and after a few days the patient has spurious offensive diarrhoea. The cycle is then repeated. There is often associated left-sided colicky abdominal pain.

In addition to the change in bowel habit the patient can present with rectal bleeding. This is always a serious symptom in the over-50s (see p. 349). As with right-sided lesions the patient may develop an iron-deficiency anaemia.

On examination

The abdomen may be distended and the caecum may be palpable. There may be a mass in the left iliac fossa or localized tenderness over the growth. On rectal examination a mass may be noted anteriorly. Palpate for an enlarged liver due to metastases.

Proving the diagnosis

The diagnosis may sometimes be proved on sigmoidoscopy. A low growth may be visible and can be biopsied. Even when the growth is not visible, blood and mucus may be seen high up in the bowel together with semi-liquid faeces, indicating a lesion higher up. The proximal colon and caecum may be distended on straight abdominal X-rays. Where a carcinoma is suspected, a barium enema is mandatory. The radiologist should also be careful to exclude other lesions such as polyps or second carcinomas in the rest of the bowel. Colonoscopy may be helpful where the barium enema findings are equivocal, and is also a method of obtaining a biopsy from a lesion higher up in the bowel. The procedure is time-consuming and uncomfortable, however, and is not recommended for the routine diagnosis of colonic carcinomas.

Management

Preoperative management
A full bowel preparation is necessary (see p. 110). Antibiotic cover may also be given as for a right hemicolectomy. The patient should be warned of the possibility of a colostomy. Colostomies are necessary either because the growth is unresectable (in which case the colostomy will be permanent), or in order to protect an anastomosis which was made under difficult conditions. In this case the colostomy will be of the loop type, usually in the transverse colon. Such a colostomy will be closed later (see below).

If a permanent colostomy is a possibility, then the site for this should be clearly marked on the patient when he is standing up. This should generally be done by a stoma therapist or by the surgeon.

Operation: left hemicolectomy
The left side of the colon is mobilized and the growth resected. An end-to-end anastomosis is usually performed. If the operation is carried out as an emergency, however, the bowel ends may be brought out as a left iliac colostomy and this may be closed later.

Codes

Blood	2 units	
GA/LA	GA	
Opn time	1−2 hours	
Stay	7−10 days	
Drains out	5−7 days	
Sutures out	7 days	
Off work........	6 weeks........................	

Operation: Paul−Mickulicz procedure
In this procedure the descending and sigmoid colon is mobilized and the growth brought out through a muscle-cutting incision in the left iliac fossa. It is then resected

outside the abdomen. This is a useful manoeuvre in an emergency operation for obstruction when no bowel preparation has been possible. In the past, continuity of the bowel was restored some days later by inserting an enterotome across the adjacent walls of the two sides of the colostomy. As the enterotome cut through the spur, it restored continuity and could be removed. The skin opening was closed later.

Codes
As for Right hemicolectomy.

Operation: anterior resection
This is a term applied to the operation required to resect growths in the upper rectum or recto-sigmoid junction. This is described in the section dealing with Carcinoma of the rectum (p. 359).

Operation: Hartmann's procedure
See p. 363 (Carcinoma of the rectum).

Postoperative care
The patient has an ileus, but a nasogastric tube is not of much value and oral fluids should be kept to a minimum until flatus is passed.

The main postoperative danger is of anastomotic leakage and the best early warning of this is the temperature chart. The development of a swinging fever, a tachycardia and faecal discharge from the drain may make the diagnosis obvious. A colonic leak in the absence of a protective colostomy can be a serious condition and it may be necessary to take the patient back to theatre to bring out the bowel ends as a colostomy.

If a temporary colostomy has been performed at the original operation, then arrangements will have to be made to close it at a suitable time.

Some surgeons perform an early limited barium enema at 10–14 days after the original resection. If this shows continuity of the anastomosis without leakage, the colostomy can be closed. Other surgeons prefer to wait longer than this and in that case a limited barium enema is usually undertaken 2–3 months after the original resection and the colostomy closed if all is well.

Operation: transverse loop colostomy
This operation is sometimes done on its own for acute colonic obstruction but it may also be part of a resection

procedure as above. The transverse colon is mobilized through a laparotomy incision and the omentum separated from it. A transverse muscle cutting incision is made in the right hypochondrium and a loop of colon brought out through it and maintained in position by passing it over a rubber tube or a glass rod. The abdominal wound is then closed and the colostomy opened by incising along the taenia. The edges of the colon are then sewn to the skin. Occasionally a loop colostomy is also formed from the sigmoid colon.

Operation: closure of colostomy
The edges of the colostomy are freed from the skin and the piece of colon is either resected or the anterior wall is closed, restoring continuity.

Codes

Blood	0 . . . .
GA/LA	GA . . . .
Opn time	1 hour . . . .
Stay	7−10 days . . . .
Drains out	7 days . . . .
Sutures out	7 days . . . .
Off work	3−4 weeks . . . .

Postoperative care
The ileus is short-lived and free fluids can be given after 24−48 hours. The wound commonly becomes infected and should be allowed to drain freely.

Other types of colostomy are shown in Fig. 65. A 'double-barrelled' colostomy is formed where part of the colon has been resected and the two ends are brought out next to each other. An 'end' colostomy is formed when the lower bowel is closed off or removed, as in an abdomino-perineal resection (p. 362) or a Hartmann's procedure (p. 363).

Carcinoma of the transverse colon

Recognizing the pattern
The patient presents with a picture intermediate between that of the right-sided lesion and the left-sided lesion, as might be expected. It is also not uncommon for the patient to notice a mass in his abdomen.

On examination
The mass may be palpable and is freely mobile in the early stages. If there is obstruction, the distended caecum may also be felt.

Management
This is identical to that described for other colonic lesions.

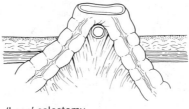

'Loop' colostomy

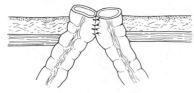

'Double-barrelled' colostomy

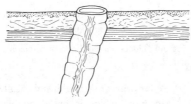

'End' colostomy

Fig. 65. Types of colostomy.

A colostomy will not usually be necessary, although, if the operation is particularly difficult, the surgeon may elect to bring out the bowel ends as a temporary colostomy rather than perform a primary anastomosis. The patient should be warned of this slight possibility.

Operation: transverse colectomy
The transverse colon is excised and an end-to-end anastomosis performed between the right colon and the left colon after full mobilization.

Codes
As for right hemicolectomy.

Postoperative care
As for other colectomies.

Carcinoma of the rectum

The condition   An adenocarcinoma of the rectum usually forms a typical malignant ulcer with a necrotic base and raised everted

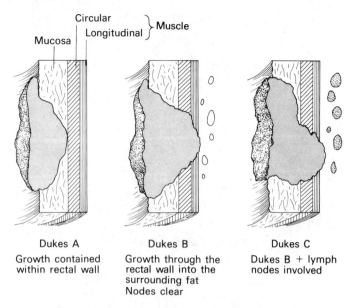

Circular
Longitudinal ⎫ Muscle

Mucosa

Dukes A	Dukes B	Dukes C
Growth contained within rectal wall	Growth through the rectal wall into the surrounding fat Nodes clear	Dukes B + lymph nodes involved

Fig. 66. Dukes' classification of carcinoma of the rectum.

edges. Growths are staged histologically according to Dukes' classification, which is based on histology and does not include distant metastases. The different stages are shown in Fig. 66.

The tumours are also classified as well differentiated (good prognosis) and averagely or poorly differentiated (poor prognosis).

The management of carcinoma of the rectum differs from that of other colonic carcinomas because much of the rectum is situated deep in the pelvis. Resection is not always possible through a laparotomy incision, and excision of the anus may be required.

Recognizing the pattern

The patient

The type of patient affected is similar to that for other colonic carcinomas.

The history

The presentation is usually in the form of bright rectal bleeding or of a change in bowel habit. The patient may experience a feeling of incomplete defaecation, which can be painful (tenesmus).

On examination

The diagnosis can often be made by rectal examination

when the characteristic irregular everted edge is felt protruding into the bowel lumen.

Proving the diagnosis

On sigmoidoscopy the lesion may be visible and should be biopsied. A barium enema is performed to look for other lesions in the colon and may also be helpful in defining the extent of the local growth.
Other investigations include the following.
1 Haemoglobin, white cell count and ESR.
2 Liver function tests.
3 Chest X-ray.
4 Liver scan.
5 Urea and electrolytes.
6 Intravenous urogram. This should be performed if there is thought to be a possibility of ureteric involvement.

Management

The management is to excise the tumour and frequently this involves creating either a permanent or a temporary colostomy. In an anterior resection the growth is excised from above and continuity is restored. In an abdomino-perineal resection the anus is also removed and a permanent colostomy made.

Preoperative management
Full bowel preparation is needed. If a permanent colostomy is a possibility, its site must be marked on the skin whilst the patient is standing. The possibility of a colostomy must be discussed with the patient and reassurance given about the implications of this procedure. It may be beneficial to introduce the patient to others who have had a colostomy performed. Prophylactic antibiotics are given and the patient is usually catheterized before the operation starts.

Operation: local resection
When the patient is too old or frail to withstand a major operation, a local resection may be performed. This is done through an operating sigmoidoscope placed in the anal canal. The lesion is excised with a diathermy. Malignant lesions recur quite quickly but palliation may be achieved for a while.

Codes
Blood . . . .   2 units . . . .
GA/LA . . . .   GA . . . .
Opn time . . . .   30 minutes to 1 hour . . . .
Stay . . . .   3–5 days . . . .
Drains out . . . . . .   0 . . . .

Sutures out ..... 0 ....
Off work........ 2−4 weeks ....

Operation: anterior resection of the rectum

This operation is indicated where the growth is more than 10 cm from the anal verge but below the recto-sigmoid junction. Mobilization of the rectum within the pelvic musculature will be necessary and this makes it a larger procedure than a left hemicolectomy. The growth is resected with a satisfactory distal margin and the anastomosis is performed between the rectal stump and the left side of the colon. This anastomosis may be difficult, particularly in males, as it is deep in the bony pelvis. The operation has been made easier with the introduction of mechanical suturing instruments. If these are used, the stapling gun is inserted through the anus and the upper and lower bowel ends are snugged down on to it using purse-string sutures. When the gun is fired the anastomosis is completed with a ring of metal staples. A protective transverse loop colostomy is frequently performed as part of the operation.

Codes

Blood	4 units ....
GA/LA	GA ....
Opn time	2−3 hours ....
Stay	About 14 days ....
Drains out	7 days ....
Sutures out	7 days ....
Off work........	6−8 weeks ....

Postoperative care

Postoperatively the care of a patient with an anterior resection of the rectum is much the same as that for a left hemicolectomy. A limited barium enema may be performed at 10−14 days and the colostomy closed if the anastomosis has healed. Alternatively, this may be done 2−3 months after the operation.

Operation: abdomino-perineal resection of the rectum

This operation is used for growths which are less than 10 cm from the anal verge. With such a low growth, adequate clearance is not possible without removing the anus. A permanent colostomy is therefore unavoidable. The necessity for this must be explained to the patient preoperatively. The site of the colostomy is marked as mentioned above.

The rectum is mobilized from above as in the anterior resection operation. In addition to this, the lower rectum and anus are also excised through a perineal incision. At the start of this the anus is closed with a purse-string suture.

The rectum is then removed and the subcutaneous fat and skin are closed, leaving a drain to the space left in the pelvis. In women this drain may usefully be brought out through the vagina as this makes the postoperative recovery easier and more comfortable.

The abdomino-perineal operation may be performed by one surgeon doing both the abdominal and the perineal resections, or by two surgeons. In the latter case it is known as a synchronous combined abdomino-perineal excision of the rectum (SCAPER). The theatre staff will need to know whether one or two surgeons will be operating.

Codes

Blood	4–6 units . . . .
GA/LA	GA . . . .
Opn time	3 hours . . . .
Stay	2–3 weeks . . . .
Drains out	Abdominal 5–7 days, perineum 7–10 days . . . .
Sutures out	Abdominal 7 days, perineum 10–14 days . . . .
Off work	2–3 months . . . .

Postoperative care
The postoperative care of an abdomino-perineal resection is slightly more complicated than for an anterior resection. There is a danger of haemorrhage in the first 24 hours and a careful watch must be kept on the perineal drain. Oral fluids can be increased when the colostomy starts to work. As far as the perineal wound is concerned, the best outcome is achieved when this heals by first intention. However, sepsis and breakdown of the perineal wound are not uncommon and in that case the sutures should be removed and free drainage established. The wound will then have to be regularly dressed until it heals from within.

The perineal drain is uncomfortable for the patient and it should be removed once drainage has become minimal. This is usually between 5 and 7 days after the operation.

Operation: Hartmann's procedure
This operation is used when a carcinoma of the rectum is found to be unresectable due to local invasion or when the patient is unfit for a more major resection. The lower end of the rectum is closed and left *in situ*. The upper end of the bowel is brought out as a descending colostomy.

Diverticular disease

The condition

Diverticular disease is a condition affecting the colon which is more common in those who eat a Western diet low in roughage. The condition is associated with muscle hypertrophy and raised intraluminal pressure. Mucosa-lined pouches are pushed out through the colonic wall, usually at the entry points of vessels (Fig. 67). These pouches are the diverticula. The condition is thought to arise because of a lack of roughage in the bowel content. Roughage is present in raw foodstuffs such as whole wheat and raw cane sugar but is removed when these are purified to make white flour and white sugar. Roughage is not normally absorbed from the bowel lumen and acts like blotting paper. The moisture it retains makes the stool more bulky and soft, and more easily propelled along the colonic lumen. Without roughage and sufficient water the stool becomes dehydrated and harder and colonic pressures are raised.

Several conditions are thought to be associated with the lack of roughage, including diverticular disease, piles, anal fissure and fistula in ano.

Diverticular disease itself may present with acute in-

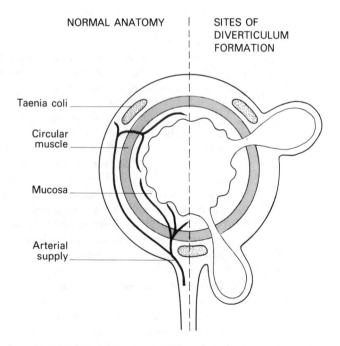

NORMAL ANATOMY | SITES OF DIVERTICULUM FORMATION

Taenia coli

Circular muscle

Mucosa

Arterial supply

Fig. 67. Diverticula are usually blown out at the entry points of vessels.

flammation in one or many pouches or as chronic disease with stricture formation due to recurrent inflammation.

Recognizing the pattern

The patient
The patient is usually over 40 and frequently obese. The condition is more common in females, although it does occur in males quite regularly.

The history
In acute diverticulitis the patient experiences a rapid onset of pain, usually in the left iliac fossa. There may be associated diarrhoea and generalized abdominal colic. The pain in the left iliac fossa rapidly becomes worse and it is exacerbated by movement such as coughing or moving. The patient develops a fever and feels generally unwell.

On examination
The patient is febrile with a tachycardia. He looks ill and is in obvious pain. The tongue may be furred and there is marked tenderness in the left iliac fossa with guarding and rebound tenderness. There may also be tenderness on rectal examination. In chronic diverticulosis the patient has often suffered from recurrent attacks of the type described above but then goes on to develop a more permanent change in bowel habit with alternating constipation and diarrhoea. There may be very little to find on general examination. He may also present with episodes of rectal bleeding.

Proving the diagnosis

In acute diverticulitis sigmoidoscopy will show the presence of inflamed mucosa, excessive mucus and loose motions high up. A straight erect and supine abdominal X-ray may show some gas in the wall of the bowel in the left iliac fossa or fluid levels in loops of small bowel adjacent to the area of inflammation. There may also be distension of the colon proximal to the area of disease. A barium enema should not be performed in the acute stage as this may exacerbate the condition or even perforate the bowel.

Once the acute episode has settled a barium enema is performed. Changes of diverticulosis are very common, however, and the presence of diverticula does not prove that these are causing the patient's symptoms. Other causes must be excluded.

When the disease becomes chronic, a narrowed area may develop in the descending or sigmoid colon and it can be difficult to decide whether this is benign or malignant. A repeat barium enema after a few weeks or a colonoscopy may decide the issue. Occasionally it is necessary to resort to laparotomy and resection in order to be sure that one is not dealing with a neoplasm.

Management

In the acute attack the patient is admitted and given a broad-spectrum combination of antibiotics such as metronidazole, gentamicin and penicillin or ampicillin. Analgesia may be needed. The condition usually settles rapidly unless there is abscess formation. If an abscess does form, it is best treated conservatively and will usually drain into the bowel. If it has to be drained externally there is likely to be a faecal fistula.

Chronic diverticular disease is treated by giving the patient adequate roughage in the diet, including wholemeal bread and bran. Bulk laxatives such as Isogel, Normacol or Fybogel may also be used. An adequate fluid intake must also be encouraged (see p. 384).

Surgery is indicated in diverticular disease where there are frequent recurrent inflammatory episodes; where complications such as perforation, stricture or fistula develop; or where there is doubt about the diagnosis.

Preoperative management
The patient should be advised to lose weight before surgery is undertaken. Patients with diverticular disease frequently have other problems, such as hiatus hernia, gall-stones or late-onset diabetes. These should be considered in the general work-up. Preparation for the colectomy is described under carcinoma of the descending colon (p. 356).

Operation: laparotomy for acute diverticulitis
Operation should be avoided in the acute stage if possible. Occasionally it becomes necessary, either because the bowel has perforated or in order to establish a cause for a generalized peritonitis. If the abdomen is opened and acute diverticular disease is found, then it is best left alone unless perforation has occurred. In the latter case a transverse defunctioning colostomy is performed and either the perforation is oversewn and drained or the affected bowel is resected. The latter involves a left hemicolectomy or Hartmann's procedure, as described on pp. 356 and 363.

Postoperative care
This is as for left hemicolectomy if the bowel has been resected. If a perforation has been closed and drained, antibiotics should be continued postoperatively and the drain removed after 5–7 days when an adequate track has formed. A decision will have to be made later about closing the colostomy and before this is done the affected piece of

bowel must be resected. This may be undertaken in either one or two stages.

Sigmoid volvulus

The condition

A sigmoid volvulus occurs in patients who have redundant sigmoid colon on a long mesentery with a narrow base. The sigmoid loop tends to twist, causing intestinal obstruction with massive dilatation of the bowel. The loop may become ischaemic. Constipation and excessive use of laxatives are common precipitating factors. This disease is more common in patients on tranquillizers and particularly occurs in mental hospitals.

Recognizing the pattern

The patient

The patient is usually elderly and may have suffered from constipation and taken laxatives for many years.

The history

The history is one of an acute onset of marked abdominal distension and colicky pain. There is complete constipation and no flatus is passed per rectum. There may be a history of repeated attacks as the colonic loop twists and spontaneously untwists.

On examination

The abdomen is grossly distended and tympanitic. There is tenderness, particularly in the left iliac fossa. Rectal examination shows an empty bowel which may be ballooned. There is tenderness high up.

Proving the diagnosis

The diagnosis is proved by straight erect and supine abdominal X-rays, which show the grossly distended sigmoid colon stretching across to the right upper quadrant. The erect film shows large fluid levels within this loop.

Management

The management in the acute stage is to perform a sigmoidoscopy and pass a large-bore flatus tube up into the volvulus. This procedure releases the flatus and faeces in the obstructed loop and gives the patient instant relief. The tube should be well lubricated before it is passed up and a bucket should be available.

The patient is then put on a high-roughage diet and if possible tranquillizers are withdrawn. The condition frequently recurs but the loop can be deflated many times if the patient is frail and not suitable for a definitive operation.

Occasionally the loop cannot be deflated and emergency laparotomy and resection may be required.

If the patient is fit and the condition becomes recurrent, then resection is also indicated. This may be done as a one-stage procedure with an end-to-end-anastomosis or two ends of the bowel may be brought out as a left iliac colostomy (see p. 356). The codes for this operation and the postoperative care are the same as for a left hemicolectomy.

Rectal prolapse

The condition

Rectal prolapse occurs in two age-groups.
1 In very young children (under the age of 2 see p. 553).
2 In elderly females (over the age of 60).

There are two anatomical types of prolapse, mucosal and complete. In *mucosal* prolapse the bowel musculature remains in position but redundant mucosa prolapses out of the anal canal. This is the type which occurs in children and also in adults with third-degree piles (see p. 383).

In *complete* rectal prolapse there is effectively an intus-susception of the upper rectum into the lower anal canal. It is associated with weakness of the pelvic musculature, often following multiple childbirth. In this case the whole bowel wall is inverted and passed out through the anus. There may be associated prolapse of the uterus. The difference between these two types of prolapse is illustrated in Fig. 68.

Complete rectal prolapse in adults

Recognizing the pattern

The patient
This usually occurs in elderly multiparous women.

The history
The rectal prolapse is of variable length and causes a profuse mucous discharge which soils the patient's underclothes. There may be associated bleeding. In advanced cases the prolapse may come down very readily and it may become impossible for the patient to get out of the house.

Proving the diagnosis

The diagnosis can be proved by asking the patient to strain and seeing the complete prolapse appear. It will be noted that the head of the prolapse is separate from the anal margins.

Management

In the early stages conservative management may be helpful but is not usually of much value once the prolapse has become well established. It consists of using stool softeners and perineal exercises. Operative measures include (i) the use of perianal sutures or wires (Thiersch wire), (ii) Delorme's operation or (iii) more radical procedures to

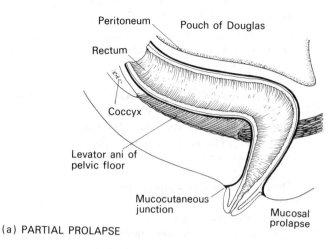

(a) PARTIAL PROLAPSE

Peritoneum

Pouch of Douglas

Rectum

Coccyx

Levator ani of
pelvic floor

Mucocutaneous
junction

Mucosal
prolapse

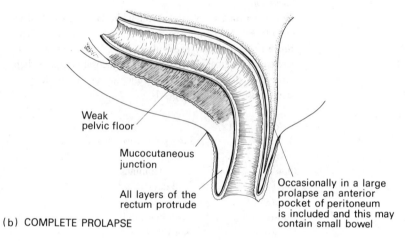

(b) COMPLETE PROLAPSE

Weak
pelvic floor

Mucocutaneous
junction

All layers of the
rectum protrude

Occasionally in a large
prolapse an anterior
pocket of peritoneum
is included and this may
contain small bowel

Fig. 68. Two types of rectal prolapse.

repair the pelvic musculature or fix the rectum to the sacral
curve (e.g. Ivalon sponge repair).

Operation: Thiersch wire for rectal prolapse
The anus is narrowed by inserting a subcutaneous suture of
Teflon or wire.

Codes
Blood . . . .   0 . . . .
GA/LA . . . .   LA or GA . . . .
Opn time . . . .   15 − 30 minutes . . . .
Stay . . . .   3 − 4 days . . . .

Drains out	0	
Sutures out	0	
Off work........	Not applicable	

Postoperative care

The limitation of this method is that the anus cannot dilate to pass a stool and faecal impaction is not uncommon postoperatively. The stool must therefore be kept soft. Alternatively, if the suture is not made tight enough, recurrent prolapse can occur.

Operation: Delorme's procedure

Preoperative management

A bowel preparation is given. Antibiotics are not required.

Operation

With the prolapse everted through the anus, a solution of 1/400 000 adrenaline is injected subcutaneously. The mucosa over the prolapse is then excised to within a centimetre of the dentate line. The upper mucosal margin is then sutured to the distal mucosa, bunching up the underlying rectal muscle within the pelvis.

Codes

Blood	Group and save serum	
GA/LA	GA	
Opn time	45 − 60 minutes	
Stay	3 − 4 days	
Drains out	0	
Sutures out	Absorbable only	
Off work........	Not applicable	

Postoperative care

Faecal softeners are given from the time of operation. The procedure is relatively non-invasive and recovery is usually rapid and uncomplicated. Recurrence is rare but if it occurs the procedure can be repeated. Patients who were incontinent before the operation may continue to be so afterwards and should be warned of this.

Operation: Ivalon sponge repair

Preoperative management

A full bowel preparation is necessary and antibiotics should be given with the premedication.

Operation

The rectum is mobilized as for anterior resection and a Teflon sponge is sewn into the presacral space and attached around the rectum anteriorly. The Teflon sponge gives rise to considerable fibrosis and the rectum is therefore 'stuck' to the sacrum preventing further prolapse. This operation can be very successful but it is essential to avoid sepsis. If the sponge becomes infected the situation can be very difficult to control.

Codes

Blood	2 units . . . .
GA/LA	GA . . . .
Opn time	60–90 minutes . . . .
Stay	5–7 days . . . .
Drains out	0 . . . .
Sutures out	7 days . . . .
Off work	Not applicable . . . .

Postoperative care

It is not uncommon for one episode of prolapse to occur in the early postoperative stages before the fibrosis has become established. It should be replaced and the patient reassured. Faecal softeners should be given as soon as the patient has recovered from ileus. A close watch should be kept for signs of developing sepsis and prolonged antibiotic treatment should be given if there is any suspicion of this.

Skeletal pain (referred pain)

The condition

'Skeletal pain' felt in the abdomen is probably due to pressure on thoracic or lumbar nerve roots as they leave the spinal column. Alternatively, the pain may radiate from one of the many joints or ligaments in the spinal column. The stimulus to the nerve root is interpreted as pain anywhere in the distribution of that nerve. Thus T8 nerve root pressure may give rise to epigastric pain and T12 root pressure to loin or suprapubic pain.

Skeletal pain is the great mimic of all abdominal conditions. Because of this there is a tendency to label any undiagnosed abdominal pain as skeletal and thus avoid trying to reach an accurate diagnosis. This tendency must be resisted.

Recognizing the pattern

The patient

The patient is of any age. There is often a history of associated anxiety or tension. With anxiety muscle tone is raised and hence the danger of nerve root pressure is increased. There may be a previous history of other skeletal pains such as sciatica or cervical spondylosis.

The history
The pain is related to posture or movement. It is usually worse in certain postures (but beware, this is also true of acute appendicitis). The patient may relate the pain to being in a fixed position such as when driving or watching television or even lying in bed. The pain is eased by certain movements and exacerbated by others. It is frequently better during the night and gets worse towards the end of the day. It may radiate to other areas supplied by the same spinal nerve.

On examination
There may be no physical signs. Tenderness over the spine or pain on femoral nerve or sciatic nerve stretching are helpful positive signs when present. The patient often feels tenderness over the area where the pain is felt even though there is no localized lesion at that site. Localized tenderness is not, therefore, very helpful in defining whether a pain is skeletal or not.

Proving the diagnosis

There is no clinical test which will prove that a pain is skeletal.

An X-ray of the spine may show spondylosis in the area of the root supplying the painful area but since such changes are very common they do not prove that the lesion found is the cause of the pain.

Management

Spinal exercises may be helpful and analgesics and re-assurance should be given as necessary. Relaxants such as Valium can be very useful to relieve both the painful muscle spasms and the overlying anxiety.

7   Perineum and Groins

7.1   **Perianal pain**
Perianal abscess
Perianal fistula
Anal fissure
Haemorrhoids
Perianal haematoma

7.2   **Lumps in the groin and other hernias**
The anatomy of the groin
General assessment
Inguinal hernia
Femoral hernia
Strangulated hernia
Incisional hernia
Umbilical hernia
Epigastric hernia
Spigelian hernia
Obturator hernia
Umbilical discharge in adults

7.1   Perianal Pain

This section deals with a number of related perianal conditions which present with pain or discomfort in the perineum. In order to understand their aetiology, it is necessary to be familiar with the anatomy of the perianal structures and these are depicted in Figs 69 and 70. The conditions include perianal abscesses, fistulae and fissures, haemorrhoids and perianal haematomata.

Perianal abscess

The condition

The most common cause of perianal abscess formation is infection arising in a perianal gland. These glands lie between the internal and external sphincters and open into the anal canal via the anal crypts at the pectinate line. The pectinate line is made up of flaps of mucosa (anal valves) above which are small recesses (anal sinuses). If the opening of the gland becomes blocked or damaged, stasis can result and lead to infection. The resulting abscess lies between the anal sphincters and tends to point towards the skin at the anal

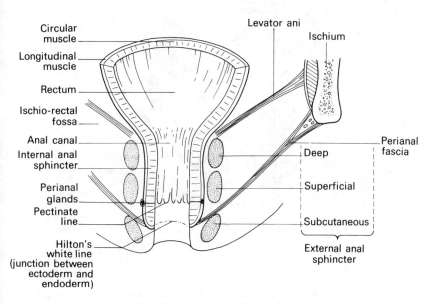

Fig. 69. The anatomy of the anal canal.

375

Sagittal section

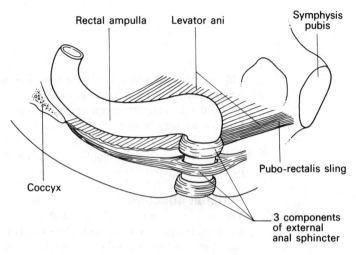

Fig. 70. The anal sphincters seen from the side.

margin (Fig. 71). It may spread laterally into the ischio-rectal fossa, or more rarely, superiorly above the levator ani into the pararectal fossa.

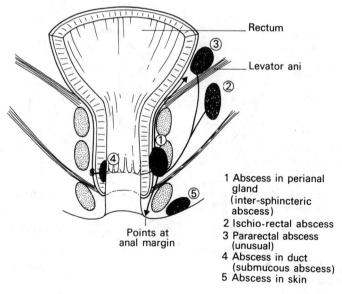

1 Abscess in perianal gland (inter-sphincteric abscess)
2 Ischio-rectal abscess
3 Pararectal abscess (unusual)
4 Abscess in duct (submucous abscess)
5 Abscess in skin

Fig. 71. The anatomical sites of abscess formation in the perianal region.

Recognizing the pattern

The patient
Patients of any age including children may be affected. The characteristic sitting posture with one buttock raised may make the diagnosis obvious.

The history
This is of gradual onset of pain around the anus, which becomes throbbing and severe. Defaecation and sitting are painful.

On examination
The abscess may be seen deep in the skin next to the anus (Fig. 72). There is much surrounding oedema. On proctoscopy the damaged opening to the affected gland may be seen and there may even be pus discharging from the opening.

Proving the diagnosis

The diagnosis is obvious on examination and no other tests are indicated.

Management

The abscess should be drained.

Operation: drainage of perianal abscess
A cruciate incision is made over the abscess next to the anus. The contents are evacuated. Loculi within the abscess are gently broken down but care must be taken not to extend the abscess upwards through the levator ani.

A proctoscopy and rectal examination are carried out and if an internal opening can be seen within the anal canal then the whole tract must be laid open as for a perianal fistula (see below).

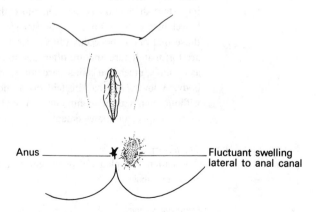

Fig. 72. The clinical presentation of a perianal abscess.

Codes
Blood . . . .   0 . . . .
GA/LA . . . .   GA . . . .
Opn time . . . .   15 minutes . . . .
Stay . . . .   3−7 days, depending on size of
                         abscess cavity . . . .
Drains out . . . . . .   48 hours . . . .
Sutures out . . . . .   0 . . . .
Off work . . . .   1−4 weeks . . . .

Occasionally perianal abscesses are secondary to pelvic abscesses above the levator ani. Such abscesses should not, if possible, be drained into the perineum as this may give rise to a high rectal fistula. The management of pelvic abscesses is described on p. 75.

Postoperative care
The abscess is dressed daily, leaving paraffin gauze in the cavity so that the wound heals without bridging over. A gauze wick should not be used, as pushing this in tends to deepen the cavity and also obstructs normal drainage. Antibiotics may be indicated if the organism is a Group A *Streptococcus*.

Perianal fistula

The condition

A perianal fistula is an abnormal connection between the lumen of the anus (or rectum) and the skin. It usually develops from a perianal abscess which bursts on to the skin or is drained surgically. If the internal opening of the original infected perianal gland remains patent, a fistula results.

Various types of fistula are described according to the level at which they transgress the anal sphincters. The important distinction is between those that open into the bowel below the deep external anal sphincter ('low') and those that open above this ('high', see Fig. 73). The latter are fortunately rare and are often due to other disease such as Crohn's, ulcerative colitis, carcinoma, trauma or a foreign body. A low fistula can be laid open and allowed to heal without endangering continence. A high fistula requires more complicated management.

Recognizing the pattern

The history
The patient complains of persistent perianal discharge and recurrent abscesses.

On examination
The external opening is usually seen lateral to the anus and

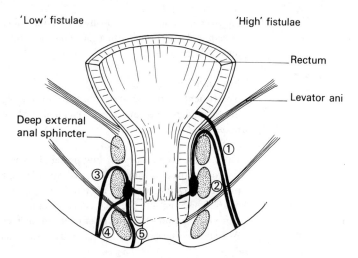

'Low' fistulae   'High' fistulae

Rectum

Levator ani

Deep external
anal sphincter

Fig. 73. The types of perianal fistula. High: 1 extrasphincteric;
2 suprasphincteric. Low: 3 high transphincteric; 4 low
transphincteric; 5 intersphincteric.

the internal opening may be palpable on rectal examination. Proctoscopy should be undertaken to try and visualize the opening. This is sometimes difficult to detect especially if it is not exuding pus at the time.

Goodsall's rule states that a fistula lying in the anterior half of the anal area opens directly into the anal canal, while a fistula lying in the posterior half tracks around the anus and opens in the midline posteriorly (see Fig. 74).

During rectal examination assess the tone of the anal sphincter. It may be weaker in the elderly, meaning that less muscle can be cut at operation.

Management

The treatment of a perianal fistula is to lay it open. Faecal continence is lost only if the deep ring of the external anal sphincter and the puborectalis sling are severed. Therefore, a low fistula may be laid open without danger of incontinence. However, a high fistula must be managed in stages to allow

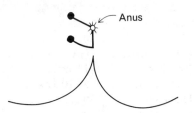

Anus

Fig. 74. Goodsall's rule.

fibrosis to develop. Occasionally a covering colostomy may be required. Any predisposing cause such as Crohn's disease must also be treated.

Preoperative management

The patient should be given a laxative on the night before the operation and the bowel emptied with enemas if necessary.

Operation: laying open of low perianal fistula

A probe is passed into the external opening and carefully passed along the fistulous tract until it goes through the internal opening into the anal canal. A knife is used to cut down on the probe and the tract thus laid open completely. Any lateral extensions of the tract must also be laid open.

Codes

Blood	0 . . . .
GA/LA	GA . . . .
Opn time	15 minutes . . . .
Stay	3–10 days, depending on size of cavity laid open . . . .
Drains out	0 . . . .
Sutures out	0 . . . .
Off work	2–4 weeks . . . .

Postoperative care

The wound is dressed daily and the patient can have regular twice-daily saline baths. The wound often takes 6–8 weeks to heal. In the final stages it is very little trouble to the patient and normal life can usually be resumed. The patient is put on a regime of bulk laxatives (e.g. Normacol or bran).

Operation: high perianal fistula

The whole tract cannot be laid open because of the danger of incontinence. The lowest part is therefore excised. A ligature may be passed through the upper tract to induce fibrosis and allow laying open 2–3 weeks later.

Codes

Blood	0 . . . .
GA/LA	GA . . . .
Opn time	1 hour . . . .
Stay	3–10 days . . . .
Drains out	0 . . . .
Sutures out	0 . . . .
Off work	4–6 weeks . . . .

Anal fissure

The condition

In this condition the anal mucosa is torn so that the circular muscle layer is exposed. Intense muscle spasm results which is worse after each bowel movement. The tear usually starts at the pectinate line when an anal valve is torn downwards by the passage of a hard stool.

The fissure is usually on the posterior aspect of the anal canal as most of the pressure during defaecation occurs at this point.

Recognizing the pattern

The patient
He can be of any age. The condition is not uncommon in babies.

The history
There is a history of pain on defaecation, often occurring first during a period of constipation. The pain then recurs each time the bowels are opened and there is often fresh rectal bleeding ('bright red blood on the paper').

On examination
A 'sentinel' pile may be visible if the anus is inspected with the buttocks gently parted. This 'sentinel' pile represents the bunched up, torn strip of mucosa at the base of the fissure. A rectal examination may be exquisitely tender or impossible because of severe pain and muscle spasm. This finding alone is enough to confirm the diagnosis.

Management

In the early stages the introduction of bran into the diet together with analgesic suppositories may give relief. If this is not successful or the condition is particularly painful, an urgent anal stretch should be performed. This gives immediate relief. The procedure weakens the anal muscle, thus relieving the pain and spasm, and the fissure then epithelializes over.

Operation: anal stretch (Lord's stretch)
The patient is put in the lithotomy position and the anal canal palpated under anaesthesia. The operation can easily be performed under a caudal or spinal anaesthetic. On palpation, with the anal sphincter relaxed, fibrous bands may be felt encircling the anal canal. The anal sphincter is stretched and the bands disrupted. Four to six fingers are inserted in the anal canal and the stretch maintained for three or four minutes. This should be done slowly and gently so as to minimize perianal haematoma formation. At

the end of the operation it is useful to insert a compressed sponge into the anal canal as this also prevents bruising.

Codes

Blood	0 . . . .
GA/LA	GA/spinal/caudal . . . .
Opn time	5 minutes . . . .
Stay	24 hours . . . .
Drains out	0, sponge removed after 1−2 hours . .
Sutures out	0 . . . .
Off work	48 hours . . . .

Operation: sphincterotomy

Where the fissure has become chronic, an anal stretch alone may not suffice to cure it. In that case it is necessary to excise the fissure and perform a sphincterotomy. The sphinctero-tomy is performed either by dividing the lower sphincter fibres through the base of the fissure or by inserting a knife laterally and dividing the lower sphincter subcutaneously (lateral subcutaneous sphincterotomy).

Codes

Blood	0 . . . .
GA/LA	GA . . . .
Opn time	15−30 minutes . . . .
Stay	48 hours . . . .
Drains out	0 . . . .
Sutures out	0 . . . .
Off work	1−2 weeks . . . .

Postoperative care

The patient should be put on regular bran. When an anal stretch has been performed many surgeons give their patients an anal dilator to use for several weeks postoperatively so as to maintain the size of the enlarged anal canal. Division of the lowest fibres of the external anal sphincter is very unlikely to cause incontinence.

Haemorrhoids

The condition

Haemorrhoids (or 'piles') are extremely common in Western civilization. The normal anal canal, just above the anal sphincter, is closed by soft 'cushions' of mucosa containing a submucosal plexus of veins. If excessive pressure is generated during defaecation, the mucosal cushions are stretched and can prolapse through the anal canal as 'piles'. The excessive pressure may be due to any of the following.

1 Hard dry stools (due to lack of roughage in the diet or inadequate water intake).

2 Failure to allow the sphincter to relax before the stool is pushed through the canal. Piles are usually worse at times of stress.

3 Excessive straining during defaecation.

4 Decreased relaxation of the anal canal due to the presence of pecten bands (fibrous bands in the upper anal canal).

In addition the veins themselves may be weak or have deficient valves. The condition is commonly associated with varicose veins in the legs and both conditions run in families.

The piles often arise or are made worse during pregnancy, when circulating progesterone makes the venous muscle relax and when intra-abdominal pressure is raised.

Once formed, piles may gradually increase in size due to congestion and hypertrophy. Three degrees of piles are described and the recognition of these degrees is important as the method of treatment is related to them.

First degree
These piles remain within the anal canal. They present with discomfort or rectal bleeding.

Second degree
These prolapse out of the anal verge but are easily replaced. They present with perianal discharge or irritation, together with discomfort and rectal bleeding. The patient may also complain of the presence of the prolapsed piles themselves.

Third degree
These are permanently prolapsed. Third-degree piles may become strangulated. The piles prolapse and the circulation is obstructed by the anal sphincter, which goes into intense spasm as the inflammation develops. The haemorrhoids thrombose.

Recognizing the pattern

The patient
The characteristic patient is a tense young executive but piles can affect people of any age and either sex. In the older age-groups the patient is frequently obese. He may also suffer from varicose veins.

The history
The history is of perianal discomfort or discharge with or without rectal bleeding. The bleeding is fresh and is noted on the paper or in the pan after defaecation. It is on the outside of the stool. The patient may also experience a

feeling of incomplete emptying of the rectum after defaecation due to the bulk of the piles in the anal canal.

On examination
With first-degree piles there is nothing visible externally or on rectal examination. Proctoscopy shows the haemorrhoids bulging over the end of the proctoscope placed just within the anal canal. Piles are never palpable on rectal examination unless they are actually thrombosed.

Second-degree haemorrhoids may be seen to prolapse out of the anal verge on straining. They are also clearly visible on proctoscopy.

Third-degree piles are visible as soon as the anus is inspected and if they can be replaced within the anal canal they rapidly prolapse again.

Strangulated third-degree piles present as inflamed bunches of tissue surrounding the anal canal. They are exquisitely painful and tender.

Management

First-degree piles may be treated conservatively or by injections or an anal stretch.

Second-degree piles can be treated either by injections or by an anal stretch, although these methods are not always successful, and the patient may eventually require haemorrhoidectomy. Second-degree piles can also be treated as an outpatient by 'banding'.

Third-degree piles require haemorrhoidectomy.

Conservative treatment
This is important, whatever other measures are indicated. The patient must be educated to modify his diet and to avoid excessive straining. Stools become bulky, soft and easy to pass if they contain enough fibre (e.g. bran). Fibre is not absorbed during digestion and acts like blotting paper keeping water in the stool. It must therefore be combined with an adequate water intake. Excessive straining may be due to nervous tension or due to a feeling of incomplete emptying associated with the bulk of the piles.

Procedure: injection of piles
The injection of piles is an outpatient procedure. The object is to cause scarring between the stretched anal cushions within the anal canal and the underlying muscle. A proctoscope is inserted in the anal canal and the piles bulge over the rim of the instrument. Injections of 5% phenol in arachis oil are put into the submucosal layer above the pectinate line. The injections should be painless. Injections should not

be put in too superficially (when blanching of the mucosa will be seen) as this will cause sloughing of the mucosa.

The patient may experience some discomfort in the first 2–3 days after injection of piles but this settles rapidly. The beneficial effect is noted after 6–10 days. It may be necessary to repeat the treatment.

Some centres use cryotherapy or photocoagulation as alternative methods of mucosal fixation. Both are relatively pain-free but the equipment is expensive and the results are not significantly better than injection therapy.

Procedure: banding of piles

The pile is grasped through a proctoscope and a tight rubber band positioned around its neck. Thrombosis and separation of the pile then follow.

Operation: anal stretch (Lord's stretch, see under Anal fissure, p. 381)

This operation is successful in the early stages of piles as it lowers the intra-anal pressure during defaecation, making the passage of the stool easier. It is not so useful for more advanced degrees of piles.

Operation: haemorrhoidectomy

Preoperative management
The bowels should be emptied using laxatives on the day before the operation.

Operation
The patient is placed in the lithotomy position and the prolapsing piles are grasped with clamps. They are excised together with the surrounding anal skin tags and the dissection is advanced to the neck of the pile in the submucosal layer. The piles are ligated within the anal canal. It is important to leave mucosal skin bridges between each group of piles excised, otherwise an anal stricture may result.

Codes

Blood	2 units . . . .
GA/LA	GA . . . .
Opn time	30 minutes . . . .
Stay	3–7 days . . . .
Drains out	0 . . . .
Sutures out	0 . . . .
Off work	3–4 weeks . . . .

Postoperative care
Reactionary haemorrhage may occur in the first few hours after the operation. Patients should always be nursed with the foot of the bed elevated. This elevation can be increased if haemorrhage does occur. Blood transfusion is then given if necessary. If the bleeding does not settle, the patient should be taken back to theatre and the individual bleeding point found, using a suitable proctoscope. It is then ligated.

The patient is given Normacol and Milpar postoperatively and encouraged to have his bowels open as soon as possible. The first defaecation is often painful but if he becomes constipated it is worse. Daily baths postoperatively are helpful in keeping the anal area clean and increasing the patient's comfort.

There is often a slight secondary haemorrhage at 7–10 days after the operation and the patient should be warned about this. It is usually minimal.

The patient may be incontinent of flatus for 2–3 weeks after the operation until the mucosal cushions have healed. He should be warned of this and reassured it will settle down.

The patient should be put on bran after any perianal operation and should remain on it indefinitely thereafter.

Management of strangulated piles
The conservative management consists of the following.
Bed rest.
Elevation of the foot of the bed.
Analgesia.
Topical icepacks.

If this produces relief, a haemorrhoidectomy is performed later. If not, an early anal stretch or haemorrhoidectomy is carried out.

Perianal haematoma (thrombosed external pile)

The condition

This is due to a ruptured superficial perianal vein which gives rise to a subcutaneous haematoma.

Recognizing the pattern

The history
The patient may be of any age. There is frequently a history of straining at stool. The condition presents with a sudden onset of severe perianal pain. Left untreated the pain gradually settles over a week or so and the haematoma resolves.

On examination
There is a cherry-like, rounded, blue haematoma in the

subcutaneous tissue next to the anal verge. It is exquisitely tender.

Management   In the first 2−3 days the treatment is to evacuate the haematoma after infiltrating with local anaesthetic. This gives immediate relief. If the haematoma has been present for longer than a week, it is probably best left to resolve naturally.

Lumps in the Groin and Other Hernias

The anatomy of the groin

A wide variety of interesting conditions can present as a lump in the groin and for this reason such lumps are popular as examination cases. Students are often confused about the anatomy of this area and hence uncertain of the interpretation of physical signs and the surgical approach to a hernia. The femoral sheath is usefully conceived as a gap between the anterior abdominal wall and the posterior abdominal wall as these two structures meet in the groin. Through this gap pass the main vessels to the leg and medial to them is the femoral canal. This part of the anterior abdominal wall consists of the external oblique, internal oblique and transversus abdominus muscles. These are all attached to the inguinal ligament. The ligament is attached to the pubic tubercle medially and the anterior superior iliac spine laterally. Behind the inguinal ligament are the muscles of the posterior abdominal wall running into the anterior thigh (psoas and iliacus) and also the pectineus. The femoral vessels lie on top of these muscles and behind the inguinal ligament (Fig. 75).

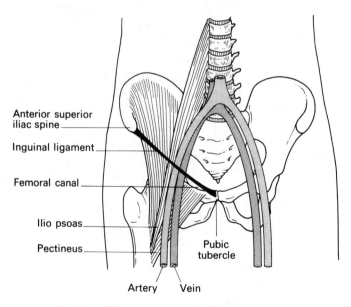

Anterior superior iliac spine

Inguinal ligament

Femoral canal

Ilio psoas

Pectineus

Pubic tubercle

Artery   Vein

Fig. 75. The anatomy of the inguinal ligament.

Inguinal hernias occur through the inguinal canal in the lower part of the anterior abdominal wall and are therefore above the inguinal ligament. Femoral hernias occur down the femoral canal and are therefore posterior to the inguinal ligament and appear in the thigh below and lateral to the pubic tubercle. Obturator hernias occur from within the true pelvis and they can be palpated within the adductor compartment of the thigh.

General assessment

In approaching a groin lump it is first necessary, therefore, to define the anatomical landmarks and thus to decide which anatomical structure is involved. It is particularly important to define the line of the inguinal ligament by palpating the bony points from which it arises (Fig. 76).

A list of possible groin lumps and their relationship to the inguinal canal is given in Table 22.

Inguinal hernia

The condition

Inguinal hernias are protuberances of the peritoneal contents through the abdominal wall where it is weakened by the presence of the inguinal canal.

Indirect hernias follow the path of the spermatic cord or round ligament down the inguinal canal. Their origin is therefore lateral to the inferior epigastric artery, which defines the medial edge of the internal ring.

Direct inguinal hernias arise from a different cause, the weakness being in the posterior wall of the inguinal canal

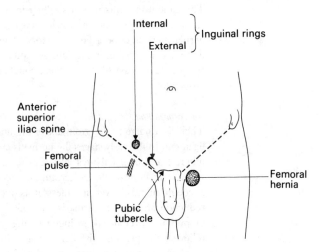

Fig. 76. The landmarks in the groin.

rather than down the canal itself. They therefore arise medial to the inferior epigastric vessels.

Strangulated hernias are described on p. 395.

Table 22. Lumps in the groin

Anatomical structure	Pathology	Above or below the inguinal ligament
In the skin	Lipoma, fibroma, haemangioma, etc. (see Section 10)	Either
Deep to the skin Femoral vein	Saphena varix (see Varicose veins, p. 505)	Below
Femoral artery	Aneurysm (see p. 493, Vascular disorders)	Below
Lymph nodes, inguinal or femoral	Primary or secondary infection or neoplasia	Either
Hernias	Inguinal, direct or indirect Femoral	Above Below

Recognizing the pattern

The patient

Indirect hernias can occur at any age and are common in children. They are more common in males than females as the inguinal canal is wider in the male.

Direct hernias are rare in children and more common in the elderly.

The history

The patient presents with a swelling in the groin that may cause some discomfort or restrict activity. In both types of hernia there may be a family history of the condition and there may also be an immediate precipitating cause such as an episode of heavy lifting or severe coughing due to chronic bronchitis.

On examination

There is a bulge in the groin above the line of the inguinal ligament. In the early stages the hernia is lateral to the pubic tubercle and as it enlarges it may protrude over the pubic tubercle and down into the scrotum or vulva. The lump has a cough impulse over it unless it is incarcerated. After reduction an indirect hernia is controlled during coughing by pressure over the deep inguinal ring (see Fig. 76). On relieving the pressure the hernia runs obliquely down the canal. A direct hernia is not so controlled and bulges straight forward.

Management

Conservative

If the hernia is indirect a truss can be used. This works by compressing the inguinal canal from front to back and thus preventing an indirect hernia protruding. A truss is not suitable for treatment of a direct inguinal hernia unless the defect is very small. Direct inguinal hernias will tend to bulge round the sides of the truss before long.

Most patients find a truss rather uncomfortable and irksome to wear but it has its place in elderly and frail patients who would prefer to avoid an operation.

Surgical

Most inguinal hernias will be repaired operatively.

Preoperative management

The patient should be advised to stop smoking and to lose any excess weight. Patients who continue smoking up to the time of a hernia repair tend to have a severe bronchitis after the operation and this puts added strain on the repair in the early stages. Obesity makes the operation more difficult and also puts more strain on the repair postoperatively.

If the patient is bronchitic, he should have a few days of physiotherapy to the chest before the operation is undertaken.

Patients with recurrent inguinal hernias may have to be warned that a satisfactory repair of the abdominal wall may only be possible if the testicle and spermatic cord are removed. Their consent must be obtained if this is being considered.

Operation: repair of inguinal hernia

The indirect hernial sac is ligated at its neck and excised after the contents have been reduced back into the abdomen. A direct hernial sac is not usually excised. It is inverted and the defect in the posterior wall of the inguinal canal is repaired. The posterior wall of the inguinal canal is then strengthened by sewing the conjoint tendon to the inguinal ligament (Bassini repair). Some surgeons also use a nylon darn which criss-crosses backwards and forwards between the inguinal ligament and the conjoint tendon.

Tanner slide. In this procedure a relaxing incision is made in the conjoint tendon close to the midline over the rectus muscle, thus relieving any tension on the repair.

In children and young adults it is only necessary to excise the sac (herniotomy) and no attention is needed to the posterior inguinal canal wall (herniorrhaphy).

Codes

Blood .... 0 ....
GA/LA .... GA or LA ....
Opn time .... 15−30 minutes ....
Stay .... 2−5 days ....
Drains out ...... 0 ....
Sutures out ..... 5 days ....
Off work .... 4 weeks ....

Postoperative care

The patient is mobilized early and can leave hospital as soon as he can walk independently. In some centres hernias are repaired as 'day case' procedures.

Strong analgesia is usually required for the first 48 hours but mild analgesics such as aspirin or paracetamol will suffice thereafter. The patient is usually advised to take things gently for two weeks from the operation date. Thereafter he should undertake gradually increasing exercise in order to regain muscular fitness. In the author's practice patients are allowed back to full activity one month after the hernia repair has been completed. There is no evidence that early return to work increases the recurrence rate.

Femoral hernia

The condition

Femoral hernias protrude down the femoral canal, which is medial to the femoral vessels and lateral to the pubic tubercle. From an understanding of the anatomy of the femoral canal, it can be seen that femoral hernias will always have a narrow neck constricted by the inguinal ligament anteriorly, the pubic bone and reflected part of the inguinal ligament (lacunar ligament) medially, the pectineal part of the pubic bone posteriorly, and the femoral vein laterally (see Fig. 77). Consequently the risk of strangulation is high. As the angle between the inguinal ligament and the pectineal part of the pubic bone is greater in females than males, the femoral canal is wider in females and femoral hernias are more common.

Recognizing the pattern

The patient

The patient is usually female and middle-aged or elderly, although femoral hernias can occur in either sex and at any age.

The history

The history is of a lump appearing in the groin which is frequently painful. Femoral hernias often present with an episode of strangulation and small bowel obstruction is not

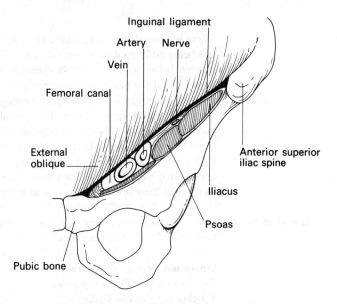

Fig. 77. The femoral canal lies behind the inguinal ligament medial to the femoral vein.

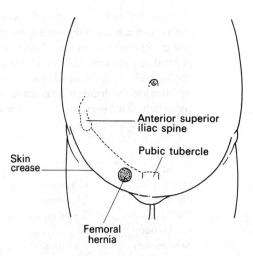

Fig. 78. The groin crease is not a guide to the position of the inguinal ligament. Always define the bony landmarks, especially in obese patients and children.

uncommon. A strangulated hernia will be missed if the groin is not adequately exposed during the general examination. Strangulated femoral hernias are frequently missed in obese patients (Fig. 78).

There is a rounded swelling tucked in medially in the groin. It is below and lateral to the pubic tubercle. It may be of any size but is frequently 2–3 cm in diameter. Even when the main bulk of the hernia has been reduced, a soft palpable lump can usually be found. If the hernia enlarges sufficiently, it tends to spread upwards over the inguinal ligament and pubic tubercle and this can be confusing. If the groin is carefully palpated, however, its origin can be determined. Definition of a femoral hernia from an inguinal one is important as the former are much more likely to strangulate and should therefore be repaired without undue delay.

Management

The management of a femoral hernia is surgical repair. A truss should never be prescribed.

Operation: repair of femoral hernia

Two main approaches are possible.

1 Below the inguinal ligament.

2 Above the inguinal ligament.

A strangulated hernia will usually have to be approached from above in order to deal with possible bowel infarction.

1 Approach from below (Lockwood's operation)

An incision is made in the groin below the inguinal ligament and the hernia found in the subcutaneous tissue. Its neck is isolated, the contents reduced back into the abdomen and the sac excised. The femoral canal is closed at its lower end by suturing the inguinal ligament to the pectineal fascia posteriorly. This operation is very minor and can be done under a local anaesthetic.

Codes

Blood	0
GA/LA	GA or LA
Opn time	15 minutes
Stay	2–3 days
Drains out	0
Sutures out	5–7 days
Off work	2–3 weeks

2 Approach from above

In this approach the abdominal muscles of the inguinal region are opened and the upper end of the femoral canal visualized within the abdominal cavity. The approach may be via either a vertical incision in the conjoint tendon (McEvedy's operation) or a transverse incision through the posterior wall of the inguinal canal (Lotheissen's operation). If the hernia is strangulated, the peritoneum is opened and the contents of the sac inspected. Non-viable bowel may then be resected. The femoral canal is then exposed in the retroperitoneal layer and closed with sutures between the inguinal ligament and the pectineal fascia.

Codes

Blood..........	0...............................
GA/LA........	GA............................
Opn time.......	30 minutes......................
Stay...........	5−7 days.......................
Drains out......	0...............................
Sutures out.....	5−7 days.......................
Off work........	4 weeks........................

Postoperative care

This is much the same as for an inguinal hernia. Where a femoral hernia has been approached from below the inguinal ligament, the recovery is rapid.

Strangulated hernia

The condition

Most types of hernia may become irreducible. Various stages are recognized.

1 In a *simple irreducible hernia*, the contents cannot be reduced but the blood supply is intact and there are no symptoms of intestinal obstruction. The usual cause is adhesions between the sac and its contents − almost certainly omentum.

2 In an *obstructed hernia*, the sac contains bowel which has become obstructed.

3 In a *strangulated hernia*, the blood supply of the contents is compromised and there is a danger of, or actual, necrosis of the tissues enclosed in the hernia. Both the preceding types of irreducible hernia predispose to strangulation.

Other terms used for irreducible hernias are as follows.

Richter's hernia. A knuckle of the side wall of the bowel is caught in the sac but the continuity of the bowel is maintained (see Fig. 79a). In this case the bowel wall is strangulated but there is no intestinal obstruction.

Reduction en masse. If a strangulated hernia is reduced the strangulation is normally relieved. Occasionally, however, it is possible to reduce the visible mass of the hernia but for the sac and its neck to be reduced as well. In this case the contents remain strangulated even though the external hernia has disappeared (see Fig. 79b). Any clinician attempting to reduce a strangulated hernia must be aware of

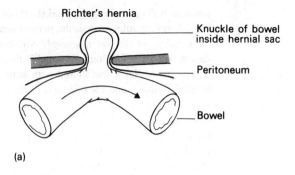

Richter's hernia

Knuckle of bowel
inside hernial sac

Peritoneum

Bowel

(a)

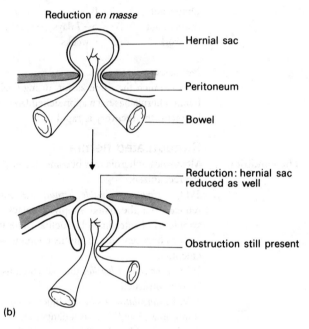

Reduction *en masse*

Hernial sac

Peritoneum

Bowel

Reduction: hernial sac
reduced as well

Obstruction still present

(b)

Fig. 79. Some terms used for special types of strangulation.

this possibility. If the patient's symptoms (e.g. of bowel obstruction and abdominal pain) persist after reduction of the hernia, it must be considered and early operation may be indicated.

Recognizing the pattern

The history

The hernia suddenly becomes irreducible, painful and tender. There may be accompanying symptoms of intestinal obstruction. Occasionally patients present only with general abdominal symptoms and have not themselves noticed the hernia.

On examination
The hernia is irreducible and tender. A distended abdomen and obstructive bowel sounds may confirm suspicions of intestinal obstruction. Similarly, an erect and supine abdominal X-ray may be helpful.

Management

Preoperative management
If the hernia cannot be reduced, urgent operation is required. The patient may need rapid rehydration first. The serum electrolytes should be within the normal range before the anaesthetic is given. Make sure the patient is shaved before the operation starts. A strangulated hernia is often infected and antibiotics (gentamicin, metronidazole and either penicillin or ampicillin) should be given with the premedication.

Operation: for strangulated hernias
The details are given under individual hernias and small bowel resection. In general, the sac is opened and the contents inspected and then the strangulation released. The affected bowel is wrapped in a warm saline swab. It may be necessary to wait several minutes in order to be sure that it is viable. If it is not, it is resected. If there is gross contamination, the wound will need to be drained. Such a drain can be removed after 3−4 days.

Codes

Blood	0	....
GA/LA	GA	....
Opn time	60−90 minutes	....
Stay	About 7 days	....
Drains out	3−5 days	....
Sutures out	5−7 days	....
Off work	4 weeks	....

Postoperative care
The patient may have an ileus for 1−2 days. Apart from this the postoperative course is as for any other hernia.

Incisional hernia

The condition

An incisional hernia occurs where there has been breakdown of the muscle closure in a previous abdominal wound. There is often a history of postoperative wound haematoma or sepsis but the hernia itself may not appear for several weeks or months after the operation.

Recognizing the pattern

The patient
He is nearly always obese.

The history
The patient notices a bulge at the side of the previous operation scar associated with discomfort. He may also suffer from more general abdominal pain associated with obstruction of loops of bowel within the hernia.

On examination
The incisional hernia is easily visible when the patient stands up or strains but it may be invisible as he lies flat. It can usually be demonstrated by asking the patient either to cough or to tense his abdominal muscles by straight leg raising. The margins of the muscular defect are palpable beneath the skin and the size of the defect should be determined. Note whether the contents of the incisional hernia are fully reducible or not.

Management

Once the muscle layers of a laparotomy wound have separated, it is difficult to be certain of obtaining a sound repair at a second closure. Frequently the tissues are poor anyway, and the patient's obesity is against obtaining a good result. A conservative approach may therefore be advocated. If an operation is advised, the patient should be told that it carries a high failure rate.

Conservative management
The patient is strongly advised to lose weight and a surgical belt is provided.

Preoperative management
The patient should stop smoking and lose weight before an operative repair is considered. The theatre staff frequently regard an incisional hernia as a minor operation and do not realize that its repair will entail a full laparotomy. The hernia cannot be repaired until the adherent loops of bowel have been freed and the edges of the muscle clearly defined. Deep instruments may therefore be necessary.

Operation: repair of incisional hernia
The stretched scar in the skin is excised. The muscle edges are defined and adhesions divided. Several different types of repair are possible and deep tension sutures will usually be used for the muscle layer.
(a) In a 'keel' repair the hernial sac is not opened. It is dissected clear and inverted. The two edges of the muscle are sewn together alongside each other using lateral mattress sutures, resulting in a 'keel' of muscle as shown in Fig. 80.
(b) Simple closure with deep-tension nylon. In this type of

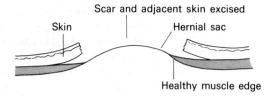

(a) Hernia

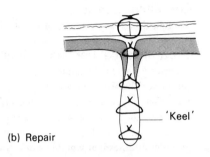

(b) Repair

Fig. 80. 'Keel' repair of an incisional hernia.

closure continuous nylon suture is inserted taking wide bites of tissue. Only the superficial layers of skin are not included.
(c) Deep tension figure-of-eight nylon sutures. These can be placed through all layers including the skin. This method of closure is also used for dehisced abdominal wounds in the postoperative period (see pp. 69−71).
(d) Relaxing incisions in the rectus sheath. In this procedure the muscle layers are closed centrally in the usual way but extra width is obtained by incising the rectus sheath laterally, thus allowing the anterior rectus sheath to slide medially to meet its opposite side.

Codes

Blood	0−2 units . . . .
GA/LA	GA . . . .
Opn time	1 hour . . . .
Stay	3−7 days . . . .
Drains out	2−4 days . . . .
Sutures out	Skin, 7−10 days; deep-tension sutures, 10−14 days . . . .
Off work	4−6 weeks . . . .

Postoperative care
If the closure is very tight the patient may develop chest problems postoperatively and chest physiotherapy will be

important. An external binder can sometimes be used to take the tension off the wound. The sutures may be left in place a lot longer than usual if the skin edges are under tension. In order to avoid abdominal distension a nasogastric tube is inserted to decompress the stomach, and oral fluids are not given until flatus has been passed. Any sign of a wound infection must be treated early and many surgeons cover these operations with antibiotics prophylactically.

Umbilical hernia

Umbilical hernias in infants are dealt with on p. 551.

Para-umbilical hernias in adults

The condition A hernia in this site in adults does not occur at the umbilicus, but rather just above it or below it, due to a weakness in the linea alba. It is commoner in women, and obesity, multiparity and weak abdominal muscles are predisposing causes. The sac may contain both omentum and bowel and in this age-group gastrointestinal symptoms of subacute obstruction are more common. The hernia may become quite large and irreducible. Strangulation may occur.

Management The patient should lose weight. Operation is usually advised because of the risk of strangulation.

Operation: para-umbilical hernia repair
The sac is dissected clear and then opened. The adhesions holding the bowel and omentum are freed and the bowel returned to the abdomen. The defect is then closed.

Codes

Blood	0 ....
GA/LA	GA ....
Opn time	45−60 minutes ....
Stay	3−5 days ....
Drains out	Subcutaneous 3−7 days ....
Sutures out	5−7 days ....
Off work........	1 month ....

Postoperative care
This is similar to that for an incisional hernia.

Epigastric hernia

The condition This is a midline hernia through a defect in the linea alba above the umbilicus. The initial weakness may be at the site of penetrating vessels. It usually contains extraperitoneal fat (epiplocoele), although if it enlarges a true peritoneal sac may protrude. In this case it may contain omentum. However, it never contains bowel.

Recognizing the pattern

The hernia may be symptomless or present as a small swelling in the epigastrium which may be painful, particularly on exercise. Occasionally it causes episodes of severe epigastric pain and vomiting. These may have been extensively investigated but no cause found.

On examination
The small epigastric mass is palpable and more prominent when the patient coughs or tenses the abdominal muscles.

Management

These hernias usually require operative repair.

Operation: repair of epigastric hernia
The hernia is excised and the defect in the linea alba closed with non-absorbable sutures. There may be other epigastric hernias present which should also be removed.

Codes

Blood	0 . . . .
GA/LA	GA . . . .
Opn time	15–30 minutes . . . .
Stay	1–3 days . . . .
Drains out	0 or 24 hours . . . .
Sutures out	5–7 days . . . .
Off work	2–3 weeks . . . .

Spigelian hernia

The condition

The hernial sac protrudes through the linea semilunaris (the lateral edge of the rectus sheath), at the level of the semicircular fold of Douglas (see Fig. 81). It usually lies underneath the external oblique. It has a narrow neck and strangulation may occur.

Recognizing the pattern

It is usually seen in obese people over the age of 50 and presents as a swelling below and lateral to the umbilicus. It may cause some discomfort which is worse on exertion and occasionally it causes nausea and vomiting.

Management

Operation: repair of Spigelian hernia
The sac is isolated, emptied and ligated, and the defect closed in layers.

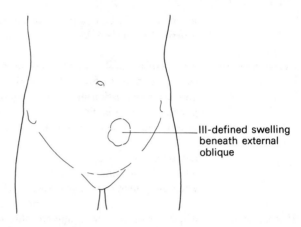

III-defined swelling
beneath external
oblique

Fig. 81. Spigelian hernia.

Codes

Blood	0 ....
GA/LA	GA ....
Opn time	30 minutes ....
Stay	3–5 days ....
Drains out	0 or 24 hours ....
Sutures out	5–7 days ....
Off work	2–3 weeks ....

Obturator hernia

The condition

This is a hernia that protrudes from the pelvis out through the obturator canal. It lies beneath the adductor muscles of the floor of the femoral triangle in the upper thigh.

Recognizing the pattern

It is commoner in women. The swelling is usually hidden, although it may be more obvious if the leg is laterally rotated, abducted and flexed. Strangulation is common and this usually causes intestinal obstruction. A Richter's hernia is quite common in this site (see pp. 395–397). Pain is often referred along the obturator nerve to the knee.

Management

Operation: repair of obturator hernia
The hernia is repaired from above, usually through a lower paramedian laparotomy incision.

Codes

Blood	0 . . . .
GA/LA	GA . . . .
Opn time	30 minutes . . . .
Stay	3−5 days . . . .
Drains out	0 . . . .
Sutures out	7 days . . . .
Off work	1 month . . . .

Umbilical discharge in adults

Umbilical discharge in children is dealt with on p. 552. In adults a vitello-intestinal or urachal cyst or fistula may also be considered.

Other causes in adults include an umbilical stone or a simple skin abscess.

An umbilical stone consists of inspissated secretions and exfoliated squamous cells which collect at the base of a deep uncleaned umbilicus. Eventually infection may occur and a persistent discharge, either through the umbilicus or through an adjoining sinus, may result.

Management

Preoperative care

The patient should lose weight. A swab is taken from the discharge and relevant antibiotic cover started with the premedication. An ultrasound examination may demonstrate a urachal cyst. A sinogram may also be useful.

Operation: exploration of the umbilicus

The umbilical scar is detached from the linea alba and the umbilical pit everted. Any deep connections can be isolated and divided. The umbilicus is cleared of all debris and its deeper part may be excised, resulting in a shallower depression. If a urachal abnormality or vitello-intestinal abnormality is present, it is excised.

Codes

Blood	0 . . . .
GA/LA	GA . . . .
Opn time	30−60 minutes (depending on extent) . . . .
Stay	2−3 days . . . .
Drains out	48 hours . . . .
Sutures out	5−7 days . . . .
Off work	1 week . . . .

8   **Urinary Tract**

8.1   Disorders of the kidney
Renal tract stones
Pyelonephritis
Renal tumours
Renal cysts
Haematuria
Renal transplantation

8.2   Conditions of the bladder and urethra
Bladder stones
Bladder diverticulum
Bladder tumours
Disorders of micturition
Acute prostatitis
Chronic prostatitis
Benign prostatic hypertrophy
Prostatic carcinoma
Urethral stricture

8.3   Male genitalia
Conditions of the foreskin
Congenital lesions of the male external genitalia
Carcinoma of the penis
Scrotal conditions

8.1 Disorders of the Kidney

Renal pain is felt in the loin between the twelfth rib and the iliac crest. The pain is usually more or less constant. Ureteric pain radiates down and forwards from the loin to the groin and on to the vulva or scrotum. Ureteric pain is usually a true colic.

Common surgical causes of renal pain are stones, pyelonephritis, and renal tumours.

Renal tract stones

The condition

Stones form in the renal tract due to increased concentration of solutes in the urine such as calcium (e.g. in hyperparathyroidism), uric acid (gout) or oxalic acid, or due to a general increased concentration of the urine during dehydration. Roughened areas within the renal pelvis and calyces may act as focal points for the formation of stones (Randall's plaques). Other predisposing factors include stasis and pooling of urine due to obstruction and urinary infection.

The commonest type of stone is composed of calcium and magnesium phosphates and carbonates. These precipitate in alkaline urine such as occurs in a *Proteus* urinary infection. The stone is soft and friable. The commonest pure stones are calcium oxalate. They are hard and rough and may cause haematuria. The formation of both calcium oxalate and uric acid stones is favoured by acid urine. Oxalate stones are radio-opaque and cystine and uric acid calculi are radio-translucent.

The stones are usually formed in the renal calyces or pelvis. They may continue growing to fill the whole of the renal pelvis (Staghorn calculus). Alternatively, they may remain small and pass down the ureter into the bladder causing ureteric colic. The stone may become stuck at any point in this passage, but particularly at the pelvi-ureteric junction, where the ureter crosses the iliac artery, and at the entrance of the ureter into the bladder.

Recognizing the pattern

The patient
The patient may be of any age, although stones are unusual before adolescence. Males are more commonly affected than females in a ratio of 2:1.

The history

Stones within the kidney give rise to pain in the loin and often present with episodes of urinary infection. If a stone passes down the ureter, the patient experiences excruciating bouts of severe colic starting in the loin and radiating round into the flank and groin. The pain is so severe that the sufferer tends to roll around in agony unable to find a comfortable position. He may vomit. Haematuria may discolour the urine after an attack of pain.

On examination

There may be tenderness in the renal angle or along the line of the ureter but the physical signs are minimal compared with the severity of the pain. Constitutional upset with fever and malaise indicate secondary infection.

Proving the diagnosis

The presence of red cells in the urine on microscopy is the most helpful finding. In the early stages these may be absent and in that case the examination should be repeated after 24−48 hours. Evidence of infection should also be sought.

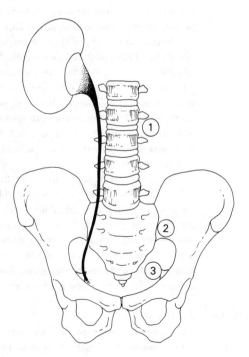

Fig. 82. The landmarks for the ureter on an abdominal X-ray. 1 Lumbar transverse processes. 2 Sacro-iliac joint. 3 Ischial spine.

A straight abdominal X-ray may show the stone lying in the kidney substance or along the line of the ureter (Fig. 82). Ninety per cent of urinary stones are radio-opaque (compared with 10% of gall-stones).

An emergency IVU will confirm the diagnosis and show the position of the stone.

Screening tests for raised serum calcium and uric acid should always be performed.

Management

This is either conservative or operative, the choice depending on the size of the stone. Try to decide whether the stone will pass spontaneously. The critical size is 0.5 cm.

If it is clearly too large to travel down the ureter, then it must be removed. If, however, natural passage is possible, then the initial management is always conservative.

Conservative management

The patient is put on a regular non-steroidal analgesic, although pethidine may be required in severe colic. The patient should be encouraged to drink plenty of fluid and the urine sieved to see if a stone has passed. If found it can be analysed.

Surgical management

The treatment of urinary calculi has advanced rapidly in the last decade. Using percutaneous renal surgery a track can be created between the skin and the intra-renal collecting system. A nephroscope can then be passed and the stone removed with forceps. If the stone is too large, it can be disintegrated by ultrasound or shattered by an electrohydraulic discharge. The fragments are then removed.

Extracorporeal shock wave lithotripsy (ESWL) was first developed in Germany. A shock wave is created by an underwater spark generator and the energy is focused on to the stone by positioning the patient in a bath and using X-ray screening to locate the stone. The shock waves generated are painful and the patient has to be anaesthetised. More modern lithotripters use electromagnetic or piezoelectric generated shock waves and the latter require minimal analgesia.

Surgical intervention is indicated if there is no significant progress of the stone down the ureter, if there is increasing renal impairment or if there is infection above the site of obstruction (a urological emergency). The surgical management of the stone depends on whether it lies in the kidney or in the ureter and, if in the ureter, at what level.

Stones in the ureter

Previously stones were removed from the ureter endoscopically by passing a Dormia basket. Rigid and flexible ureteroscopes are now available and allow the stones to be removed under direct vision. They may first be disintegrated by ultrasound or electrohydraulic shock waves.

Stones in the upper ureter may be pushed into the renal pelvis and treated as a renal stone by percutaneous renal surgery or by ESWL.

Operation: endoscopic stone removal

Stones in the lower third of the ureter may be removed by passing a cystoscope into the bladder through which a Dormia basket is passed beyond the stone. The basket is opened and pulled back, hopefully engaging the stone. Several passes of the basket may be required.

If the above procedure fails, or the stone is above the lower third of the ureter, the ureteric orifice is dilated and a ureteroscope is passed into it. The instrument is carefully advanced until the stone is encountered and extracted.

Codes

Blood	0 . . . .
GA/LA	GA . . . .
Opn time	Variable . . . .
Stay	3−5 days . . . .
Drains out	0 . . . .
Sutures out	0 . . . .
Off work	Variable . . . .

Rarely, if non-invasive methods fail, open surgery is performed.

Operation: uretero-lithotomy

The ureter is exposed through a muscle-cutting or muscle-splitting transverse abdominal incision lateral to the rectus muscle. The retroperitoneal area is exposed and the peritoneum and its contents retracted medially. The ureter is found and slings passed above and below the stone to prevent it displacing upwards or downwards. The ureter is incised and the stone removed. The ureterostomy is closed with absorbable sutures and the wound drained.

Codes

Blood	2 units . . . .
GA/LA	GA . . . .
Opn time	30−60 minutes . . . .

Stay	7–10 days	
Drains out	3–5 days	
Sutures out	7 days	
Off work........	4–6 weeks	

Postoperative care
There is usually very little ileus and no nasogastric tube is required. The patient is encouraged to drink 2–3 litres a day after the first 24 hours. The drain is removed once it is clear that there is no ureteric fistula. If a urinary leak does occur, the drain is left *in situ* and the leak will usually close. If leakage continues longer than a week, the passage of a ureteric catheter will usually solve the problem.

Stones in the kidney
Ninety per cent of renal stones can be treated by percutaneous renal surgery and/or ESWL. For the rest, open surgery is required.

Preoperative management
If the urine is infected, antibiotics are commenced preoperatively. The stone or stones must be adequately demonstrated radiologically. The radiographers should also be warned that they may be required during the operation.

Operation: removal of renal stones
The kidney is exposed via a postero-lateral incision over the 12th rib. The stone may be removed from the renal pelvis (pyelolithotomy), the renal substance (nephrolithotomy) or both (pyelonephrolithotomy). An intraoperative X-ray may be taken to ensure that all the stones have been removed. Occasionally, if the stones are numerous or there is associated renal damage, a partial or even total nephrectomy is required. A drain is put down to the kidney bed and occasionally, if the operation has been difficult, a nephrostomy tube is inserted to remove any blood clot that may form in the renal pelvis.

Codes

Blood	2 units	
GA/LA	GA	
Opn time	60–120 minutes	
Stay	10 days	
Drains out	3–5 days, nephrostomy 48 hours	
Sutures out	7 days	
Off work........	4 weeks........................	

This is similar to that after uretero-lithotomy.

Prevention of recurrence
The patient should be encouraged to drink as much as possible. Any cause of renal stones found on screening must be treated.

Pyelonephritis

The condition

This is due to parenchymal infection of the kidney secondary either to ascending infection from the bladder or problems in the kidney itself such as renal stones or pelvi-ureteric obstruction. Occasionally the kidney may become infected via the bloodstream as a complication of septicaemia. The organism is usually a Gram-negative *Bacillus*. Pyelonephritis in the presence of urinary tract obstruction is a urological emergency and should be diagnosed without delay. The progression to septicaemia and shock can be rapid.

Recognizing the pattern

The patient
The patient is of any age but more frequently female and of childbearing age.

The history
There is a sudden onset of illness with a high fever and vomiting. The systemic symptoms are often dominant and the patient may not complain of any symptoms referable to the urinary tract in the early stages. On questioning, however, there may be pain in the loin and this can be severe.

On examination
There may be a tachycardia and a high fever (up to 39.5°C) often with rigors. There is localized tenderness over the affected kidney.

Proving the diagnosis

The diagnosis is confirmed by finding bacteria and pus cells in the urine, and growing the organism. Pus cells may be absent in the early stages if the affected kidney shuts down and fails to excrete infected urine into the bladder. One negative mid-stream urine specimen (MSU) should not, therefore, be taken as excluding the diagnosis but must be repeated.

An IVU is performed and it may show a temporarily non-functioning kidney on the affected side. Where pyelonephritis and obstruction is present, a plain X-ray may show a stone and an ultrasound may demonstrate a dilated collecting system.

Management	If the kidney is obstructed it is urgently decompressed by inserting a percutaneous nephrostomy tube. Antibiotics are given in high dosage, intravenously if necessary. It is important to set up urinary cultures before treatment is commenced. The patient should be confined to bed until the systemic symptoms and localized tenderness settle. Analgesia with opiates may be needed, and the patient is encouraged to drink at least 3 litres of fluid daily. Open operative treatment is not required unless a peri-nephric abscess forms, in which case it is drained through a loin incision.

Renal tumours

Renal tumours may be either benign or malignant. Benign tumours include cysts and true benign neoplasms. Malignant tumours may be primary or secondary. Primary renal tumours arise either from the urothelium of the calyces and pelvis (pelvi-ureteric tumour) or from the kidney substance itself (hypernephroma).

Pelvi-ureteric tumours

The condition	Urothelial tumours can arise anywhere where there is transitional cell epithelium. They are associated with the ingestion of carcinogens (transitional cell carcinomas) or the presence of chronic renal calculi (squamous cell carcinoma) (see p. 407).
Recognizing the pattern	The patient is usually over the age of 40. He presents with a history of painless haematuria or occasionally ureteric colic associated with the passage of a clot. There are usually no physical signs.
Proving the diagnosis	An IVU shows a filling defect in the renal tract. Urinary cytology may show carcinoma cells.
Management	As a urothelial tumour represents an instability in the epithelium of the renal tract, it is usually considered necessary to remove the whole of the renal tract on the affected side. The need for this must be explained to the patient. Occasionally two incisions are necessary, one in the loin to remove the kidney and a second in the lower abdomen to remove the pelvic part of the ureter.

Operation: nephro-ureterectomy

The kidney is explored and its vessels isolated and ligated. The kidney is removed and the ureter is followed down into the pelvis and excised together with a patch of the bladder mucosa. The bladder muscle is repaired. A urinary catheter is left *in situ* and the renal bed drained.

Codes

Blood	2 units	
GA/LA	GA	
Opn time	1–2 hours	
Stay	7–10 days	
Drains out	48 hours	
Sutures out	7 days	
Off work	4 weeks	

Postoperative care

In the early stages there is a danger of haemorrhage in the renal bed and the vital signs must be carefully monitored. The urinary catheter should not be removed until it is clear that the bladder repair has healed. This usually occurs within 7 days. If there is any doubt, a cystogram is helpful.

The patient should be followed up by cystoscopy and with regular review of the other kidney by intravenous pyelography. This is in order to detect the development of further tumours.

Hypernephroma

The condition

Hypernephroma is an adenocarcinoma arising from the substance of the kidney. The tumour may grow very large and metastasize both to local lymph nodes and via the bloodstream. It tends to spread up the renal vein and grow into the inferior vena cava. Metastasis occurs via the bloodstream and secondaries may occur in lung, bone and brain. It may be clinically silent until it has grown to a large size, and systemic symptoms often divert attention away from the local disease.

Recognizing the pattern

The patient

The patient is usually over 50 years old and more commonly male. However, the disease can affect young people and may be seen in anyone between the ages of 20 and 60.

The history

The patient can present with a wide variety of symptoms. The typical triad is a palpable mass, loin pain and haematuria.

There may be generalized ill-health or changes in personality. It may present as a pyrexia of unknown origin associated with night sweats or with anaemia. The tumour may bleed into the renal tract producing 'clot colic'. Patients may also present with symptoms from metastases (e.g. pathological fracture). A hypernephroma spreading along the renal vein sometimes obstructs the testicular vein on the left, causing a varicocoele. Finally, hormonal secretion from the growth may cause hypertension (renin), polycythaemia (erythropoietin) or hypercalcaemia (parathormone). Not infrequently a hypernephroma presents as an incidental 'cannon ball' metastasis found on a chest X-ray.

On examination
The lump in the loin may be easily palpable. It is usually only possible to feel the lower pole, which may be ballotted, and moves down on respiration. It is resonant to percussion due to the overlying colon.

Proving the diagnosis

Investigation of the urine will often show microscopic haematuria. An ultrasound of the renal area shows a solid mass arising from the kidney. The ultrasound may also be used to investigate whether or not there is growth in the renal vein and vena cava. An IVU shows a renal mass distorting the calyces. Renal angiography demonstrates the characteristic tumour circulation within the mass. Recently CAT scanning has replaced angiography. During these investigations the state of the opposite kidney should also be determined. Bilateral hypernephromas are not unknown and congenital absence of a second kidney must be recognized.

Management

During the preoperative work-up a careful search should be made for the presence of metastases. This will include liver function tests, a chest X-ray, a liver scan and a bone scan. A venogram may be undertaken to determine whether the tumour has spread into the vena cava. If this has occurred, a much more extensive operation will be required. In some centres where the facilities are available, the vascularity and size of the tumour may be reduced by therapeutic intra-arterial embolization. This should be done immediately before the operation as pain and pyrexia are common complications. This is also a possible way to treat patients unfit for major surgery or those with widespread metastases.

Operation: nephrectomy
The tumour may be very bulky and this can make the operation difficult and increase the blood loss. Occasionally it is necessary to open the chest and divide the diaphragm in order to get adequate exposure.

The kidney is explored through either an anterior or a loin incision. You should determine which approach is intended by the surgeon and inform the theatre staff and anaesthetist. When the approach is through the bed of a rib, a pneumothorax is not uncommon. A chest drain may be needed postoperatively.

If the tumour is invading the inferior vena cava, then the surgeon will have to control that vessel in order to effect an adequate removal. He may open the chest to achieve this. Once the tumour and kidney have been mobilized the renal vessels are clamped and the ureter tied and divided. The kidney and tumour are then removed. A drain is left in the renal bed.

Codes

Blood	4–6 units . . . .
GA/LA	GA . . . .
Opn time	2–3 hours . . . .
Stay	5–10 days . . . .
Drains out	48 hours, chest 24–48 hours . . . .
Sutures out	5–7 days . . . .
Off work.	4–6 weeks . . . .

Postoperative care

Where a pneumothorax has occurred, a post-operative chest X-ray should be carried out in the erect position in the first few hours after the operation to check that the lung has fully re-expanded.

There is a danger of haemorrhage in the first 24 hours and careful monitoring is necessary during this period. There may be an ileus but this is not usually prolonged beyond 48 hours. Very occasionally surrounding organs are damaged during the removal of a large tumour. Examples of this are damage to the tail of the pancreas on the left side (pancreatic fistula) and damage to the stomach, colon or spleen.

Radiotherapy may be given to the renal bed if residual carcinoma is present. It is very useful for relieving pain from bony metastases. Systemic chemotherapy is not helpful, although hormonal treatment with medroxyprogesterone acetate (Provera) produces a good response in 20% of patients with metastatic disease. Interferon has been reported to produce tumour regression.

Renal cysts

The condition Renal cysts may be single or present as part of polycystic disease of the kidney. The latter is a familial condition and may affect both kidneys and be associated with cysts in other organs. A single cyst is quite common and usually produces no symptoms. It may be found during investigations for other renal conditions.

Management

Polycystic kidneys may progress to renal failure and there is little that can be done to prevent this. Eventually renal transplantation may be needed.

If a single renal cyst has been detected on ultrasound, it can be aspirated under ultrasound control and the fluid sent for cytology. Radio-opaque contrast is then injected to outline the cyst wall. Occasionally a cyst and a carcinoma may coexist. This is excluded if:

1 cytology is negative;
2 the aspirated fluid is clear;
3 the cyst wall is smooth;
4 the lesion avascular; and
5 there is no calcification.

Haematuria

Haematuria is a common presenting complaint and a routine series of investigations is undertaken.

Making the diagnosis

The history
There are three important points to establish.

1 Is it true haematuria?
Other causes of red urine include the following:
(a) drugs, i.e. rifampicin, para-aminosalicylic acid (PAS), nitrofurantoin and phenindione;
(b) foodstuffs such as beetroot;
(c) porphyria.

The differentiation can be made on the history and on urine microscopy. Ward testing 'stix' for blood are also helpful.

It is also important to make certain that the blood is not coming from the vagina or rectum and this can be discovered by a careful history and examination.

The causes of true haematuria are listed in Table 23.

2 The timing of the bleeding in the urinary stream
Blood at the start of the urinary stream suggests a urethral lesion. Blood at the end of the urinary stream suggests a localized bladder lesion. Blood showing throughout micturition suggests a renal, ureteric, or diffuse bladder disorder. The presence of clots points towards a renal tumour.

3 Is the haematuria painful or not?

Painful haematuria
The bleeding is usually secondary to a cystitis, which may itself be secondary to other problems such as bladder neck obstruction or stones. You have to remember, however, that infection is a common complication of urothelial tumours.

Table 23. Causes of haematuria

General	Bleeding disorders Anticoagulants Haemoglobinopathy
Local Kidney	Glomerulonephritis Carcinoma Trauma Infarction Papillary necrosis
Ureter	Tumours Stones
Bladder	Cystitis Trauma Foreign body Tumours
Urethra	Prostatic disease Carcinoma of the penis

A diagnosis of cystitis can be confirmed by examining the urine, when an excess of red and white cells will be found and there may be a positive growth on culture.

Painless haematuria
Further investigation is mandatory in order to exclude a carcinoma. An IVU may show a cause in the upper genito-urinary tract such as a hypernephroma or pelvi-ureteric tumour. Cystoscopy must be undertaken to visualize the bladder mucosa and search for a papilloma or carcinoma of the bladder.

Routine investigations

1 Microscopy and culture of a midstream specimen of urine. Red cell casts or protein indicates glomerular disease. Pus cells are present in an acute infection. If they are present and the urine is sterile, the possibility of tuberculosis, tumour or calculi must be considered.

2 Exfoliative cytology of a fresh specimen may show tumour cells.

3 An intravenous urogram is mandatory in all cases of

painless haematuria and in most cases of painful haematuria. Ultrasound and renal angiography may also be needed.
4 Cystoscopy is nearly always necessary in adults.

Management

The treatment of cystitis is with antibiotics, and, if it is the first episode in a young woman, no further investigation may be needed providing the haematuria settles. If it persists, if the infection recurs or if the patient is male, further investigation of the urinary tract by cystoscopy and IVU is required. This is in order to exclude causes such as urothelial tumours, calculi or prostatic hypertrophy.

The management of hypernephroma is dealt with on p. 414, pelvic-ureteric tumours on p. 413 and bladder tumours on p. 427.

Recurrent bleeding due to enlarged veins on a benign prostate may necessitate prostatectomy (pp. 437–439).

Renal transplantation

This operation is indicated for the treatment of terminal renal failure, commonly as an end result of chronic glomerulonephritis, chronic pyelonephritis, obstructive uropathy, hypertensive or diabetic renal failure, or rare metabolic diseases affecting the kidney such as oxalosis. Such patients are usually maintained on a chronic dialysis regime and after full counselling their name may be placed on a transplant waiting list.

Preoperative management

The patient is grouped, tissue typed and screened for antibodies. The donor may either be a living relative or a 'brain-dead' cadaver. Once a donor becomes available and the potential recipient is known to have a negative cross-match, arrangements are made to admit him to hospital.

Donor operation

Removal of a kidney from a living donor is similar to a nephrectomy for other reasons (see p. 415). Great care is taken not to damage the renal vessels and the kidney is then perfused as below. This procedure carries the disadvantage of the risk to the health of the donor. It is preferable that the donor is looked after by a separate team of surgeons from the recipient.

When a living donor kidney is not available, a cadaveric kidney is used. Once the diagnosis of brain death is established, and once permission has been obtained from the relatives, the kidneys are removed through a cruciate or subcostal incision. This operation is often combined with the removal of other organs, including the heart and liver.

The renal artery, vein and ureter are all carefully dissected out. The aorta is then cannulated and the kidney perfused with a preserving solution. All renal arteries are included in a patch of aorta and the kidney removed. It is stored in a preserving solution in a sterile plastic bag surrounded by ice.

Recipient operation

The recipient may be dialysed immediately preoperatively. The kidney is transplanted into the retroperitoneal tissues of the iliac fossa. The renal vein is usually anastomosed to the external iliac vein and the renal artery to the external iliac artery. The ureter is implanted into the bladder.

Codes

Blood	2 units	. . . .
GA/LA	GA	. . . .
Opn time	2 hours	. . . .
Stay	Variable	. . . .
Drains out	48 hours	. . . .
Sutures out	10 days	. . . .
Off work	Variable	. . . .

Postoperative management

If necessary dialysis is maintained until the kidney function is satisfactory. Standard immunosuppression is given. A full blood count, electrolytes, urea, creatinine and cyclosporin levels are measured each day. Common complications include rejection, infection, ureteric obstruction, and fluid collections around the kidney. Long-term immunosuppression and follow-up are mandatory.

Conditions of the Bladder and Urethra

Bladder stones

The condition
Bladder calculi have the same aetiology as renal calculi. A stone in the bladder may have originated in the renal pelvis, although if a stone can pass down the ureter it usually manages to pass out through the urethra. In most cases bladder stones form primarily in the bladder. Stone formation is favoured by urinary stasis, infection or the presence of a foreign body.

Recognizing the pattern
The patient
Bladder stones can occur in any age-group. Males are more commonly affected than females.

The history
The typical pattern of symptoms is pain, frequency and haematuria. The pain is felt in the suprapubic area, perineum and tip of the penis or labium majora. It is worse when the patient is upright and the stone is lying on the trigone. The pain increases with any jolting movements or at the end of micturition. Urinary frequency is also more troublesome during the day and there may be a feeling of incomplete emptying after micturition. Haematuria commonly occurs at the end of the stream. Occasionally there may be intermittent obstruction to urinary flow.

On examination
The prostate may be enlarged. In women it may be possible to feel a bladder stone on bimanual vaginal examination.

Proving the diagnosis
1 Test the urine for blood, pus cells and evidence of infection.
2 Request a plain abdominal X-ray. Ninety per cent of bladder stones are radio-opaque.
3 Cystoscopy. This enables one to see the bladder stone and also to look for any predisposing pathology (e.g. prostatic hypertrophy or bladder diverticulum).

Management
Once the diagnosis has been made, metabolic causes of stone formation should be excluded by the appropriate blood and urine tests. Stones elsewhere in the urogenital tract must be excluded by plain X-ray or IVU.

421

A very small stone may be managed conservatively in the hope that it may pass. Larger stones are removed. This may be done either by crushing the stone with a lithotrite, by using ultrasound or electrohydraulic probes to shatter the stone or by open operation.

Operation: crushing the stone — litholapaxy

This involves passing an optical lithotrite (an instrument to crush the stone) up the urethra. The stone is crushed under direct vision and the bladder then irrigated to remove all the fragments. If there is a urethral stricture or enlarged prostate, this is usually treated at the same time, e.g. by dilatation or trans-urethral resection of the prostate (TURP) (see pp. 444 and 437).

Codes

Blood	0 . . . .
GA/LA	GA . . . .
Opn time	1 hour . . . .
Stay	3–7 days . . . .
Drains out	0 . . . .
Sutures out	0 . . . .
Off work	1–2 weeks . . . .

Litholapaxy is not suitable for hard stones, or stones formed round a foreign body. In these cases, or if there is another lesion which will require open operation (e.g. a very large prostate or a bladder diverticulum), open cystostomy is preferred.

Operation: cystostomy

The stone is removed by open operation. In a male a transvesical prostatectomy is done at the same time (see p. 437).

Codes

Blood	2 units . . . .
GA/LA	GA . . . .
Opn time	1–2 hours . . . .
Stay	10 days . . . .
Drains out	Wound 3–5 days, suprapubic catheter 1–2 days, urethral catheter 5–10 days . . . .
Sutures out	7 days . . . .
Off work	4 weeks . . . .

Postoperative care
The bladder wound heals in 5−7 days and the catheter is then removed. It is important to avoid urinary infection and prophylactic antibiotics are given over the early postoperative course.

Bladder diverticulum

The condition

This is an extrusion of bladder mucosa through the hypertrophied muscle of the bladder wall. It is most often acquired as a pulsion diverticulum secondary to outflow obstruction and is usually close to the ureteric orifice. Very occasionally it is congenital, arising from remnants of the urachus in the midline.

Symptoms are due to urinary stasis and secondary infection, with calculus formation. A diverticulum may cause a hydronephrosis by compressing the ureter. Occasionally a carcinoma develops in a diverticulum and, because of the lack of a muscle coat, extravesical spread occurs early.

Recognizing the pattern

The patient
The patient is usually male and over the age of 50.

The history
Haematuria or recurrent cystitis may occur. Sometimes there is a history of double voiding of urine (*pis-en-deux*), the first batch being clear and the second batch being cloudy as the diverticulum drains its contents into the bladder. Diverticula are not infrequently found inadvertently on an IVU and may be symptomless.

On examination
Usually no signs are found. Rectal examination may reveal a large prostate.

Proving the diagnosis

1 An IVU or retrograde cystogram will demonstrate the diverticulum by filling it with contrast.
2 Cystoscopy with the bladder distended demonstrates the opening of the diverticulum.

Management

Provided any outflow obstruction of the bladder is treated, and provided the diverticulum itself is asymptomatic and uninfected, it can be left alone. However, if symptoms or the complications listed above ensue, then the diverticulum must be removed.

Preoperative management
The patient should be given a course of antibiotics and, if necessary, bladder washouts for 4 days before operation.

Operation: resection of diverticulum
The bladder is approached extraperitoneally. The ureter is catheterized for identification. The diverticulum is dissected out, separated from the ureter, and then excised and the hole in the bladder closed.

Codes

Blood..........	0..............................
GA/LA........	GA............................
Opn time.......	90 minutes.....................
Stay...........	7–10 days......................
Drains out......	Catheter 10 days, extravesical drain 3 days........................
Sutures out.....	7 days.........................
Off work........	4 weeks........................

Postoperative care
A short course of antibiotics may be given to cover the operation and the first few days afterwards, e.g. ampicillin or co-trimoxazole. The only major complications to watch for are urinary tract infection and urinary fistula (see p. 66).

Bladder tumours

The condition

Ninety-eight per cent of primary bladder carcinomas are transitional cell carcinomas. The remainder are rare and are either squamous cell carcinomas (associated with chronic irritation and squamous metaplasia due to bilharzia or bladder stones) or adenocarcinomas (arising from persistent urachal remnants).

The majority of bladder neoplasms have no known aetiology. However, there is an increased incidence of transitional cell carcinomas in those working in the dye, rubber and printing industries. β-Naphthylamine and benzidine have been implicated as the carcinogens. Cyclophosphamide can cause bladder carcinoma. Smokers have a high incidence of recurrence although it has not been proved that smoking can cause bladder tumours.

Staging (see Fig. 83)
Bladder carcinomas are staged as follows:

T_{is} *In situ* carcinoma affects multiple areas in the bladder and has a tendency for anaplastic change.

T_a Papillary, no invasion of basement membrane.

T_1	Invades lamina propria.
T_2	Invades superficial muscle.
T_{3a}	Invades deep muscle.
T_{3b}	Invades perivesical fat.
T_4	Invasion of adjoining organs.

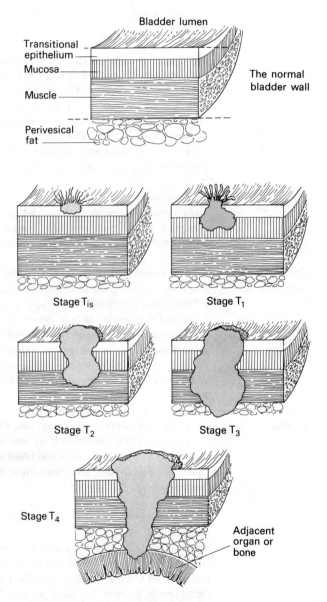

Fig. 83. The staging of bladder tumours.

Tumours are also graded on histological appearances.

G_1 Well differentiated
G_2 Moderately differentiated
G_3 Poorly differentiated

Recognizing the pattern

The patient
The patient is elderly and the disease is four times more common in men.

The history
Ninety per cent of patients present with painless haematuria, occasionally passing blood clots. Fifteen per cent have frequency and dysuria due to associated infection. Obstruction of the bladder neck may cause the symptoms of retention of urine. Involvement of the ureteric orifices can cause hydronephrosis and loin pain. Bilateral ureteric obstruction will present as uraemia. Nerve involvement causes continuous suprapubic pain radiating to the groin and perineum.

On examination
Usually there are no signs. In advanced cases abdominal examination may reveal a palpable mass in the pelvis, enlarged lymph nodes in the groin or a palpable liver.

Proving the diagnosis

1 Urine cytology. Sixty per cent of bladder tumours can be diagnosed and the grade of tumour assessed.
2 Intravenous urogram. The tumour may appear as a filling defect and the function of both kidneys can be assessed.
3 Cystoscopy. Every patient presenting with painless haematuria must have a cystoscopy and a bimanual examination under anaesthesia. The tumour is biopsied and stages T_a and T_1 can be treated during this procedure.

Assessment and staging

This is gauged by cystoscopy and biopsy of the growth and bimanual examination under anaesthesia. For stage T_3 and T_4 tumours a CAT scan and a bone scan are performed.

A chest X-ray is performed and blood taken for a full blood count and urea and electrolytes, to assess renal function.

Operation: cystoscopy and examination under anaesthesia
Typical well-differentiated non-invasive tumours look like a sea anemone and may be multiple. An invasive tumour appears solid and may be ulcerated. The lesion is biopsied, taking normal tissue at the base if possible. Multiple lesions are removed or diathermied at the same time.

Following cystoscopy, the bladder is emptied and a bi-manual examination performed. Superficial bladder tumours are not palpable. Stage T_2 tumours cause induration of the bladder wall. Larger tumours can be staged depending on the size and degree of fixation.

Codes

Blood	Group and save . . . .
GA/LA	GA . . . .
Opn time	20–30 minutes . . . .
Stay	1–2 days . . . .
Drains out	Catheter 24 hours . . . .
Sutures out	0 . . . .
Off work.	Variable . . . .

Management

T_a tumours can be treated by repeated cystodiathermy. Larger T_a tumours to T_2 tumours are treated by trans-urethral resection. Multiple tumours can be given intra-vesical chemotherapy (adriamycin, mitomycin). Radiotherapy is given for high-grade T_2 tumours and a cystectomy is performed if recurrence occurs.

T_3 and T_4 tumours are treated with radiotherapy and a cystectomy is performed if tumour recurrence occurs.

Adenocarcinomas are treated by partial cystectomy with or without post-operative radiotherapy. Metastases occur early with squamous cell carcinoma. They are treated by radiotherapy followed by cystectomy.

All patients with superficial bladder tumours need to have a repeat cystoscopy initially at 3 months and thereafter at regular intervals as recurrence is likely. Five per cent of superficial tumours become invasive.

Surgery for bladder tumours

Operation: trans-urethral resection of tumour (TURT)
The tumour is excised completely including the superficial layer of bladder wall muscle in its base. The specimens are sent for histological staging. The main danger of this procedure is bladder wall perforation. If the decision is taken at cystoscopy to proceed to a TURT, two units of blood should be requested.

Codes

Blood	2 units . . . .
GA/LA	GA . . . .
Opn time	60 minutes . . . .
Stay	3–4 days . . . .

Drains out	Urinary catheter 3−5 days . . . .
Sutures out	0 . . . .
Off work	1−2 weeks . . . .

Postoperative care
The catheter is removed once the urine is clear of blood. The patient is followed up as below.

Operation: Helmstein's procedure
This operation is rarely performed now but may be used for intractable bleeding from invasive bladder tumours.

A balloon is inflated inside the bladder until the pressure inside equals the patient's systolic blood pressure. Any tumour projecting into the bladder is therefore flattened against the bladder wall, and by maintaining the balloon pressure for 4−6 hours (under epidural anaesthesia) the tumour will necrose.

Codes

Blood	0 . . . .
GA/LA	Epidural . . . .
Opn time	4−6 hours . . . .
Stay	Variable . . . .
Drains out	0 . . . .
Sutures out	0 . . . .
Off work	Variable . . . .

Postoperative care
The patient is warned that following the removal of the catheter he may pass blood and pieces of necrotic tumour.

Operation: partial cystectomy (for adenocarcinoma of the bladder vault)
The tumour is removed together with a 3 cm rim of normal, full-thickness bladder wall. The ureter is preserved or re-implanted. The local recurrence rate is high.

Codes

Blood	2 units . . . .
GA/LA	GA . . . .
Opn time	2 hours . . . .
Stay	10 days . . . .
Drains out	Perivesical drain 3−5 days, urethral catheter 10 days . . . .
Sutures out	7 days . . . .
Off work	6 weeks . . . .

Postoperative care
Frequency of micturition is almost inevitable in the post-operative period. This does improve as the bladder remnant expands.

Operation: total cystectomy
A lower midline incision is made and a full laparotomy performed. If distant metastases or gross local invasion has occurred, the operation is abandoned. Otherwise the ureters are divided close to the bladder and the distal ends ligated. The bladder, prostate and urethra (and uterus in females) are removed *en bloc* with the iliac and obturator lymph nodes.

The ureters are diverted into an ileal conduit or less commonly into the sigmoid colon. Drains are left in the bladder bed and to the ureteric anastomosis.

Codes

Blood	6 units ....
GA/LA	GA ....
Opn time	4 hours ....
Stay	2–3 weeks ....
Drains out	5 days ....
Sutures out	10 days ....
Off work........	2 months ....

Postoperative care
There are many problems following this procedure. Breakdown of the urinary anastomosis may result in a urinary fistula (see p. 66). Long-term problems associated with implantation of the ureters into the colon include chronic pyelonephritis and absorption of chloride and urea in the colon, resulting in hyperchloraemic acidosis. If the ureters are diverted into the small bowel, which is a more popular procedure, patients also suffer from chronic urinary infections and, in the long term, pyelonephritis.

It is important to keep a close eye on the serum electrolytes after this procedure, both early on and during follow-up.

Palliation
Radiotherapy is given to advanced carcinoma to relieve the symptoms of haematuria, local pain, persistent frequency and incontinence. A 'salvage' cystectomy is performed in some cases not responding to radiotherapy. Radiotherapy is effective in the treatment of bone pain.

Disorders of micturition
The commonest cause of disordered micturition is outflow

obstruction due to diseases of the prostate and urethra. This will cause symptoms of poor urinary stream, frequency, and eventually acute and chronic retention of urine.

A less common symptom is urge incontinence due to over-stimulation of the sensory nerves of the bladder caused by cystitis, stones and carcinoma.

Disorders of micturition can be investigated by carrying out urodynamic studies. These involve measurement of bladder pressures during filling and voiding and measuring the urinary flow rate. In some centres a video-cystometrogram is performed using contrast material and the bladder observed under X-ray screening during filling and voiding.

Certain patients require further investigation by urethro-cystoscopy.

Operation: urethro-cystoscopy

Preoperative management
It is common practice, on completion of this examination, to proceed to definitive treatment under the same anaesthetic. If this is intended, make sure that theatre know and that the appropriate instruments are ready (e.g. a resectoscope or urethrotome).

Operation
The urethra is examined on the way into the bladder. A forward-viewing cystoscope is used. This is later changed to a side-viewing cystoscope to examine the bladder. Biopsies can be taken of inflammed bladder mucosa.

Codes

Blood	0/group and save . . . .
GA/LA	GA . . . .
Opn time	30–40 minutes . . . .
Stay	Outpatient/Inpatient 24 hours . . . . . .
Drains out	0 . . . .
Sutures out	0 . . . .
Off work	Variable . . . .

Acute retention of urine

The condition This is painful complete inability to pass urine of sudden onset. Postoperative retention of urine is described on p. 63. A second cause is 'acute on chronic' obstruction occurring in an elderly man with an enlarged prostate. This is often precipitated by drinking or cold weather.

Other rarer causes of acute retention are stones or blood clot in the urethra, urethral stricture, constipation, pregnancy or pelvic tumour. Trauma causing acute retention is considered on pp. 602 and 603.

Recognizing the pattern

The patient presents complaining of an inability to pass urine and suprapubic pain which characteristically comes in spasms. 'Acute on chronic' retention may be painless. There may be a history of prostatism, urethral disease or stones.

On examination
The bladder is enlarged and tender. The urethra should be palpated for stones or stricture and a rectal examination should be done to assess the size of the prostate and to exclude constipation (particularly in the elderly).

Proving the diagnosis

The diagnosis is proved by catheterization (see below).
   Further investigations should be arranged to try and discover the cause.
1 Test the urine for blood or signs of infection.
2 Perform a white cell count and haemoglobin.
3 Measure the urea and electrolytes to assess renal function.
4 Perform an abdominal X-ray to look for bladder calculi. This may also show bony secondaries from carcinoma.

Management

The patient should be admitted. First give some strong opiate analgesia. Conservative measures include privacy, the sound of running water, and standing the patient up. A hot bath also helps.
   If these conservative methods fail, then the patient must be catheterized. This is a technique that every medical student must learn properly. Although it appears easy, if it is done badly or carelessly, urinary tract infection and urethral damage may result.

Procedure: catheterization
A 12- or 14-gauge Foley catheter is usually large enough and is inserted with strict, aseptic technique. An assistant should be available. Firstly prepare the trolley and make sure that everything you require is there. After cleansing the penis or vulva, squeeze plenty of local anaesthetic lubricant gel (1% lignocaine with 0.25% chlorhexidine) into the urethra. Poor lubrication is a frequent cause of failure to catheterize. After allowing time for the anaesthesia to work, pass the catheter gently but firmly. If resistance occurs, maintain this gentle firm pressure. Do not force the catheter

as this may cause further spasm and oedema. As the bladder is entered, urine flows. This may take a few seconds as the lubricant is cleared from the inside of the catheter. Pass most of the catheter up into the bladder and then inflate the balloon (if present). Connect the catheter to a bag. If you encounter difficulty passing the catheter, call someone with more experience before you damage the urethra. After catheterizing a male, pull the foreskin over the glans again or a paraphimosis may result. After catheterization the urine is drained into a bag. Failure to pass a catheter may be evidence of a urethral stricture.

Procedure: suprapubic catheterization

If urethral catheterization is not successful, supra-pubic catheterization is required. Local anaesthetic is infiltrated above the symphysis pubis and a catheter is inserted through a small incision via a trocar. It is important to keep in the midline. Make sure that you can feel the bladder and that you aspirate urine with the needle used for infiltrating the local anaesthetic. The catheter is then secured with a stitch. Remember to push enough catheter into the bladder to allow it to remain inside once the bladder has emptied. If the catheter does come out, it must not be reintroduced when the bladder is empty as the trocar may enter the peritoneum and damage the bowel.

Further management

Postoperative or bedridden patients who have gone into acute retention can have the catheter removed once they are mobile. If acute retention recurs, the catheter is reinserted for 24−48 hours. Once the patient is up and in less pain, the problem usually resolves.

Patients with acute retention due to prostatic enlargement and who are fit can be treated by early prostatectomy.

With 'acute on chronic' retention time must be allowed for a general assessment and the detection and treatment of any chronic renal failure before a prostatectomy can be undertaken.

In a very elderly patient who is quite clearly unfit for operation, the only solution may be long-term catheter drainage. Small, soft, silastic catheters are available for this and the patient may either change this himself or have it done by a district nurse at home.

Antibiotics and catheter management

1 When antibiotic prophylaxis is required on a patient with chronic obstruction and probable infection, either ampicillin

with gentamicin i.v. or cefotaxime i.v. can be used. If the organism is known to be resistant to these, try ciprofloxacin i.v.

2 If the patient is asymptomatic or has local symptoms only, even in the presence of urinary growth, do not treat until the catheter is removed. Gram-positive organisms (e.g. faecal streptococci and coagulase-negative staphylococci) are then likely to clear spontaneously whereas Gram-negative bacilli (e.g. *Escherichia coli*) often require 3 days' oral antibiotic to clear. (Prescribe according to susceptibility.)

3 If the catheter has to be removed and then replaced because of blockage, then use a chlorhexidine washout. (Inject 100 ml of 0.02% aqueous chlorhexidine solution, hold for 30 minutes, then release and change catheter.)

4 If the patient's catheter is functioning and should not be removed, but there are systemic symptoms including pyrexia, then the drug of choice is probably oral ciprofloxacin 100–250 mg b.d. Also check the organism's susceptibility.

The management of prostatic carcinoma is dealt with on p. 441 and urethral stricture on p. 443.

Acute prostatitis

The condition
This is acute inflammation of the prostate gland. It may follow bacteraemia or direct infection after urethral instrumentation. The organisms commonly involved are *Escherichia coli*, *Streptococcus faecalis*, *Staphylococcus aureus* or *albus*, and *Neisseria gonorrhoeae*.

Recognizing the pattern
The patient
He may be an adult of any age but is usually over 35.

The history
The history is of symptoms of general infection including malaise, fever, rigors and muscle pain. There is pain in the perineum and frequency of micturition, dysuria or occasional haematuria. An abscess may cause acute retention or pain on defaecation.

On examination
The patient is pyrexial and rectal examination reveals a very tender, swollen, boggy prostate. Occasionally there is an abscess and the prostate is hot, tender and fluctuant and projects into the rectum. Palpate the testicles to exclude epididymo-orchitis.

Proving the diagnosis
An attempt should be made to isolate the causative organism from the urine. The patient is asked to micturate and the

first urine passed is collected separately from the rest and examined.

Management

Treatment consists of bed rest and the patient is encouraged to drink as much as possible. Not all antibiotics gain good access to the prostate but erythromycin (500 mg 6-hourly), trimethoprim (200 mg 12-hourly), cinoxacin (500 mg 12-hourly) or tetracycline (250–500 mg 6-hourly) is effective.

Prostatitis is a difficult infection to eradicate completely so antibiotics are continued for at least 6 weeks.

If an abscess is present, it must be drained. This may either be performed per urethra with a resectoscope or through the perineum.

Chronic prostatitis

The condition

This is a condition characterized by recurrent mild episodes of acute inflammation of the prostate gland or by constant pain in the perineum. The usual cause is failed treatment of acute prostatitis. The gland has many small ducts and infection is difficult to eradicate completely. Another cause is genito-urinary tuberculosis.

Recognizing the pattern

The patient
He is middle-aged to elderly.

The history
The history is one of persistent episodes of perineal pain varying in severity and frequency and often causing great distress. Other symptoms include low backache, mild bouts of fever and dysuria.

On examination
The prostate is enlarged, firm and irregular. Massage of the prostate will produce purulent discharge. This contains pus cells and may grow organisms such as *Chlamydia*, faecal streptococci, coliforms or anaerobes.

Proving the diagnosis

This is essentially clinical with laboratory confirmation of the infective organism.

Management

Treatment is with antibiotics but the condition is difficult to eradicate. Resection of the prostate does not usually help. Changing the antibiotics and giving them long term may help and regular prostatic massage is beneficial.

Benign prostatic hypertrophy

The condition This is a benign nodular or diffuse proliferation of both the musculofibrous and glandular elements in the prostate gland. It involves the inner zone of the gland, unlike carcinoma. The rest of the gland is compressed to form a capsule. It occurs to a varying degree in all men over the age of 50. The cause is uncertain but possible factors are an imbalance between androgens and oestrogens in later life or a benign neoplastic process.

The enlargement causes elongation, narrowing and kinking of the prostatic urethra. There is no relation between the size of the prostate on examination and the degree of obstruction. The obstruction results in hypertrophy of the detrusor muscle, producing a trabeculated appearance of the bladder wall. The mucosa may protrude between bands of muscle, forming saccules or diverticula. Eventually the muscle may become atonic, leading to chronic urinary retention, infection and stone formation. Engorged veins at the base of the bladder may burst and cause haematuria. Back pressure may eventually cause ureteric obstruction with hydronephrosis and eventually renal failure.

Recognizing the pattern *The patient*
He is usually aged between 55 and 75.

The history
The history is of a poor urinary stream with hesitancy and terminal dribbling. Micturition is incomplete, resulting in a gradually increasing volume of residual urine. As the bladder hypertrophies, the detrusor becomes excitable, resulting in urinary frequency and nocturia. There may be associated urgency of micturition. The patient may present with an episode of acute retention, commonly precipitated by drinking, bed rest or being trapped in a situation where he has to hold on too long due to lack of toilet facilities.

Eventually the bladder distends and chronic retention results, the residual urine becoming infected and predisposing to stone formation. Excess residual urine causes overflow incontinence. Haematuria may occur, characteristically at the end of micturition. Finally there are symptoms such as loin pain, thirst, malaise or mental impairment due to renal involvement and chronic renal failure.

On examination
The prostate is examined through the rectum. Make sure the patient's bladder is empty. Assess the following:
(a) shape,

(b) symmetry,
(c) surface,
(d) size,
(e) sulcus of the prostate.

The sulcus is the median groove on its posterior surface. It is preserved in benign hypertrophy but may disappear in malignant disease. In a normal prostate it is possible to slide the finger forward round each side of the convex surface of the gland. It is 2−3 cm across. In benign prostatic hypertrophy the gland is smooth but symmetrical, the surface is flattened and it is difficult or impossible to get the examining finger forward round each side.

There may be general evidence of chronic renal failure and uraemia, e.g. dehydration, anaemia, skin pallor or hypotension. Abdominal examination may reveal loin tenderness and a palpable bladder.

Proving the diagnosis

Investigations performed to confirm the diagnosis of benign prostatic hypertrophy are as follows.

1 An intravenous urogram. This looks for evidence of obstruction.

2 Urodynamic studies (see p. 430).

3 Urethro-cystoscopy (see p. 430).

4 Serum acid phosphatase to exclude carcinoma of the prostate.

5 Test a specimen of urine for blood and send samples off for cytology and bacteriology.

6 Send blood off for haemoglobin, ESR and urea and electrolytes to assess renal function.

Management

Medical

Phenoxybenzamine: This is an alpha-adrenoceptor antagonist and should relax the proximal urethra by blocking the alpha-receptors in the internal sphincter and so improve urinary flow. The dose is 10 mg 12-hourly. Side-effects include dizziness and tiredness. The best use of this drug may be for patients awaiting prostatectomy and who are at risk of developing retention.

Surgical

The usual treatment of this condition is surgical removal of the prostate gland. This may be done by:

(a) transurethral resection;

(b) transvesical prostatectomy;

(c) retropubic prostatectomy.

The indications for prostatectomy include the following:

(a) acute retention;

(b) ureteric obstruction and uraemia;

(c) urinary frequency and flow problems provided there is definite urodynamic evidence of bladder neck obstruction. If not, these symptoms are treated conservatively;

(d) heavy haematuria.

Preoperative management

If the urine is infected, this must be sterilized with antibiotics before operation. Any uraemia is improved by a few days of catheter drainage. Dehydration and anaemia must also be corrected.

The patient should be told that one result of prostatectomy is to reduce the quantity of ejaculate on sexual intercourse. In younger patients this may mean a reduction in fertility and this should be discussed with them preoperatively.

Operation: transurethral resection of the prostate

The operation is a specialist procedure requiring experience with a resectoscope. The whole of the lateral and middle lobes of the prostate are resected. On completion a urethral catheter is inserted. The prostatic chippings must be sent for histology to exclude a prostatic carcinoma.

Codes

Blood	2 units . . . .
GA/LA	GA . . . .
Opn time	30–90 minutes . . . .
Stay	7 days . . . .
Drains out	Urethral catheter 2–3 days . . . .
Sutures out	0 . . . .
Off work	4 weeks . . . .

Postoperative care

See below.

Operation: transvesical prostatectomy

In this operation the prostate is removed through the bladder using a suprapubic abdominal incision.

The bladder is opened and after a general survey the surgeon looks down on the top of the prostate gland identifying the enlarged lateral and median lobes. The mucosa of the bladder neck is incised and the adenoma is enucleated. Haemostasis is achieved, a catheter is passed through the urethra, and then the bladder closed. This operation is now performed if there is associated bladder disease such as stones.

Codes

Blood	2 units . . . .
GA/LA	GA . . . .
Opn time	60−90 minutes . . . .
Stay	10−14 days . . . .
Drains out	Urethral catheter 2−5 days, wound drain 3−5 days . . . .
Sutures out	7 days . . . .
Off work	4−6 weeks . . . .

Postoperative care
See below.

Operation: retropubic prostatectomy (Millin's)
Here the anterior abdominal wall is opened and the rectus muscles retracted. The peritoneum is displaced and the prostate approached retroperitoneally behind the pubic symphysis. The prostatic capsule is opened transversely and the adenoma identified and enucleated. The veru montanum and external sphincter are carefully preserved.

Codes

Blood	2 units . . . .
GA/LA	GA . . . .
Opn time	60−90 minutes . . . .
Stay	10−14 days . . . .
Drains out	Irrigating urethral catheter 3−5 days, retropubic drain 24 hours . . . .
Sutures out	5−7 days . . . .
Off work	4−6 weeks . . . .

Postoperative care
Ensure that the catheter drains satisfactorily. This may require constant irrigation through a three-way catheter, or intermittent irrigation using a bladder syringe.

A bladder irrigation system is usually set up, using either a triple-lumen urethral catheter or a separate suprapubic catheter. Three to four litres of normal saline or sterile water are instilled daily. This is left running for 48 hours or until the urine is sufficiently clear of clots to drain freely.

Should clot retention occur, it is relieved by syringing the bladder with 50−100 cm^3 of normal saline (do not withdraw the syringe too forcefully as this causes the catheter to collapse). Occasionally it may be necessary to take the patient back to theatre and pack the prostatic capsule to control severe bleeding.

The catheter is removed once the urine is clear of blood.

Do not remove it too soon as it may be difficult to reintroduce in the early postoperative period. The catheter may be left *in situ* longer after transvesical prostatectomy to cover bladder healing.

Complications include primary or secondary haemorrhage, deep vein thrombosis, urinary incontinence and, in the long term, urethral stricture. These problems are less common after transurethral resection than open prostatectomy.

Prostatic carcinoma

The condition
This is an adenocarcinoma. There is no known aetiological factor, although it often coexists with benign prostatic hypertrophy. It is commoner in those patients with blood group O. The tumour is usually androgen dependent.

It arises in the outer zone of the gland (unlike benign prostatic hypertrophy). It can still occur, therefore, after a prostatectomy for benign prostatic hypertrophy. Local direct spread may involve the bladder, the ureters or the urethra. Direct invasion posteriorly is hindered by the fascia of Denonvilliers and involvement of the rectum is unusual.

Blood-borne spread occurs to bone, particularly the pelvis, lumbar vertebrae or greater trochanter of the femur via the communications of the prostatic venous plexus. Bony secondaries are characteristically osteosclerotic and appear on X-ray film as areas of increased density.

The stages of the tumour's development are shown in Fig. 84.

Recognizing the pattern
The patient
He is usually over the age of 65.

The history
Prostatic carcinoma usually presents with a disturbance of flow similar to benign prostatic hypertrophy. The history of flow disturbance is usually shorter. Other presentations are with back pain or bilateral sciatica (due to vertebral secondaries), neurological lesions due to compression of the spinal cord, or the general symptoms of carcinomatosis.

On examination
Rectal examination characteristically shows asymmetrical, nodular enlargement of the prostate, which feels hard and irregular with obliteration of the posterior median sulcus. There may be evidence of spread, with enlarged lymph nodes in the groin or an enlarged liver. Metastases in bone may cause areas of tenderness, particularly in the pelvis, femur and lumbar region of the back.

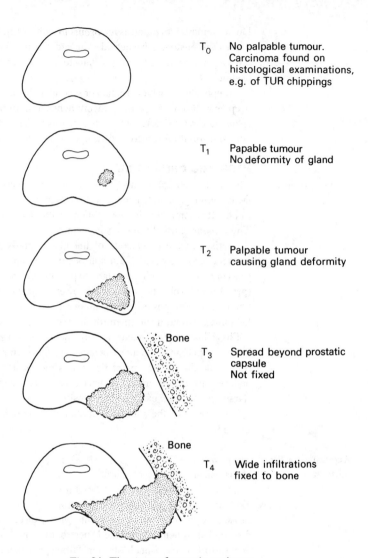

	T_0	No palpable tumour. Carcinoma found on histological examinations, e.g. of TUR chippings
	T_1	Papable tumour No deformity of gland
	T_2	Palpable tumour causing gland deformity
Bone	T_3	Spread beyond prostatic capsule Not fixed
Bone	T_4	Wide infiltrations fixed to bone

Fig. 84. The stages of prostatic carcinoma.

Proving the diagnosis

The diagnosis is proved by the following investigations.

1 *Biopsy.* This may be done with a 'Tru-cut' needle either transrectally or perineally. Alternatively, a biopsy may be obtained if a cystoscopy is performed.

2 *Acid phosphatase.* This is elevated in 40% of prostatic carcinomas when there are widespread metastases. It is not elevated in benign prostatic hypertrophy. The blood should be taken before breakfast as serum lipids can affect the result. Many people believe that the acid phosphatase is raised by rectal examination but there is no good evidence

for this. False positives can occur in prostatitis, Paget's disease or cirrhosis of the liver.

3 *Urethro-cystoscopy.* This is indicated if there is haematuria or any outflow obstruction (see p. 429). A biopsy may be performed at the same time.

Other investigations to assess and stage the disease are as follows.

1 Test the urine for signs of infection.

2 Haemoglobin and ESR.

3 Urea and electrolytes to assess renal function.

4 Alkaline phosphatase (raised if there are bony secondaries).

5 Chest X-ray and X-ray of lumbar spine to look for metastases.

6 Perform an IVU. This will demonstrate any impaired renal function or evidence of ureteric or bladder outflow obstruction.

7 Technetium bone scan. This demonstrates the presence of bony metastases.

8 Bimodal transrectal ultrasound is also used for detection of early prostatic carcinoma.

9 CAT scanning may have a role in staging the disease.

Management

The mainstay of treatment is to decrease androgen activity either by orchidectomy or by medical castration with cyproterone acetate or an LHRH (luteinizing hormone releasing hormone) agonist e.g. Zoladex and buserelin. Oestrogens are rarely used due to the high incidence of thromboses (coronary thrombosis, strokes and DVT) associated with the drug.

Bilateral orchidectomy performed for the endocrine control of prostatic carcinoma is usually done by the subcapsular method (described below).

An alternative to hormonal therapy is radiotherapy, which is effective. Surgery plays a very small part in the treatment of this disease but a TURP is performed if there is outflow obstruction.

Operation: subcapsular orchidectomy

Preoperative management
The clotting time should be checked. Prostatic carcinoma can cause fibrinolysis.

Operation
The scrotum is opened by a transverse incision and the testes exposed. The capsule of each testicle (tunica

albuginea) is incised vertically and the testicular tissue inside removed. The tunica is then resutured after careful haemostasis, and the testicle replaced in the scrotum. Occasionally a silastic prosthesis is placed inside the tunica albuginea.

Codes

Blood	Group and save ....
GA/LA	GA ....
Opn time	30–60 minutes ....
Stay	5–7 days ....
Drains out	0 ....
Sutures out	7 days ....
Off work........	1 month ....

Postoperative care
A scrotal support helps to alleviate discomfort from scrotal swelling or bruising.

Operation: radical prostatectomy
This operation may be performed in the early stages of prostatic carcinoma. This is rarely done these days as trials have shown that the results are no better than radiotherapy.

Preoperative management
Any urinary infection must be treated. A clotting time must be sent off.

Operation
The prostate is approached either through the retropubic space (see Millin's prostatectomy) or through a perineal incision. The prostate gland and the seminal vesicles are isolated and removed and the bladder outflow refashioned and joined to the membranous urethra using a catheter as a splint. Care is taken not to damage the external urethral sphincter.

Codes

Blood	2–4 units ....
GA/LA	GA ....
Opn time	2–3 hours ....
Stay	2–3 weeks ....
Drains out	Retropubic space 5–7 days, catheter 7–10 days ....
Sutures out	7–10 days ....
Off work........	4–6 weeks ....

Postoperative care
The main risk with this procedure is of urinary incontinence or faecal fistula.

Urethral stricture

The condition
This is narrowing of the urethra causing obstruction to urine flow followed by back pressure on the bladder, ureter and kidney. The signs are identical to those discussed under prostatic hypertrophy.

It is usually caused by either inflammation or trauma. An inflammatory stricture is caused by *Neisseria gonorrhoeae*, *Chlamydia* or other causes of non-specific urethritis. A traumatic stricture may follow a previous urethral operation or instrumentation (e.g. a large catheter may result in pressure necrosis of the urethral epithelium). A stricture may also result from external trauma. Rare causes of urethral stricture are carcinoma of the prostate or bladder invading the urethra.

Recognizing the pattern
The patient
The patient can be of any age and is usually male.

The history
There may be a history of catheterization, prostatectomy, trauma or urethral infection. The patient presents with flow problems including a poor stream and dribbling. The flow can often be increased by abdominal straining (unlike prostatic hypertrophy where the flow is usually worsened by straining). Fibrosis and narrowing may cause painful ejaculation and very occasionally distortion of the erect organ (chordee) which may make intercourse impossible.

On examination
The urethra should be carefully palpated along its length and the stricture may be felt. Abdominal examination may reveal a palpable bladder.

Proving the diagnosis
The diagnosis is confirmed by the following.
1 *Urethrography*. This is a radiological technique using contrast medium to outline the urethra.
2 *Urethroscopy*. This is carried out as part of a general cystoscopy (see p. 430).

Management
A stricture is usually a chronic condition requiring regular follow-up. The initial treatment is commonly by internal urethrotomy and this is followed by regular dilatation. A

urethroplasty may occasionally be performed for strictures which remain a problem in spite of these measures.

Preoperative management
If the urine is infected, antibiotics should be given and bladder washouts performed. Prophylactic antibiotics (e.g. gentamicin 80 mg) are given at induction and oral broad-spectrum antibiotics for 5 days postoperatively.

Operation: internal urethrotomy
A urethrotome is passed under direct vision. The stricture is viewed and incised to the required depth. This is followed by dilatation.

Codes

Blood	0
GA/LA	GA
Opn time	15–30 minutes
Stay	3 days
Drains out	Urinary catheter 1–4 weeks
Sutures out	0
Off work	1 week

Postoperative care
In all but the smallest strictures a catheter is left in position afterwards for 1–4 weeks. The patient is followed up regularly and usually requires urethroscopy and dilatation on one or two occasions. If the obstruction continues to recur, then dilatation is performed regularly.

Operation: urethral dilatation
This procedure is performed using specific urethral dilators called bougies or urethral sounds. After applying lubricant gel they are inserted into the urethra and allowed to enter using minimal pressure. Bougies of gradually increasing diameter are passed, the aim being to stretch the urethra without tearing the mucosa.

Codes

Blood	0
GA/LA	GA or LA
Opn time	20 minutes
Stay	Outpatient
Drains out	0
Sutures out	0
Off work	1–2 days

Postoperative care

Gram-negative bacteraemia is a common complication and can be very severe. Any patient whose blood pressure remains low and is confused following the operation, perhaps with an abnormally low temperature, requires urgent administration of the appropriate antibiotics.

Other complications include a urethral tear with haematuria and scarring, which may worsen the stricture.

Operation: open urethroplasty

There are many types of operation that are performed using skin flaps to enlarge or refashion the urethral lumen. This procedure has now largely been replaced by internal urethrotomy described above.

Prevention

Avoidance of excessive instrumentation of the bladder, care at prostatectomy and the use of narrow, soft catheters for as short a time as possible will all help in cutting down the incidence of this condition.

Male Genitalia

Conditions of the foreskin

The care of the foreskin remains a mystery to most parents. Generally speaking it should be left alone for the first year or two of life. Thereafter it can be gently but firmly retracted, usually at bath time. Adhesions gradually separate and the glans becomes fully visible. This process is usually complete by the age of 1–5 years.

In young boys the foreskin is often relatively long and the tip tends to be slightly tight causing a groove as it is retracted on to the penile shaft. This will stretch up by natural processes as development occurs. It must be distinguished from a scarred stricture which can result in a paraphimosis, non-retractile foreskin, or even a 'pinhole meatus'.

Non-retractile foreskin

The condition

The patient is usually brought along by his parents, who are concerned that the foreskin does not retract. There may be a history of recurrent balanitis.

On examination
The foreskin is adherent. Check how far it can be retracted and whether there is any stricturing at the tip.

Management

There is no need for surgical treatment until after the age of 4 unless complications such as balanitis or phimosis occur. Before this time the only management is to reassure the parents and give advice about the care of the foreskin as above. After the age of 4, examination under an anaesthetic is performed (see below). The preputial adhesions are separated and a circumcision performed if there is a phimosis.

Balanoposthitis (balanitis)

The condition

This is acute inflammation of the glans and foreskin, usually caused by pyogenic organisms (*Staphylococcus*, *Streptococcus* and coliforms) or fungal infection (*Candida*). It occurs commonly in young boys with a non-retractile foreskin. In elderly patients there may be a predisposing cause such as carcinoma or diabetes.

In adults there is a chronic fibrosing condition of the foreskin, called balanitis xerotica et obliterans, of unknown aetiology. It is cured by circumcision.

Recognizing the pattern	*The history* The patient with acute balanitis may be of any age and presents with either irritation or pain in the penis, and a discharge from beneath the foreskin. Recurrent balanitis may cause a phimosis with disturbance of micturition. *On examination* The inflammation is visible.
Management	The management is to give antibiotics and treat the cause. Frequently this means a circumcision once the inflammation has settled down. In older patients the urine should be tested for sugar.

Phimosis

The condition	This is a narrowing of the opening of the foreskin. It can follow trauma or recurrent infection. It may be caused by the parents trying to force adhesions apart too early.
Recognizing the pattern	*The history* The patient is usually young and there is a history that the foreskin balloons out on micturition, causing a spraying stream. Adults often complain of pain on intercourse. *On examination* The foreskin is usually long with a small, tight opening.
Management	Management is by circumcision (see below).

Paraphimosis

The condition	This condition occurs when a tight foreskin is forcibly retracted back off the glans and cannot be pulled forwards again. The tight band causes obstruction of venous return followed by swelling of the distal foreskin and glans. It can occur at any age. It is especially common in the elderly patient who after catheterization has not had his foreskin pulled forwards again.
Management	Unless reduced quickly the distal foreskin rapidly becomes so swollen that reduction is impossible. The swollen glans and foreskin are wrapped in a swab and squeezed gently to reduce the oedema. Once this has been achieved pressure is applied to the glans to push it back through the tight band. This procedure can, if necessary, be carried out with a dorsal penile nerve block. In some cases a dorsal slit may be required to obtain reduction. Circumcision is performed at a later date when the oedema has settled.

Trauma to the foreskin

The condition A torn frenulum is usually seen in young men following intercourse. Occasionally the foreskin may be caught in the zip of trousers resulting in tears or superficial lacerations.

Management A torn frenulum usually requires no treatment other than reassurance to the patient and advice about intercourse. A catgut stitch may be required if there is bleeding from the torn frenula artery. A lubricant such as 'KY' jelly may be helpful. If the problem becomes recurrent, a circumcision may become indicated.

Operation: circumcision
The indications for circumcision are as follows.
1 Phimosis.
2 Recurrent balanitis.
3 Balanitis xerotica et obliterans.
4 Religious reasons. Some people or religious groups practise the rite of circumcision and these ritual circumcisions are usually carried out between the ages of 6 months and 1 year.

Preoperative management
Circumcision should not be done in the presence of ammoniacal dermatitis as this can cause ulceration of the meatus. Balanoposthitis should be treated with antibiotics before surgery.

Operation
The foreskin is lifted from the glans by carefully freeing any adhesions. Preputial adhesions are separated. A dorsal split is made in the foreskin down to the predetermined level and the foreskin then carefully removed, preserving sufficient epithelium next to the glans (5 mm). The preputial layer of skin is sutured to the skin of the penile shaft using absorbable sutures. Care is taken to align the skin correctly. The wound is dressed and some surgeons place a dressing of anaesthetic jelly around the base of the glans. Alternatively, a suprapubic block of the dorsal nerve of the penis using a long-acting anaesthetic, or a caudal nerve block, is effective.

Codes

Blood	0 . . . .
GA/LA	GA . . . .
Opn time	15–30 minutes . . . .
Stay	24–48 hours . . . .
Drains out	0 . . . .
Sutures out	0 . . . .
Off work	Up to 1 week . . . .

Congenital lesions of the male external genitalia

The male external genitalia are formed by the fusion of the external genital folds around the urethra and its surrounding erectile tissue. Failure of this fusion results in a urethra that opens either at the base of the glans or further down the penile shaft, underneath the body of the penis. This condition is known as hypospadias and requires reconstruction of the penis, usually using the skin of the foreskin. This is usually carried out by paediatric or urological surgeons and is not discussed further here.

Rarely the urethra forms a gutter on the upper surface of the penis. This condition is usually associated with major abnormalities in the structure of the bladder and is known as epispadias.

Carcinoma of the penis

The condition
This is a squamous cell carcinoma. It is rare in the UK but occurs more frequently in the Far East and Africa.

It is associated with an intact foreskin with retained smegma. Jews who are circumcised at birth do not get the condition. In other religions where circumcision is practised at puberty there is a decreased incidence of carcinoma of the penis although it is still more common than in the Jews, implying a prepubertal influence. Carcinoma of the penis may also be precipitated by *Herpes genitalis*.

The condition may start as leucoplakia on the glans. Erythroplasia of Queryat is the name given to carcinoma *in situ* of the penis. It consists of a persistent red, raw area on the glans.

With advanced disease the whole penis may be engulfed with malignant growth and the urethra may be invaded. Lymphatic spread occurs to the inguinal nodes. Blood-borne spread is late and rare.

Malignant melanoma can rarely affect the skin of the penis and this differential diagnosis should be borne in mind.

Recognizing the pattern

The history

The patient is usually elderly. The presenting complaint is one of a lump or discharge and irritation. Later the discharge becomes bloody and offensive. The foreskin is usually non-retractile. Advanced disease presents with an ulcerated, fungating lesion destroying the whole penis or a mass in the groin. Urethral obstruction with retention of urine is rare.

On examination

The lesion is visible if the foreskin can be retracted. If not, it is usually possible to feel it beneath the foreskin. Most commonly it is an indurated ulcer at the base of the glans penis, although it may be a papillary growth. In 60% of cases the nodes in the groin are enlarged but only half of these are malignant. The rest are due to reactive changes secondary to the inflammation and infection.

Proving the diagnosis

The diagnosis is proved by taking a biopsy, and a circumcision may be required to reveal the growth.

Other investigations are as follows.

1 A chest X-ray is performed to look for secondary growths.

2 A CAT scan of the pelvis may be useful to assess spread of the tumour along the iliac vessels if block dissection is contemplated.

Management

Even in the presence of enlarged nodes in the groin, it is usual to treat the primary growth first and then only treat the nodes if they are still enlarged after 3 to 4 weeks.

Radiotherapy is used in early-stage disease with no urethral involvement or for palliation. It can be given either by radio-active implants, by external X-rays or as a radio-active mould fitted around the shaft of the penis. The results are good, with a 60–70% 5-year survival rate. Radiotherapy is also used in the treatment of fixed malignant nodes in the groin.

Surgical treatment is used in the following conditions.

1 When the urethra is involved.

2 If the growth has failed to respond to radiotherapy.

3 If the groin lymph nodes are persistently enlarged 1 month after the surgery, a block dissection or deep X-ray therapy (DXT) to the inguinal lymph nodes is performed.

Operation: partial amputation of the penis

This operation is performed if there is at least 2 cm of uninvolved penile shaft available at the base. The new urethral meatus must be carefully fashioned to avoid ensuing stricture.

Codes

Blood	0	
GA/LA	GA	
Opn time	1–2 hours	
Stay	14 days	
Drains out	Urethral catheter 7–10 days	
Sutures out	7 days	
Off work	1 month	

Postoperative care
Once the catheter has been removed, regular meatal dilatations may be required. The patient is followed up regularly to assess the inguinal nodes and to look for local recurrence.

Operation: complete amputation of the penis
This operation involves complete removal of the penis from the perineal membrane and ischio-pubic ramus. The stump of the urethra is brought out through an incision in the perineum behind the scrotum. Occasionally the testicles and scrotum are also removed as they will get in the way of a urethrostomy.

Codes

Blood	2–4 units	
GA/LA	GA	
Opn time	2–3 hours	
Stay	2 weeks	
Drains out	Urethral catheter 7 days	
Sutures out	7 days	
Off work	6 weeks	

Postoperative care
As for partial amputation.

Scrotal conditions
The following conditions in the scrotum commonly present to the general surgeon.
1 Absent testis.
2 Lump in the scrotum.
3 Painful testis.
These will be dealt with in this section.

Absent testis (cryptorchidism)
The testis may be absent from the scrotum either because it is undescended or because it is retractile. The testis develops as a retroperitoneal organ at the lower pole of the kidney and during development descends caudally through the inguinal

canal and into the scrotum. Its descent may be either incomplete or abnormal. If it is abnormal the testis is ectopic and can lie in a pubic, inguinal, femoral or perineal site.

A *retractile* testis has descended normally but is pulled up into the inguinal canal by an active cremasteric reflex.

A true *undescended* testis is frequently abnormal and may never undergo spermatogenesis. There is evidence, however, that bringing the testis down into its correct place early in life can improve the chances of fertility. There is also an increased danger of malignant change in an undescended testis. Neither of these problems occurs with a retractile testis.

It is therefore important to differentiate clinically between these two causes of absent testis.

Retractile testis

The condition

In these boys the cremaster is unusually active and the testis readily retracts up into the groin.

Recognizing the pattern

The history

Although the parents may not have seen the testes in the scrotum, close questioning often reveals the fact that the testis does occasionally appear, particularly during a warm bath. Testes may also have been seen in the scrotum earlier in life, during a routine medical examination.

On examination

The scrotum is well developed and looks 'as if it could contain a testis'. The clinician must develop a good examining technique to make the diagnosis. Warm hands, a warm examination room and a warm personality all help. One hand is placed in the groin to occlude the inguinal canal and moved down towards the scrotum so as to 'milk' the testis into the external ring. The testis is then gently trapped by the index finger of the other hand as it emerges. Gentle pressure with the finger and thumb can then pull the retractile testis into the scrotum. If the above manoeuvre fails, getting the patient to squat on the examination couch may reveal the testis.

If the testis does descend to the base of the scrotum, its presence there should be demonstrated to the parents. They can be reassured that it will eventually descend normally and nothing further needs to be done. If the testis only comes part of the way down to the scrotum, it probably is un-descended and in this case an orchidopexy will be required.

	Undescended testis
The condition	An undescended testis should be spotted early in life at a routine medical examination. This will enable plans to be made to bring the testis into the scrotum before the age of 5. Frequently, however, the condition is first diagnosed later than this. There is some evidence to suggest that the longer the testis remains undescended, the more danger there is of infertility and malignancy.

Occasionally the condition presents with torsion of the undescended testis and this must be considered in the differential diagnosis of abdominal pain in young boys if the testis is found to be absent from the scrotum. |
| Recognizing the pattern | *The patient*
He can present at any age from newborn to between 20 and 30 years old, although the usual age of presentation in the UK is between the ages of 2 and 5.

On examination
The scrotum is underdeveloped and flattened. The condition may be unilateral or bilateral and the position of both testes should be determined. The undescended testis may be palpable in the groin or inguinal canal and should be located if possible. |
| Management | As mentioned above it is important that the undescended testis is brought down early, preferably before the age of 5. Some surgeons advocate operation in the first year of life. However, the testicular vessels and vas are very small at that age and there may well be an increased risk of damaging them if the operation is carried out too early. The age of 4−5 seems optimal to the authors as the vessels are better developed by then and this is before the child starts school.

Undescended testes in the late teens and early twenties are unlikely ever to be fertile. Where the testis is undescended on one side only, it is probably best excised to obviate the danger of later malignancy. Where both testes are undescended in the older age-group, they should be brought down into the scrotum for cosmetic reasons and also because it makes them easier to examine later on.

Operation: orchidopexy (dartos pouch procedure)
This is at present probably the most popular operation for undescended testis. An incision is made in the groin and the testis found and mobilized together with its vessels. The latter are freed right up into the deep inguinal ring, and further into the abdomen if necessary. They are separated |

453 SECTION 8.3

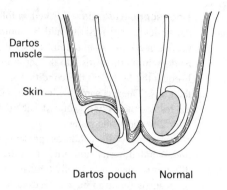

Dartos
muscle

Skin

Dartos pouch   Normal

Fig. 85. Dartos pouch orchidopexy.

from the processus vaginalis and any small inguinal hernial sac. A subcutaneous pouch is then made in the scrotum between the skin and the dartos muscle. The testis is pulled down through a small hole in the dartos muscle (see Fig. 85). Once the bulk of the testis is through this hole it is unable to retract back and hence it becomes fixed in the scrotum.

Codes

Blood . . . . 0 . . . .
GA/LA . . . . GA . . . .
Opn time . . . . 30 minutes per side . . . .
Stay . . . . 2−3 days . . . .
Drains out . . . . . . 0 . . . .
Sutures out . . . . . 5−7 days . . . .
Off school or
    work . . . . 2 weeks . . . .

Postoperative care

The scrotum may be bruised and swollen for a while and the parents may need some reassurance that this will settle down. When a dartos pouch has been made and where the testicular vessels are short the scrotum will be pulled well up into the groin. This should not cause concern providing the testis remains within the scrotal tissues. Apart from these points the postoperative course is usually straightforward.

Lumps in the scrotum

Patients with lumps in the scrotum are common cases in surgical examinations. It is important to develop a disciplined technique for examining them as there is frequently embarrassment on the part of both the patient and the student, making logical thought more difficult.

A routine should be established as follows.

1 Can you get above it? That is to say, is the lump truly scrotal or is it a continuation of a lump in the groin (e.g. an inguinal hernia)?

2 What is its relation to the testis? Which anatomical structure does it arise from?

3 Is the lump tender or not?

4 Does it transilluminate? Scrotal lumps lend themselves to the technique of transillumination. Use a good torch with a narrow beam and observe the other side of the swelling in a darkened environment. A paper tube can be useful for this.

5 Define the characteristics of the lump, e.g.:
   (a) shape,
   (b) size,
   (c) surface,
   (d) consistency,
   (e) mobility.

The features of individual types of lump will be dealt with below.

Hydrocoele

The condition A hydrocoele is a collection of fluid in the tunica vaginalis. Hydrocoeles may be either primary or secondary. In the primary type there is no predisposing cause in the scrotum, but there may be a persistent processus vaginalis (congenital or infantile hydrocoele — see pp. 548—551).

Secondary hydrocoeles represent a reaction to some pathology in the testis or its covering (e.g. testicular infections, tumours, torsion of the testis or hydatid of Morgagni). In adults the possibility that a hydrocoele is secondary to an impalpable tumour of the testis must always be considered.

Hydrocoele of the cord. This is a condition in which the hydrocoele arises in part of the processus vaginalis in the spermatic cord above the testis (p. 550, Fig. 100). A rounded lump slips up and down the inguinal canal. The abnormality here is that the processus has not closed off fully and the operative repair is the same as for an inguinal hernia in children.

Cysts of the canal of Nuck. This is a similar condition occurring in females.

Recognizing the *The patient*
pattern He may be of any age. Primary hydrocoeles are common in young boys; secondary hydrocoeles are more common in adults.

The history

The patient usually presents because he has noticed a swelling in the scrotum. Occasionally the hydrocoele is large enough to cause discomfort. If it occurs secondary to underlying disease of the testis, there may also be symptoms due to the primary cause such as pain or weight loss.

On examination

You can get above the swelling. It has a smooth surface and is of any size. It transilluminates well. The testis is within it and not palpable separately.

Management

Hydrocoeles in children are treated as a patent processus vaginalis and should be dealt with operatively in the same way as an inguinal hernia (see p. 550).

A hydrocoele in an adult may be treated:

(a) conservatively,
(b) by tapping, or
(c) by operation.

Conservative treatment consists of reassurance and possibly providing the patient with a scrotal support. This may be all that is necessary for a small hydrocoele where it is the development of the swelling that usually bothers the patient rather than any symptoms from it. Beware, however, of reassuring a patient who may have a hydrocoele secondary to a tumour. If in doubt, these are best explored.

Hydrocoeles may be tapped using a sterile needle and syringe. A sclerosing agent such as tetracycline may be injected after aspiration to prevent reaccumulation of fluid which is common with this procedure. This type of management may be indicated where the patient is not thought fit for surgery.

Operative treatment is indicated where there is doubt about the diagnosis (see secondary hydrocoele above), where the hydrocoele is very large, or where there are repeated recurrences after tapping.

Operation: removal of hydrocoele

An incision is made in the scrotum, and the hydrocoele and its immediate coverings are separated by gentle finger dissection. If this is carried out in the correct layer, very little bleeding occurs. The hydrocoele is then delivered out of the scrotum and incised, releasing its fluid. The testis is inspected for abnormalities. The coverings of the tunica fall behind the testis and cord and can be fixed there with sutures. In this way the hydrocoele cannot refill. The testis plus the everted coverings are then replaced in the scrotum and the skin is closed over them. Accurate haemostasis is essential. The skin is closed with catgut. A good scrotal support is applied.

Codes

Blood	0 ....
GA/LA	GA ....
Opn time	15 – 30 minutes ....
Stay	1 – 3 days ....
Drains out	0 ....
Sutures out	Absorbable sutures in the scrotum are not removed ....
Off work	1 – 2 weeks ....

Postoperative care
The patient should rest quietly for 12 – 24 hours. Haematoma formation is the main complication to be avoided. If a haematoma does occur, convalescence will be prolonged and there is a danger that it may become infected. Large haematomas should be evacuated under sterile conditions in theatre.

Epididymal cysts

The condition

Epididymal cysts are very common and often multiple. They may be of any size and contain either clear or milky fluid.

Recognizing the pattern

The patient
He is usually post-pubertal and the condition seems to be more common in the middle-aged and elderly.

The history
The patient has usually noticed a lump which may have become large enough to cause trouble by its size. Occasionally the cyst is painful or the patient may be experiencing pain on direct pressure over it.

On examination
It is possible to get above the swelling, which is situated above and behind the testis in the epididymis. The testis is palpable separate from it. Cysts are frequently multiple and several cysts next to each other give rise to a lobulated swelling. The condition is often bilateral. The cysts are fluctuant but only transilluminate if they contain clear fluid.

Management

Conservative management is followed where possible. Patients should be reassured that the cysts are nothing to worry about.

If the cysts are causing trouble because of pain or their

size, they can then either be tapped (as for hydrocoeles) or excised.

Operation: excision of epididymal cyst

The testis is exposed within the tunica vaginalis and delivered out of the scrotum. Either the individual cysts or the affected part of the epididymis can then be excised. The epididymis has a good blood supply and a lot of time must be spent securing full haemostasis.

Codes

Blood	0 ....
GA/LA	GA ....
Opn time	15–30 minutes ....
Stay	1–3 days ....
Drains out	0 ....
Sutures out	Absorbable sutures in the scrotum are not removed ....
Off work........	1–2 weeks ....

Postoperative care

This is much the same as for a hydrocoele.

Testicular neoplasms

The condition

Ninety-two per cent of testicular neoplasms are malignant but they only account for 1 or 2% of all male malignancies. They are, therefore, uncommon.

Benign neoplasms are even more rare. Leydig (interstitial) cell tumours account for 7% of testicular tumours and they may secrete androgens. In young boys they may produce early puberty and the 'infant Hercules' syndrome. Sertoli cell adenomas (<1%) secrete oestrogens and produce feminization.

Malignant neoplasms of the testis are commonly either seminomas (40% of testicular tumours) or teratomas (30%); 15% are of a mixed type. Undescended testes have a 30-fold increased risk of neoplastic change, although the overall incidence is still very low.

Seminomas probably arise from the primordial germinal cells in the testicular tubule. This is a solid tumour and tends to be slow-growing. It is usually very radiosensitive. In the absence of metastases there is a 90% 5-year survival rate.

Teratomas may have solid or cystic components and are less radiosensitive than seminomas. Ninety per cent of teratomas will secrete human chorionic gonadotrophin and/or alpha-fetoprotein, which can be measured in the serum and used as a tumour marker.

The prognosis of seminomas and teratomas depends on the stage of the growth and in the case of a teratoma its degree of differentiation.

Staging of testicular tumours

Stage I	Disease confined to the testis.
Stage II	Abdominal lymph node involvement.
Stage III	Supra- and infra-diaphragmatic lymph node involvement.
Stage IV	Extralymphatic spread (e.g. lung and liver).

Degree of differentiation of teratomas

TD	Teratoma differentiated.
MTI	Malignant teratoma intermediate.
MTU	Malignant teratoma undifferentiated.
MTT	Malignant teratoma trophoblastic.

The less differentiated the teratoma the worse the prognosis.

With the advent of combination chemotherapy 100% 5-year survival can be achieved for Stage I or Stage II teratomata. If hepatic metastases are present the 5-year survival falls to 10%. Stage I seminomas have a 90% 5-year survival. The overall 5-year survival for Stage II seminomas is 50%.

Both these tumours spread either locally to the scrotum or through the bloodstream and the lymphatics. Bloodstream spread occurs earlier in teratomas and metastases appear in the lungs and the liver. Lymphatic spread is common in both seminomas and teratomas. The lymph drainage of the testis follows its arterial supply and spread therefore occurs to the para-aortic lymph nodes at the level of the umbilicus. Inguinal lymph node involvement is rare and occurs when the scrotal skin is invaded.

Lymphomas comprise a further 7% of testicular tumours. They are more common in the elderly and are usually of the non-Hodgkin's type. Treatment is by combination chemotherapy but the overall results are poor.

Recognizing the pattern

The patient
Seminomas tend to occur between the ages of 20 and 45 and teratomas occur in a slightly younger age-group between 15 and 35 years.

The history
The patient or his partner may notice a small painless lump

in the testis or that one testis is larger than the other. Alternatively, these findings may be noted at a routine medical examination. Other presenting symptoms are unexplained pain in one testis, haemospermia or the development of a secondary hydrocoele. Occasionally the first presentation is an abdominal mass due to enlarged para-aortic lymph nodes, cervical lymphadenopathy or pulmonary metastases.

On examination
A hard swelling is felt within the testis, and it is possible to get above it. The tumour does not transilluminate. The examination should include the abdomen, liver, chest and left supraclavicular fossa, feeling for evidence of metastatic spread.

Proving the diagnosis

The tumour may be proved to be solid by an ultrasound examination. However, a mass arising in the testis is a malignant neoplasm until proved otherwise and must be explored and biopsied.

Management

A chest X-ray is performed and blood taken for alpha-fetoprotein and beta-HCG levels before the operation. Other investigations may be performed in the postoperative period. These include a CAT scan of the chest, abdomen and pelvis in order to stage the disease. An intravenous urogram may show distortion of the ureters by para-aortic nodes.

The patient must be warned of the possibility of an orchidectomy and consent for this obtained. It should be explained that the testis will be explored through the groin. Percutaneous biopsy through the scrotal skin should never be carried out because of the risk of seeding along the needle track. The groin is shaved as for a hernia operation.

Operation: exploration of testicular mass
— ? orchidectomy
The groin is explored through an oblique incision as for an inguinal hernia and the spermatic cord isolated. A soft vascular clamp is placed on the cord at the internal ring. This prevents the venous spread of malignant cells while the testis is being manipulated. The testis is delivered into the groin, inspected and if necessary transected to look for a tumour. If it is normal it can be repaired with chromic catgut sutures. If a tumour is found, it is biopsied and a frozen section obtained. If this shows malignancy, the clamp on the cord is replaced by a tie and the testis plus the spermatic cord are excised. No drains are necessary.

Codes

Blood	0 . . . .
GA/LA	GA . . . .
Opn time	30–60 minutes . . . .
Stay	3–5 days . . . .
Drains out	0 . . . .
Sutures out	5–7 days . . . .
Off work	Varies according to the need for further treatment . . . .

Postoperative care

The patient requires a scrotal support and his recovery is much the same as for an inguinal hernia (see. p. 392). Further treatment then depends on the histology and the clinical staging. Serum tumour markers are measured 1 week postoperatively and if they remain elevated this indicates the presence of metastases.

Seminomas. Radiotherapy is given postoperatively, although some omit this in Stage I disease. Stage IV seminomas are rare and are treated with chemotherapy (usually cisplatin).

Teratomas. Combination chemotherapy is given post-operatively.

Radiotherapy

The dose and field of radiation depend on the histological type and the presence or absence of metastases. Radiotherapy is given over a 5–6-week period. The minimum field includes the retroperitoneal lymphatics, and runs from the scrotum to the 10th thoracic vertebra (see Fig. 86). Even in the absence of proved secondary deposits, micrometastases are assumed to have occurred. Mediastinal and supra-clavicular fields are irradiated in the presence of metastases in these sites (see Fig. 86). Metastases in the lung are not usually irradiated due to the discomfort and pneumonitis that often results.

Chemotherapy

Chemotherapy is used when the disease has spread beyond the regional nodes, particularly when it has gone above the diaphragm into the mediastinal or supraclavicular nodes. The exception to this is with undifferentiated or trophoblastic teratoma when it is used from the start, whatever the stage of the disease. Alkylating agents (e.g. cyclophosphamide) are used against seminoma. Teratoma is usually treated by combination therapy including actinomycin, bleomycin, methotrexate, etoposide and cisplatin.

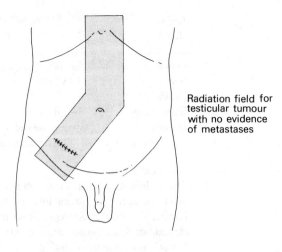

Radiation field for
testicular tumour
with no evidence
of metastases

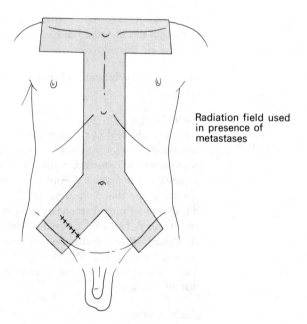

Radiation field used
in presence of
metastases

Fig. 86. Radiotherapy for testicular tumours.

Painful testis

A painful testis can follow direct trauma and haematoma
formation but in the absence of this history two important
diagnoses must be considered and excluded. One is torsion
and the other is a developing tumour. In the first case the
pain is very severe and in the second it is usually of lower

intensity. More often than not, however, the painful testis turns out to be due to epididymo-orchitis.

Epididymo-orchitis

The condition Epididymo-orchitis is an inflammation of the epididymis and testis due to either bacterial, chlamydial or viral infection. The most common viral cause is mumps and it may then be associated with the characteristic parotitis.

Bacterial infections may be gonococcal or due to other bacteria such as coliforms. The infection is thought to arise through reflux of infected urine or prostatic fluid along the vas. It used to be common after open prostatectomy unless the vasa were tied. Chlamydial infection is becoming more common. The epididymis alone may be infected or the inflammation may occasionally spread to involve the testis as well.

Recognizing the pattern *The patient*
Bacterial epididymo-orchitis usually occurs in the elderly whereas viral infections are more common in the younger age-group.

The history
The typical picture is of an acute onset of very severe pain in the testis. There is swelling of the scrotum and the testis becomes hard and very tender. The patient is ill with a fever, and rigors are not uncommon. There may or may not be associated dysuria and frequency.

Proving the diagnosis The main differential diagnosis is torsion of the testis. The presence of a urinary infection, demonstrated on a midstream specimen of urine, may be helpful, although it does not, of course, rule out a torsion. In epididymo-orchitis the pain is said to be relieved by elevating the organ where this is not so with a torsion. The large, hot, swollen testis of epididymo-orchitis is characteristic, as are the systemic signs of infection. When there is difficulty in deciding whether or not the testis is twisted, the scrotum should be explored. No harm is done by exploring an infection but much harm can follow conservative treatment of a torsion.

Management The treatment is to give antibiotics, a scrotal support and bed rest. The epididymis frequently remains very hard and indurated for several weeks.

Chronic infections of the testis and epididymis

Two chronic infections which may affect the epididymis are

tuberculosis and syphilis. Both are now extremely rare thanks to adequate early antibiotic treatment. Because of this rareness, however, the diagnosis is liable to be missed.

A gumma of the testis is commonly seen in examination specimens but fortunately not in clinical practice any more. The treatment of syphilis is penicillin.

Tuberculosis may affect the epididymis as part of an infection involving the urinary tract. The chronically indurated epididymis is not usually painful. The inflammation may slowly progress to sinus formation.

The diagnosis is made either by finding acid-fast bacilli in the urinary tract or by culturing them from sinuses. The treatment is with antituberculous drugs and this may be combined with excision of the affected epididymis.

Torsion of the testis

The condition The testis and epididymis are normally fixed within the scrotum by a 'bare area' which is outside the tunica vaginalis. Part of the epididymis and testis are involved in this 'bare area'. Torsion of the testis can occur when this attachment is minimal and the organ is on a 'mesentery' (Fig. 87). Occasionally the epididymis and testis are more separated than usual and in this case torsion can occur between the two. As these abnormalities are usually bilateral the opposite testis should usually be fixed when a torsion has occurred on one side. The actual twist occurs due to the action of the cremaster muscle. The fibres of this muscle run from the inguinal region downwards and medially across the front of the testis. When they contract the testis tends to rotate with its medial side moving forwards. Torsions not infrequently occur at times of excessive strain or exercise. Undescended testes have a higher incidence of torsion than those which are fully descended.

Recognizing the pattern

The patient
Torsion can occur at any age but is more common between the ages of 15 and 30.

The history
There is a sudden onset of very severe scrotal pain, often associated with right iliac fossa pain radiating into the loin. The patient may feel ill and faint and experience nausea and vomiting.

On examination
The patient looks pale and ill and is in pain. The testis is swollen and hard and exquisitely tender. Because of this

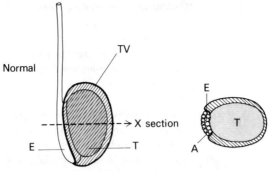

Normal

Tunica vaginalis (TV) enveloping testis (T)
and anterior half of epididymus (E). Broad bare area (A)

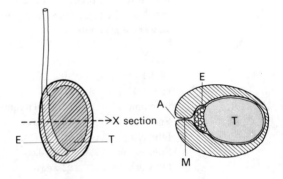

Tunica vaginalis includes epididymis. Small bare
area (A) and mesentery (M)
Testis prone to torsion

Fig. 87. The anatomy of testicular torsion.

tenderness the twist in the cord may not be palpable.
However, the testis rides higher than its fellow and this sign
is helpful in making the diagnosis. Elevation of the twisted
testis does not relieve the pain in contrast to the findings in
epididymo-orchitis.

**Proving the
diagnosis**

Where torsion is suspected the scrotum should be explored
under a general anaesthetic without delay. If the testis is
twisted for more than 4 hours irreversible damage is likely to
occur. At operation the diagnosis is confirmed by seeing the
twist in the spermatic cord.

Operation: correction of torsion of the testis

Preoperative care
The patient or his parents must be warned of the slight possibility of the testis needing to be excised.

Operation
The scrotum is incised laterally and the tunica opened. If this is done carefully, the testis is not rotated and the twist may be demonstrated. It is corrected and the colour of the testis observed. A non-viable testis will have to be removed. If viable, the tunica is fixed back behind the cord as in a hydrocoele. The exposed testis is then placed subcutaneously. A chromic catgut suture may be used to fix it to the skin. The contralateral testis may then also be fixed in a subcutaneous pouch.

Codes

Blood	0	
GA/LA	GA	
Opn time	30−60 minutes	
Stay	3−5 days	
Drains out	0	
Sutures out	5−7 days	
Off work	2 weeks	

Postoperative care
Where the testis has proved viable a scrotal support is supplied. This and bed rest for 24 hours will assist the testicular swelling to settle. Where the testis has been excised early mobilization and discharge are the rule.

Varicocoele

The condition
A varicocoele is a collection of varicose veins in the pampiniform plexus of the cord and scrotum. It carries a higher than average incidence of infertility and this is thought to be due to the higher scrotal temperature associated with the abnormality. Varicocoeles can be secondary to lesions causing obstruction to the testicular veins in the abdomen.

Recognizing the pattern

The patient
He is usually a young adult. The varicocoele may have been spotted at a routine medical examination (e.g. for the Forces).

The history
The usual complaint is of a dull ache, especially at the end of

the day or after exercise. The varicose veins themselves may also have been noted and caused the patient concern.

On examination
The varicocoele is usually plainly visible when the patient stands up. On palpation the typical 'bag of worms' feel is easily recognized. The left side is more commonly affected than the right. The swelling diminishes or even disappears when the patient lies flat.

Management

The patient is reassured that no harm is likely to come from this lesion. Indications for operation are if the pain is persistent in spite of adequate support or if there is associated infertility.

Operation: for varicocoele
The cord is explored in the groin and all the veins in the spermatic cord are divided leaving only one to conduct blood from the testis. The artery and vas are also preserved.

Codes

Blood	0 ....
GA/LA	GA ....
Opn time	60 minutes ....
Stay	1−3 days ....
Drains out	0 ....
Sutures out	5−7 days ....
Off work........	2 weeks......................

Postoperative care
The patient wears a scrotal support and early discharge is the rule.

9   Vascular Disease

9.1 Chronic ischaemia of the leg
Assessment of the ischaemic leg

9.2 Management of the ischaemic limb
General management
Vascular operations
Types of procedure
Amputation

9.3 Aneurysms, emboli and arterio-venous fistulae
Arterial aneurysms
Acute arterial embolism
Arterio-venous fistulae

9.4 Other arterial conditions
Carotid artery disease
Raynaud's phenomenon

9.5 Venous disorders
Varicose veins
Venous ulceration

9.6 Lymphoedema

9.1   Chronic Ischaemia of the Leg

Introduction

This section will deal with the problem of recognizing and investigating the patient who presents with an ischaemic leg. The management is dealt with in Section 9.2.

Assessment of the ischaemic leg

In the initial assessment three questions have to be answered before decisions about management can be made. These are as follows.

1 *Is the leg ischaemic or not?* Does the patient have the pattern of symptoms and signs which suggest ischaemia? The differential diagnosis includes referred pain (sciatica), cauda equina syndrome, and pain due to venous congestion secondary to venous thrombosis or varicose veins.

2 *Site of the lesion.* What is the site of the lesion causing the ischaemia?

3 *Severity.* How severe is the ischaemia?

1 Is the leg ischaemic?

Recognizing the pattern

The patient

The patient is more often male than female and almost always beyond middle age. The disease is more common in smokers.

The history

The main complaint is of pain in the limb and this may be:

(a) Intermittent claudication,

(b) Rest pain, or

(c) Painful ulceration.

Intermittent claudication is a cramp-like pain which comes on in the muscle masses of the leg on walking, especially if going uphill. The pain comes on after a certain distance (known as the exercise tolerance) and is relieved by resting. When resuming exercise the tolerance is often decreased.

Rest pain is a more severe symptom. Pain at rest is particularly noticed at night when it may keep the patient awake. It may be very severe and is relieved by making the leg dependent. The patient may get up and walk about or hang the leg over the edge of the bed. Elevating the leg makes the pain worse. This is useful in differentiating the pain from that of venous congestion where the pain is worse when the leg is dependent.

Trophic changes occur finally. These changes consist of discoloration of the foot followed by dry gangrene and eventually ulceration. This is seen particularly over pressure points. Ischaemic ulcers are usually extremely painful.

There is frequently a family history of vascular disease such as coronary thrombosis or strokes, and the patient may himself have had such a problem in the past. The disease is common in diabetics.

On examination

The characteristic features of ischaemia are the following.

1 *Absent pulses.* Feel carefully for the femoral, popliteal and foot pulses. Absent pulses in one limb are good evidence of an arterial block. If no pulses are palpable on either side there may be bilateral disease or the vessels may be constricted for other reasons such as a cold environment.

2 *Loss of texture and hair on the distal limb.*

3 *Cold extremity.* Compare the temperature of the good side with the bad side. The back of the examiner's fingers is more sensitive to temperature difference than the flat of the hand.

4 *Postural colour change* (Buerger's test). To elicit this sign raise both the legs up in the air with the patient supine. Observe the colour of the soles. If the leg is ischaemic, there is insufficient head of pressure to perfuse the elevated leg and the foot becomes pale.

After a period of a minute or two ask the patient to sit up and hang the legs down over the edge of the couch. The colour will return slowly in the ischaemic leg, and the skin will turn dusky blue. This is because the blood is being deoxygenated in its slow passage through the ischaemic tissue. If the opposite leg has a normal circulation the difference will be very obvious.

5 *Persistent venous guttering.* This sign can be elicited at the same time as postural colour change. As the legs are elevated the foot veins empty. When the legs are dependent the veins at first remain collapsed as a 'gutter'. The time taken for this venous gutter to fill up is an indication of the rate of perfusion through the foot. The greater the degree of ischaemia, the more slowly the venous gutters fill.

6 *Visible gangrene.* Ischaemic tissue necrosis is usually well demarcated with dusky tissue around the edge. Arterial ulcers are punched out with little sign of active healing.

In addition to these signs there may be more general signs of vascular disease such as carotid artery bruits, cardiac irregularities and hypertension.

You should now be in a position to know whether the patient's pain is due to ischaemia or not. If it is, you need to define the site and severity of the lesion.

2 Anatomical site of lesion

This can usually be diagnosed with considerable accuracy before an arteriogram is undertaken. Such an accurate assessment then makes the interpretation of the X-rays more meaningful. A knowledge of the normal anatomy of the vascular tree is necessary (see Fig. 88).

The site of the lesion is determined by the following.

The history

The level of the claudication must be determined. Aorto-iliac disease causes buttock as well as thigh and calf claudication. With such high disease there may also be a history of impotence (Leriche's syndrome). Femoral disease gives rise to calf claudication only.

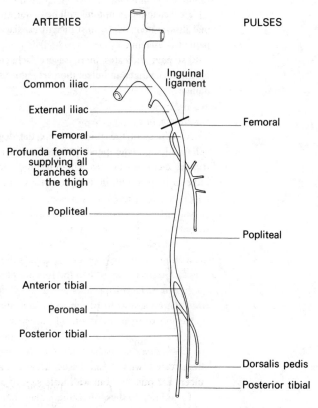

Fig. 88. The arterial supply to the lower leg: the named arteries and the palpable pulses.

On examination

The level of the pulse deficit will usually be diagnostic of the level of the block. An absent femoral pulse indicates disease in the iliac system or above, and so on.

Listen for bruits. Even when distal pulses are present a proximal bruit in the abdomen or groin can tell you there is narrowing at that site. Proximal stenoses are more significant than distal ones, and therefore important to diagnose. A bruit in mid-thigh can tell you the superficial femoral artery is patent at that level even though the distal popliteal pulse is impalpable (see Fig. 89).

3 Severity of ischaemia

The severity is determined by the following.

The history

Intermittent claudication represents the least severe symptom of ischaemia and the longer the exercise tolerance the more minor the problem.

Any ischaemic symptoms will be made worse if the proximal flow is poor due to insufficient cardiac output or if the patient is anaemic.

Rest pain indicates more severe ischaemia. The onset of trophic changes and ulceration are signs that the limb is in danger.

On examination

The coldness of the affected limb, the degree of postural colour change, the persistence of venous guttering, and trophic changes such as gangrene and ulceration will all indicate how severe the ischaemia is.

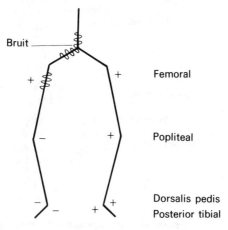

Fig. 89. A method of recording pulses and bruits.

Proving the diagnosis

The opinions formed in the above assessment may be strengthened or weakened by a variety of tests, the most important of which remains the arteriogram.

Arteriography

Arteriograms can be obtained through a variety of routes and you should be aware of these when you request the X-ray.

1 *Direct femoral arteriogram.* In this technique the needle is inserted directly into the femoral artery and the distal arterial tree only is visualized. Generally speaking, however, one would require a picture of the proximal vascular tree in every case.

2 *Retrograde femoral arteriography.* The femoral artery is punctured and a cannula fed up into the aorta. A patent iliac system is necessary for this technique.

3 *Translumbar aortogram.* The aorta is punctured by a needle placed in the lumbar region and the distal arterial tree visualized.

4 *Trans-axillary aortogram.* The axillary or brachial artery is punctured and a catheter fed antegradely down to the abdominal aorta. This technique is invaluable where both iliac arteries are blocked.

The hazards of arteriography

Arteriograms do carry a complication rate and this must always be kept in mind before they are ordered. Complications include the following.

1 Detachment of an arterial plaque and intimal dissection due to damage by the catheter, causing distal ischaemia.

2 Haematoma formation and thrombosis at the site of the needle puncture.

Look out for signs of these when the patient has returned from the X-ray department. Because of these risks, arteriograms are not usually performed unless the intention is to proceed to surgical reconstruction.

Digital subtraction angiograms

Pictures are obtained by injecting contrast intravenously and enhancing the pictures digitally. This requires special equipment and has the advantage of being no more invasive than an intravenous injection. The pictures are not as clear as direct angiograms but can be of great value, particularly in follow-up studies.

Other methods of investigating arterial disease

Ankle-brachial pressure index
The arterial blood pressure is normally measured by inflating a cuff around the limb and noting the pressure at which distal pulses disappear. This is not possible when the main artery is blocked as any circulation only arrives through collaterals and the distal pulse is impalpable. Flow within the distal artery can, however, be detected with a Doppler ultrasound probe in these circumstances and this instrument enables the occlusion pressure at various levels in the leg to be measured. The actual pressure in the leg is related to the mean systolic arterial pressure in the patient and it is conventional to standardize the measurement by expressing the limb pressure as a fraction of the central pressure (measured in the arm). This index is known as the ankle-brachial pressure index (ABPI). It can be correlated with the patient's clinical status (see Table 24).

Table 24. The relation of ankle-brachial pressure index to symptoms (Yao S.T. (1970) *British Journal of Surgery*, **57**, p. 761)

Clinical status	ABPI
Normal	1
Claudication	0.5
Rest pain	0.3
Impending gangrene	0.2 or below

Plethysmography
In this technique the venous output of the limb is obstructed by a cuff and the rate of increase in the size of the limb distally is used as a measure of arterial inflow. In volume plethysmography the volume of the limb is measured. In gravimetric plethysmography the increase in weight of the distal limb is measured.

Isotope clearance
A radioactive isotope is injected either systemically or directly into the artery supplying the limb. The rate of clearance is measured using a counter and this is related to the flow through that region of the limb.

Electromagnetic flow meter
The limb is placed in a magnetic field. The blood moving within the limb creates an electric potential and this can be monitored with a suitably placed electrode. The deflection produced is an indicator of flow.

The effect of exercise
All these tests can be carried out before and after a standardized form of exercise. Popular methods include the treadmill and using a step test. In general, the normal foot pressure rises with exercise but will fall if there is an arterial obstruction. Various patterns of change in flow can be detected and related to the severity of the arterial obstruction.

Other routine investigations
Table 25 shows some of those to be considered.

Table 25. Routine investigations in arterial disease

Investigation	Reason
Haemoglobin, white cell count, ESR	? Anaemia
Serum proteins	? Collagen diseases
	? General nutritional state
Urea and creatinine	? Ischaemic or other renal disease
Electrolytes	? Low potassium on diuretics
ECG	? Cardiac ischaemia
Wassermann reaction	Exclude syphilitic arterial disease
MSU	? Proteinuria
Urine for sugar	? Diabetes
Chest X-ray	? Lung disease
	? Enlargement of the heart
Abdominal X-ray	? Calcification of major vessels

Management of the Ischaemic Limb

General management

If the patient continues smoking, the prognosis for the ischaemic limb is grave. All patients should therefore be told that smoking will endanger their limb, and advised to stop. Weight reduction also helps in the overall perfusion of the limb.

Attention should be given to improving the cardiac output, correcting anaemia, and also treating infection in the limb.

Apart from these general measures, the management will be determined by the severity of the lesion.

Management of claudication only

The management is generally conservative. The patient should be encouraged to exercise as much as possible to open and develop the collateral circulation. Care should be taken not to injure the limb as healing may be very poor and injury may be the first step towards persistent ulceration. Chiropody should be undertaken with extreme caution, realizing that painful toes and pressure points may be due to ischaemia.

Patients with claudication should be regularly followed up and further investigation and operation may be indicated in the following circumstances.

1 The claudication distance is decreasing.

2 The patient's symptoms persist and are interfering with life or work to an intolerable degree.

3 The patient develops rest pain.

Management of rest pain

The onset of pain at rest is an indication for active measures. An arteriogram is performed with a view to planning reconstructive arterial surgery or other treatment.

Factors in favour of a reconstructive operation are the following.

1 Proximal disease (above inguinal ligament).

2 A relatively fit patient.

3 Good distal 'run-off'. There must be an adequate arterial tree distal to the block in order that a bypass or reconstruction can be successful.

Conversely, an operation is less likely to be worthwhile in the presence of the following.

1 Distal disease.
2 Claudication only.
3 An unfit patient.
4 A poor distal run-off.

Vascular operations

Preoperative care
Attention to general fitness is more important in an arteriopath about to undergo surgery than in most other cases. A careful record of the preoperative state of pulses and pressures should be made as this will be invaluable in monitoring progress post-operatively.

If there is a possibility that the surgeon may wish to use the long saphenous vein in the reconstruction operation, this should be marked pre-operatively. This is done by standing the patient up, waiting for the vein to fill, and then marking its position carefully on the skin.

If a prosthesis is likely to be inserted, antibiotics should be given with the premedication. These should be broad-spectrum and cover staphylococci (see p. 108).

Operative techniques available

There are various techniques which can be used to help these patients.

Endarterectomy

The atheromatous lining of the narrowed artery is cored out. This procedure is particularly suitable for short stenoses in the larger vessels above the inguinal ligament, and also for the removal of plaques in the internal carotid arteries in patients with transient ischaemic attacks (see p. 500).

Bypass

In this technique a new vessel is anastomosed above and below the block. The best graft material is the patient's own long saphenous vein, but because of its diameter it is usually only suitable for procedures involving smaller arteries such as a femoro-popliteal bypass or a renal artery bypass. Synthetic grafts of small diameter have a significant incidence of thrombosis. Above the inguinal ligament, problems with graft thrombosis are not so common because of the larger diameter of the vessels and the higher flow rate. In this situation prosthetic grafts can be used successfully and these are usually made of Dacron or Teflon.

Replacement

The diseased artery is taken out of the circulation and replaced by a prosthetic graft. The technique is particularly used in the replacement of aortic or other aneurysms.

Profundaplasty

The narrowed origin of the profunda femoris artery is widened by sewing in a vein patch, usually of the long saphenous vein, at the site of the narrowing. This technique can also be used on localized narrowings elsewhere.

Balloon angioplasty

Some localized stenoses in arteries can be dilated by a balloon placed within the lumen of the artery. The method has the advantage of being relatively 'non-invasive' and may give long-term success. This technique is carried out by a specialist radiologist but it should always be done in conjunction with an arterial surgeon, as a reconstructive procedure will be necessary if the angioplasty fails.

Sympathectomy

Division of the sympathetic nerve supplying the limb results in a dilatation of the vessels in the skin and diversion of the blood towards the skin. This can be beneficial if the ischaemia is superficial, but is of no benefit when the deep tissues of the limb are short of blood. Sympathectomy can only redistribute the blood in the limb and cannot increase the total amount which can enter by the narrowed main arteries. The procedure is, therefore, of no value in patients with intermittent claudication, where the problem is a lack of blood supply to the muscle. It is of value to patients with peripheral ischaemia due to small vessel disease, such as Buerger's disease or diabetic angiopathy. It may also be helpful in some cases of Raynaud's phenomenon (see p. 500).

Sympathectomies may be carried out either by injection or by a direct surgical approach.

Postoperative care

The distal pulses should be recorded at the end of any direct arterial operation and checked regularly thereafter. If the pulses disappear the surgeon should be informed. If a prosthesis or reconstructed artery blocks in the immediate postoperative period, it may be possible to unblock it provided the situation is not left undetected too long.

In all direct vascular procedures it is important to maintain an adequate cardiac output postoperatively. If the flow through the vessel falls, the roughened arterial surfaces are likely to precipitate thrombosis. For this reason it is important to maintain the circulating volume by adequate transfusion. Where the patient has a coexisting cardiac condition, it may be wise to monitor this carefully by inserting a central venous line. Vasoconstriction on the part of the patient in order to maintain the circulation must be avoided.

Types of procedure

Each particular vascular operation tends to be a one-off exercise using a combination of the above techniques to suit the particular situation found in the patient. The procedure may be named by the proximal and distal vessels to be dealt with, e.g. aorto-iliac endarterectomy, aorto-femoral bypass, aorto-popliteal bypass. Some of the more common types of procedure are described below.

Operation: injection sympathectomy

A needle is passed through the back into the sympathetic chain under radiographic control. Its position is confirmed by injecting contrast medium and phenol is then injected. This can be carried out under a general or local anaesthetic.

Operation: lumbar sympathectomy

The lumbar sympathetic chain is approached retroperitoneally through an oblique incision in the anterior flank. The peritoneum is retracted medially and the sympathetic chain exposed on the vertebrae lateral to the aorta or vena cava. The lower lumbar ganglia are removed.

Codes

Blood	2 units . . . .
GA/LA	GA . . . .
Opn time	60–90 minutes . . . .
Stay	5–7 days . . . .
Drains out	24 hours . . . .
Sutures out	7 days . . . .
Off work	About 4 weeks . . . .

The operation of cervical sympathectomy is described in the section on Raynaud's phenomenon, p. 500.

Operation: aorto-iliac endarterectomy or bypass

In these operations the aorta and iliac vessels are exposed and disobliterated or bypassed as necessary (see Fig. 90).

It is frequently necessary to expose the femoral arteries in both groins, and the groins and thighs should be shaved

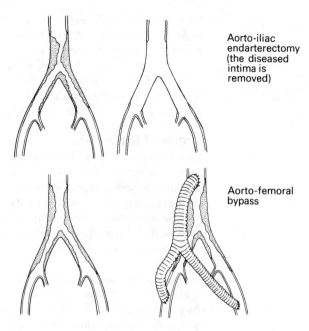

Aorto-iliac
endarterectomy
(the diseased
intima is
removed)

Aorto-femoral
bypass

Fig. 90. Two procedures for improving aortic flow.

preoperatively. The aorta may be approached transperitone-
ally or retroperitoneally. The former causes a longer postoperative ileus, but gives a better exposure of the upper
aorta.

Codes

Blood	10 units	. . . .
GA/LA	GA	. . . .
Opn time	2 – 5 hours	. . . .
Stay	10 – 14 days	. . . .
Drains out	48 hours	. . . .
Sutures out	7 – 10 days	. . . .
Off work	4 – 6 weeks	. . . .

Operation: femoro-popliteal bypass (Fig. 91)
In this operation the femoral artery is exposed in the groin
and the popliteal artery in the popliteal fossa. The long
saphenous vein is excised along its length in the thigh and
used to bypass the blocked superficial femoral artery. The
vein is inverted so that the valves do not obstruct the arterial
flow.

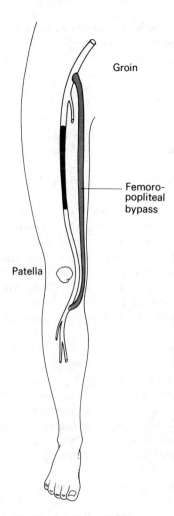

Groin

Femoro-
popliteal
bypass

Patella

Fig. 91. Femoro-popliteal bypass.

Codes

Blood	6 units	. . . .
GA/LA	GA	. . . .
Opn time	2–3 hours	. . . .
Stay	7–10 days	. . . .
Drains out	48 hours	. . . .
Sutures out	7–10 days	. . . .
Off work	4–6 weeks	. . . .

Operation: profundaplasty

This operation can be a very minor procedure carried out
under a local anaesthetic. A suitable piece of long saphenous

vein is isolated and removed and used as a patch to widen the profunda femoris origin.

Codes

Blood	4 units ....
GA/LA	GA or LA.......................
Opn time	1–2 hours ....
Stay	5–10 days ....
Drains out	48 hours........................
Sutures out	7 days..........................
Off work........	Variable ....

Operation: axillo-femoral bypass (Fig. 92a)

This operation is used to bring blood to the ischaemic lower limbs when there is an aortic block or an infected prosthesis in the abdomen. A long prosthetic graft is sutured to the axillary artery under the clavicle and routed subcutaneously down to the common femoral artery in the groin. If both legs are ischaemic an inverted 'Y'-shaped graft may be used to bring blood to both femoral arteries.

Codes

Blood	6 units ....
GA/LA	GA ....
Opn time	1–2 hours ....
Stay	7–10 days ....
Drains out	24 hours........................
Sutures out	7 days..........................
Off work........	Variable ....

Operation: femoro-femoral bypass (Fig. 92b)

A long saphenous vein or prosthetic graft is sutured from one common femoral artery in the groin to the other femoral artery. The graft is routed across the suprapubic region, usually behind the rectus abdominis. This procedure is valuable where only one iliac artery is blocked and the patient is unsuitable for a more major reconstruction.

Codes

Blood	4 units ....
GA/LA	GA or spinal ....
Opn time	2 hours.........................
Stay	7–10 days ....
Drains out	24 hours........................
Sutures out	7 days..........................
Off work........	Variable ....

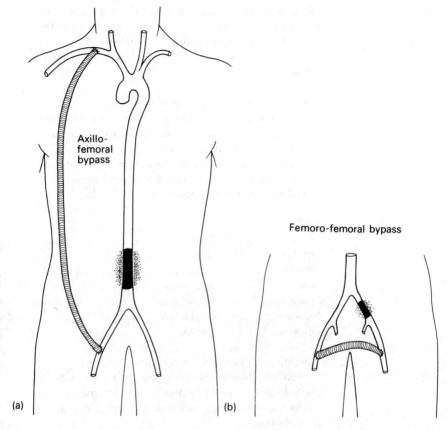

Fig. 92. Two forms of 'extra-anatomical' bypass.

Amputation

Where attempts to save an ischaemic limb have failed, amputation may become necessary to relieve the patient's symptoms. The level of amputation will have to be high enough to ensure adequate healing of the stump. In patients with major vessel disease (aorta, iliac or femoral arteries), this usually means amputation just below the knee or higher. In patients with distal small vessel disease (diabetic arteriopathy, Buerger's disease) or those who have had a successful proximal reconstruction, a more distal amputation may be possible. Amputation operations at seven different levels in the lower limb are described here.

Preoperative management
The question of amputation is best introduced slowly to the patient against the background of failure of other measures.

Always leave the final decision to him. Once he has accepted that nothing else can be done he will usually decide that amputation is preferable to continued suffering. As soon as a decision has been made, the operation should rapidly be arranged.

Operation: above knee amputation

The site of elective bone division is 40 cm below the greater trochanter. The skin flaps are cut approximately 5 cm distal to this and are of equal size anteriorly and posteriorly. Once the bone has been divided, the muscles are closed over the cut end and the skin flaps closed with loose sutures. The wound is drained and the stump carefully bandaged.

Codes

Blood	2 units . . . .
GA/LA	GA . . . .
Opn time	90 minutes . . . .
Stay	2–3 weeks . . . .
Drains out	48 hours . . . .
Sutures out	10–14 days . . . .
Off work	Variable . . . .

Operation: through knee amputation

The limb is divided through the knee and a long anterior flap fashioned and sutured around behind the condyles. The patella may or may not be removed. This type of amputation is weight-bearing.

Codes

As for above knee amputation.

Operation: below knee amputation

The blood supply to the tissues of the lower leg is better posteriorly than anteriorly, and this amputation is therefore designed to use a long posterior flap of skin and muscle. The anterior incision is made 12 cm below the tibial tuberosity and the posterior one above the Achilles tendon. The latter is folded forwards across the bevelled cut ends of the bone and sutured to the short anterior flap. This amputation has the advantage of preserving the knee joint and thus making rehabilitation easier. It can usually be carried out providing the profunda femoris artery remains patent.

Codes

As for above knee amputation.

Operation: Syme's amputation

In this amputation the forefoot is excised together with the calcaneum and the lowest part of the tibia and fibula. A flap is fashioned from the heel pad and folded forwards to be sutured to the skin on the anterior aspect of the lower tibia. This is a weight-bearing stump.

Codes

Blood	Group and save . . . .
GA/LA	GA . . . .
Opn time	60−90 minutes . . . .
Stay	10−14 days . . . .
Drains out	24−48 hours . . . .
Sutures out	10−14 days . . . .
Off work	Variable . . . .

Operation: ray amputation

Where there is necrosis of a digit accompanied by necrosis of the muscles of the foot, a ray amputation of the metatarsal may be necessary. The affected toe is excised together with a wedge of tissue based on the metatarsal. The metatarsal is removed. The effect is to narrow the forefoot. The amputation produces a cosmetically satisfactory result. The wound is usually left open and dressed daily.

Codes

Blood	Group and save . . . .
GA/LA	GA . . . .
Opn time	30−60 minutes . . . .
Stay	10−14 days . . . .
Drains out	24−48 hours . . . .
Sutures out	0 . . . .
Off work	Variable . . . .

Operation: transmetatarsal amputation

In this operation the forefoot is amputated removing the metatarsals. The sole of the foot is formed into a flap which is sutured to the skin dorsally over the tarsal bones.

Codes

Blood	Group and save . . . .
GA/LA	GA . . . .
Opn time	30−60 minutes . . . .
Stay	2−3 weeks . . . .
Drains out	0 . . . .
Sutures out	10−14 days (may be left open) . . . . . .
Off work	Variable . . . .

Operation: amputation of the toe

The toe is amputated together with either all or part of the proximal phalanx. The dorsal and ventral skin flaps are sutured together over the bone.

Codes

Blood	0 ....
GA/LA	GA or LA.......................
Opn time	30–60 minutes ....
Stay	10–14 days ....
Drains out	0 ....
Sutures out	10–14 days ....
Off work........	Variable ....

Postoperative care

In the first 8 hours you should check that the bandages are not too tight. Otherwise, where the stump has been sutured, they are best left strictly alone for a week. The drains are not usually sutured in place and can be gently pulled out without disturbing the dressing. Generally, only half the sutures are removed at 7–10 days and the rest when healing is complete. Unsutured amputation wounds will require daily dressings. The physiotherapist should ensure that contractures do not occur at the proximal joint. The limb fitting centre should be informed and, as the patient recovers, arrangements made for a prosthesis to be fitted.

Aneurysms, Emboli and Arterio-venous Fistulae

Arterial aneurysms

Aneurysms arise as a result of weakness in the arterial wall, usually secondary to *arteriosclerosis*.
Other causes can be the following.

1 *Congenital*. The best example is the Berry aneurysm in the cranial arteries.

2 *Traumatic*. The arterial wall may be damaged during a surgical operation, by direct trauma during an accident or by gunshot injury.

3 *Inflammatory*. Syphilis is perhaps the most famous cause of aneurysms but other organisms also give rise to this problem as part of subacute bacterial endocarditis.

4 *Cystic medial necrosis*. This degenerative lesion of the media may occur as part of Marfan's syndrome.

Aneurysms can occur anywhere in the vascular tree but are particularly common in the abdominal aorta below the origin of the renal arteries. They also occur in the thoracic aorta and the femoral and popliteal arteries.

Aortic aneurysms

The condition

The abdominal aorta usually dilates distal to the origin of the renal arteries as the aortic wall is poorly supported below this level. A small aneurysm is usually asymptomatic but once the elasticity of the wall is weakened it tends to enlarge steadily. Above 6 cm in diameter there is a danger that it may rupture.

The chances of a cold aneurysm rupturing have been estimated at about 20% per year. If it is dealt with once it has ruptured, the operative mortality is 50%. If the aneurysm is dealt with as a cold procedure in a good unit, the operative mortality should be of the order of 5%. By and large, therefore, it should be replaced before it ruptures.

Aortic aneurysms also tend to be lined with thrombus and distal embolism and ischaemia may occur.

An aneurysm of the abdominal aorta is frequently associated with aneurysms elsewhere (e.g. iliac, femoral or popliteal).

Recognizing the pattern

The patient

The patient is usually over 50 and males are more frequently affected than females. There may be other stigmata of atheromatous disease such as a history of myocardial infarction or hypertension.

The history
The patient sometimes notices the mass or abdominal pulsation ('my heart has slipped'). Alternatively the aneurysm is found by the examining physician either as an incidental finding or when it causes abdominal pain or distal ischaemia.

On examination
The pulsatile swelling is usually easily felt in the epigastrium and central abdomen. The fact that the pulsation is true rather than transmitted is confirmed by palpating it from side to side. A true pulsation is expansile, and the examining hands move apart with each pulse. In thin elderly patients with a prominent lordosis the normal aorta may be easily palpable and somewhat tortuous and feel like an aneurysm. Nevertheless, careful bimanual palpation of its lateral and medial margins should disclose the fact that it is not in fact widened.

The state of the distal pulses must be recorded at the initial examination.

Proving the diagnosis

A straight abdominal X-ray may show the characteristic curved line of calcification of the aneurysm wall and in that case a lateral view also helps to define its size. The best method of measuring the aneurysm is by ultrasound. A CAT scan is more expensive but very accurate. It may also be helpful in showing how much thrombus there is and whether there is any surrounding haematoma.

Arteriography is not always indicated in aneurysms and may be dangerous. The advantage of performing an arteriogram is that the relationship of the renal vessels to the neck of the aneurysm can be defined preoperatively, as can its distal extent.

Management

The indications for surgery are the following.
1 An expanding aneurysm.
2 An aneurysm over 6 cm in diameter.
3 The onset of abdominal and back pains. These may be the first signs of impending rupture.

The patient should be informed of the dangers of living with an unresected aortic aneurysm. If the aneurysm is small, a policy of waiting may be adopted but in that case regular 3-monthly visits should be arranged to check whether it is enlarging.

Preoperative management

The relatives should also be informed about the dangers of the untreated aneurysm. The patient should be told that it will be necessary to insert a prosthesis to replace it.

In the preoperative work-up the patient's cardiac state and renal function are assessed. Antibiotics are usually given with the premedication. A catheter should be passed, usually in the anaesthetic room at the beginning of the operation, in order to monitor urinary output during and after the procedure.

Operation: replacement of aortic aneurysm

The aorta is exposed and the extent of the aneurysm defined. The easiest procedure is simply to replace the abdominal aorta between the renal arteries and the aortic bifurcation. Occasionally it is necessary to bring a bifurcated trouser graft down to both femoral regions. Once the aneurysm has been controlled it is opened and the lumbar vessels are sutured from within. The Dacron prosthesis is then sewn into the upper aorta and a similar anastomosis made either to the bifurcation or to the femoral arteries. The aneurysm walls are used to cover the graft.

Codes

Blood	6 – 10 units . . . .
GA/LA	GA . . . .
Opn time	2 – 3 hours . . . .
Stay	10 – 14 days . . . .
Drains out	Abdomen 0, groin 24 hours . . . .
Sutures out	7 – 10 days . . . .
Off work	Variable, 4 – 6 weeks . . . .

Postoperative care

Immediately after the operation you should check whether the pulses in the leg are present as they were preoperatively. Absent femoral pulses are an indication for early embolectomy. There is usually an ileus, which may be prolonged. In the early stages careful assessment is necessary to make sure that blood replacement is accurate and that bleeding is not continuing. The danger of continued haemorrhage is usually over after the first 24 hours.

Renal failure is a complication of this operation. The kidneys may previously have been damaged by hypertension or atheroma and additional ischaemia in the perioperative period due to high aortic clamping or hypotension can result in failure. Careful monitoring of hourly urinary output is therefore needed.

The patient is mobilized after the third or fourth day. Anti-coagulants may be given during the operation but are not usually continued postoperatively unless there is a specific indication for it. The groin and foot pulses should be checked on a daily basis during the first week or 10 days after the operation.

Once the patient has left hospital, prolonged follow-up is advisable. Occasionally the aortic suture line may become infected or it may become adherent to a loop of bowel, eventually resulting in an aorto-enteric fistula. Any evidence of pain or tenderness in the region of the prosthesis should be taken seriously and is probably now best investigated by performing a CAT scan. Any suggestion of infection in the region of the prosthesis should be treated energetically with broad-spectrum antibiotics for several weeks.

Ruptured aortic aneurysm

This is one of the more dramatic problems the surgical team may be called upon to deal with. Once an aortic aneurysm has burst the patient is likely to die unless the aorta can be replaced before he exsanguinates. Fortunately, the rupture is usually temporarily controlled by the surrounding tissues and this gives a little time to get an operation organized. Rapid action is required, however, if the patient is to be saved.

Recognizing the pattern

The patient usually experiences a sudden onset of very severe pain in the flank or back. The pain is more commonly on the left than the right. He feels faint, cold and sweaty. Occasionally the presentation is less dramatic.

On examination

The aneurysm is tender. Avoid palpating it more than is absolutely necessary. The patient is pale and shocked with a low blood pressure and a tachycardia. Make a quick note of the distal pulses for future reference.

Proving the diagnosis

Time should not be wasted on investigations if the patient is shocked. A tender aneurysm and a shocked patient are an indication for surgery. If the situation is less acute and the diagnosis is in doubt, an ultrasound may confirm the presence of the aneurysm and a CAT scan can show whether it is leaking or not.

Management

Warn the surgeon and theatre as soon as possible that a leaking aneurysm has been admitted. Take blood for cross-matching (10 units at least) and for base-line investigations such as haemoglobin, urea and electrolytes. Set up at least one and possibly two good intravenous lines. Institute regular blood pressure and pulse recording. Once the surgeon has confirmed the diagnosis or even before, contact the anaesthetist. Then transfer the patient to the theatre suite.

Pass a catheter and give preoperative antibiotics (e.g. gentamicin and flucloxacillin).

Once in the anaesthetic room there is usually time to reflect and consolidate the situation. Complete the history and the full examination if the initial one was hurried.

Check how long it will be until blood is available. Check the stability of the patient's blood pressure and pulse on the chart. If the patient's condition is stable, there is no immediate hurry to proceed with the operation until everyone is ready.

The patient will usually be induced on the operating table in theatre once the surgeon and the rest of the team are ready to start operating. The relaxation of the abdominal muscles associated with anaesthesia and resulting loss of tamponade frequently precipitates more major bleeding.

Operation: repair of ruptured aortic aneurysm
The abdomen is opened and a massive retroperitoneal haematoma is usually encountered. The common iliac arteries and the aorta above the graft are controlled and once this has been done the main danger is over. The aneurysm is opened and a Dacron graft sewn inside it as in a 'cold' procedure (p. 491).

Codes

Blood	10−12 units	
GA/LA	GA	
Opn time	2−5 hours	
Stay	10−21 days	
Drains out	Abdomen 0, groins 24 hours	
Sutures out	7 days	
Off work	Variable, 8−12 weeks	

Postoperative care
This is as for a cold aneurysm and is described on p. 491. There is, however, usually a more prolonged period of intensive care as the patient has almost certainly been hypotensive and has lost a lot of blood.

Femoral aneurysms
These may require resection or replacement with a graft if they enlarge markedly.

Popliteal aneurysms

These frequently thrombose, with loss of the distal limb. The presence of a popliteal aneurysm is therefore an indication for surgery. The aneurysm may be tied off and a saphenous vein bypass graft inserted.

Acute arterial embolism

The condition

In this condition there is an acute block of an artery due to an embolus arising from thrombus formation proximally.

Sources of emboli include the following.

1 Atrial fibrillation.
2 Myocardial infarction with mural thrombosis.
3 Subacute bacterial endocarditis.
4 Thrombus formation on an ulcerated atheromatous plaque.
5 Thrombus formation within an aneurysm.

Because there is no time for a collateral circulation to develop, the effects of an acute arterial block are more dramatic than a block in a similar place coming on slowly due to atheroma.

Recognizing the pattern

The patient

Arterial emboli can occur in either sex and at any age but are much more common in the elderly.

The history

Symptoms which occur in the limb are characterized by four P's.

1 Pain.
2 Paraesthesia.
3 Paralysis.
4 Pallor.

The characteristic history is of a very sudden onset of these symptoms. If there is a previous history of intermittent claudication, you should consider the possibility of acute thrombosis of the artery rather than an embolism. The paraesthesia and paralysis are due to acute ischaemia of nerves.

On examination

The limb is pale, cold and immobile. Distal pulses are absent. There is loss of pin-prick and light touch sensation in a 'stocking' distribution over the distal leg. The pulse may be irregular, and the patient may have other signs suggesting a possible source (e.g. a heart murmur, an aortic aneurysm or a localized arterial bruit).

| **Proving the** | Acute arterial embolism must be distinguished from |
| **diagnosis** | thrombus on a previously existing atheromatous plaque. The |

Proving the
diagnosis

Acute arterial embolism must be distinguished from thrombus on a previously existing atheromatous plaque. The history is the most reliable guide. An arteriogram may be helpful where the issue is in doubt.

Management

The treatment of an acute arterial embolus is urgent operation to remove the block and restore the circulation. The patient is anti-coagulated with heparin (see p. 107).

Fogarty embolectomy should not be attempted where the embolus is long-standing or where the diagnosis is of acute thrombosis on previous atheroma. There is a danger of trauma to the diseased artery in these circumstances and later reconstruction may be rendered difficult or impossible by the arteriotomy made in the femoral artery. An arteriogram should be performed and either thrombolytic therapy (p. 60) or reconstructive surgery planned.

Finally, the cause of the thrombosis must be treated if possible.

Operation: Fogarty catheter embolectomy
Where the embolus has affected the femoral artery, the vessel is isolated in the groin and controlled with clamps. An arteriotomy is made and any visible clot removed. The embolus and propagated clot is then extracted using a Fogarty catheter. This is a narrow-gauge arterial catheter with an inflatable balloon at its tip. The catheter is passed beyond the embolus and the balloon inflated. When the catheter is pulled back towards the arteriotomy, the clot precedes the balloon and is removed. Great care must be taken not to over-inflate the balloon as this may cause damage to the vessel wall, with resultant stricture formation and permanent obstruction to the blood flow.

Codes

Blood	4 units	....
GA/LA	GA	....
Opn time	1−2 hours	....
Stay	Variable	....
Drains out	48 hours	....
Sutures out	7 days	....
Off work........	Variable	....

Postoperative care
This is similar to that following other arterial operations (p. 480).

Arterio-venous fistulae

The condition

An arterio-venous fistula is a condition in which there is an abnormal connection between the arterial and venous circulations. The major causes are the following.

1 Congenital — often associated with haemangioma or hamartoma formation.

2 Post-traumatic — arterio-venous fistulae may follow damage done to vessels during operations or by other forms of trauma such as penetrating wounds.

3 Iatrogenic — arterio-venous shunts are created, usually in the forearm, as a route of access to the circulation for those on dialysis (Cimino fistula).

The high pressure in the vein causes it to dilate and become tortuous. There is an increased cardiac output and a high pulse pressure if the shunt is large.

Recognizing the pattern

The patient

Arterio-venous fistulae are rare but can occur at any age from birth onwards.

The history

The patient may have noticed the mass of the haemangioma, or the appearance of a 'throbbing swelling' at the site of previous trauma. Occasionally they complain of 'buzzing' associated with the flow disturbance through the fistula.

On examination

A subcutaneous fistula presents as a swelling beneath the skin. On palpation there is an expansile pulsation. An old wound in the skin suggests previous trauma.

The characteristic sign is the audible machinery murmur over the lesion. This is a continuous systolic and diastolic murmur. It can be abolished by occluding the arterial inflow to the fistula either by direct pressure on the feeding artery or by a proximal arterial cuff. In addition to the audible murmur there may be a palpable 'thrill'.

When the condition has occurred early in life the affected limb may grow larger than its fellow. The presence of dilated veins may be noted over the site of an haemangioma. One of the commonest forms of arteriovenous fistula seen (particularly in medical examinations) is the Cimino fistula. In this case a surgical scar in the skin is visible.

Proving the diagnosis

The diagnosis is mainly proved on the clinical findings. The fistula can be demonstrated by an arteriogram when early venous filling will be noted.

Management

Small arterio-venous fistulae do not require intervention. Larger ones can be dealt with in the following way.

1 *Embolization.* This is a technique in which the radiologist first performs an arteriogram and then selectively injects a substance via an arterial catheter on to the fistula, blocking its arterial supply. Emboli used include the following:

(a) absorbable synthetic emboli such as gelatin sponge ('Sterispon');

(b) emboli derived from natural materials such as dura mater or blood clot;

(c) emboli made from plastic particles, or coiled stainless steel wire.

2 *Direct arterial surgery.* In this case the feeding vessels are carefully defined by preoperative angiography.

Operation: for arterio-venous fistula

The feeding vessels are dissected out and tied off and the fistula removed. The operation can be very difficult. Congenital arterio-venous fistulae often have multiple feeding vessels and the blood loss can be considerable. For this reason arterial embolization has become a popular method of treatment. It can, if necessary be combined with direct arterial surgery.

Codes

Blood	6–10 units . . . .
GA/LA	GA . . . .
Opn time	2–5 hours . . . .
Stay	1–2 weeks . . . .
Drains out	2–5 days . . . .
Sutures out	7 days . . . .
Off work	4 weeks . . . .

Other Arterial Conditions

Carotid artery disease

The condition

An atheromatous plaque affecting the carotid artery presents a special problem because of its effect on the blood supply to the brain. Plaques are commonly formed at the bifurcation of the carotid arteries or at the origin of the internal carotid artery. These may then affect the cerebral circulation either by cutting down the total flow or because the plaque undergoes ulceration, thrombus formation and distal embolization. If the artery occludes totally, a complete hemiparesis may result. Before this happens there are often minor episodes of cerebral ischaemia (transient ischaemic attacks, TIAs).

The brain is supplied by four major arteries, the two internal carotid arteries and the two vertebral arteries. Where several of these are diseased the effects of a critical lesion in one of them is not so well localized. The frequency of TIAs is very variable and quite unpredictable. Patients may have several such attacks in a short period of time and then none for many months or years. Some go on rapidly to develop the full picture of a stroke but this is not inevitable. This variation in pattern makes for difficulties in assessing different forms of treatment.

Recognizing the pattern

The patient

The patient is a typical 'arteriopath', middle-aged or elderly and usually a heavy smoker. He may already have had other vascular problems.

The history

There is a history of recurrent transient ischaemic attacks. These consist of symptoms of focal cerebral or retinal dysfunction of short duration, usually followed by complete recovery. The nature of the symptoms depends on the area supplied by the diseased artery. Emboli from an internal carotid plaque can cause transient blockage of the retinal artery on the same side as the lesion with symptoms of 'amaurosis fugax'. The patient suffers from transient blindness, which occurs as a shutter descending over the eye. If the embolus affects the cerebral cortex the symptoms arise in the opposite side of the body, and minor paralysis of the arms and legs, paraesthesiae, or difficulties with speech may occur.

On examination
A characteristic sign to look for is a localized bruit over the lateral side of the neck arising from the narrowed carotid artery. The neurological and eye signs secondary to the emboli may be transient. There may be a peripheral visual field defect and evidence of previous arterial emboli seen on the fundus.

Proving the diagnosis

The diagnosis of a localized narrowing in the internal carotid artery is proved by performing an angiogram. It is also advisable to obtain a picture of the opposite carotid for comparison and because the disease is frequently bilateral.

Less invasive techniques have been developed and these include ultrasound imaging of the artery (MAVIS imaging). These methods are entirely safe but as yet they lack the definition of arteriograms.

Other methods used in vascular laboratories include ocular plethysmography and methods to determine the difference in pressure between the ocular vessels (supplied by the internal carotid artery) and the superficial temporal vessels (supplied by the external carotid artery).

Management

Asymptomatic bruit
Where a bruit is found in the neck but the patient has no symptoms, most clinicians in the UK would agree that investigation and treatment are not indicated.

Transient ischaemic attacks
There are two possible methods of management.
1 The use of anti-platelet agents, such as aspirin or dipyridamole, and/or anti-coagulants, such as warfarin.
2 Direct arterial surgery to remove the plaque.

There is some controversy about the value of each of these methods of treatment. In the author's view the patient who has transient ischaemic attacks and who is found to have a localized bruit over the relevant carotid artery should have a carotid angiogram. If a localized lesion is then found in the artery, it should be removed surgically.

Where a patient has transient ischaemic attacks and a bruit but no localized lesion is found, anti-platelet agents should be used.

Where a patient has transient ischaemic attacks and no bruit, an angiogram is not usually undertaken.

Preoperative management
The patient should be fully informed of the nature of the operation and the dangers of developing a stroke from the

existing disease. He must also be warned that there is a slight danger of developing a stroke as a result of the operation. Such postoperative hemiplegias are fortunately rare and usually transient.

The neck should be shaved from the ear downwards. If the patient is already on anti-coagulants, the surgeon must be asked whether he wishes these to be stopped, wishes them to be continued right up to the operation, or wishes the therapy to be changed on to intravenous heparin.

Operation: carotid artery endarterectomy
The carotid is exposed through a longitudinal incision in front of the sternomastoid muscle. The common, internal and external carotid arteries are controlled. The surgeon may decide to use a shunt. This is a tube placed between the common carotid artery and the internal carotid artery to maintain blood flow while the operation is carried out. The patient is heparinized before the arteries are clamped and the effect of the heparin is usually allowed to wear off postoperatively. Once the artery has been opened the localized plaque is removed by endarterectomy. The artery is closed and a vein patch may be used to widen it.

Codes

Blood	2 units ....
GA/LA	GA ....
Opn time	2 hours ....
Stay	5−7 days ....
Drains out	48 hours ....
Sutures out	5 days ....
Off work........	4−6 weeks ....

Postoperative care
As in other cases of direct arterial surgery, it is important to maintain an adequate blood pressure postoperatively. Patients tend to drop their peripheral resistance when the baroreceptors in the internal carotid artery are perfused at a relatively increased pressure after the operation. They may therefore require a transfusion of 500 cm^3 of plasma expander even though they have lost very little blood.

The patients often complain of severe headache after the operation but this is an indication that the cerebral flow has been improved. Patients should be reassured and given adequate analgesia.

Raynaud's phenomenon

The condition   Raynaud's phenomenon is the name given to the sequence of colour changes seen in the fingers in response to cold. Less commonly it occurs in the toes. The colour changes are caused by vasospasm of the digital arteries with peripheral ischaemia and cyanosis, followed by arteriolar dilatation and hyperaemia.

It occurs occasionally as a disease of unknown aetiology (Raynaud's disease) where the vessels appear to be over-responsive to a fall in temperature. More usually it is seen in organic diseases, particularly scleroderma, systemic lupus erythematosus and other connective tissue diseases. Other causes include a cervical rib, Buerger's disease, atherosclerosis, cryoglobulinaemia, and certain drugs (e.g. the contraceptive pill). It may occur in workers using vibrating tools.

Recognizing the pattern

The patient
The patient is usually a woman aged around 30.

The history
There is a history of colour changes following exposure to cold. The episode begins with pallor, coldness and numbness of some or all of the fingers of one or both hands. After a few minutes the fingers become blue. Then after a variable time the spasm wears off and the fingers become tense and red. Pain of variable degree is present in all stages.

On examination
During an attack the characteristic changes are seen. The hand may be normal between attacks. In chronic disease there may be evidence of ischaemia, e.g. dry gangrene, superficial ulceration or loss of finger pulp. The peripheral pulses are normal. An attack may sometimes be induced by immersing the hands in cold water.

Proving the diagnosis

The diagnosis is based on the history. An arteriogram may show narrowing of the digital arteries, particularly in chronic cases. Serological investigations should be carried out to identify any underlying cause, e.g. full blood count and ESR, antinuclear antibodies, rheumatoid factor and cryoglobulins.

Management

Conservative measures include keeping the extremities warm (gloves, socks and boots) and the avoidance of sudden exposure to cold. Any infection in the hands and feet should be treated promptly. The patient should not smoke. Severe attacks are occasionally relieved by reserpine (1 mg in 10 ml saline intra-arterially) or a slow intravenous infusion of dextran 40 (500 ml daily for 5 days).

In severe cases a sympathectomy may be indicated. This

provides relief in 50−70% of cases but the results are not always long-lasting. Distal amputation may be required if the finger tip is gangrenous.

Operation: cervical sympathectomy

The sympathetic chain may be exposed by a supraclavicular or trans-axillary approach. In the former an incision is made above the clavicle and deepened to expose the stellate ganglion lying on the neck of the first rib. The second and third sympathetic ganglia are excised.

In a trans-axillary approach access is gained through the third intercostal space or after resection of part of the third rib. The lung is expanded as the pleura is closed to express all the air. If a bilateral procedure is performed, then chest drains may be used. The anaesthetist must be told whether the operation is going to be unilateral or bilateral.

Codes

Blood . . . .   Group and save . . . .
GA/LA . . . .   GA . . . .
Opn time . . . .   1−2 hours . . . .
Stay . . . .   5−7 days . . . .
Drains out . . . . . .   Chest drain 24 hours (if inserted) . . . .
Sutures out . . . . .   4−7 days . . . .
Off work . . . .   2 weeks . . . .

Postoperative care

A chest X-ray is performed within 1−2 hours of operation to exclude a pneumothorax. The patient may be in some pain for the first 48 hours and adequate analgesia should be prescribed. Following a supraclavicular operation, a transient Horner's syndrome (due to traction of the stellate ganglion) may occur. Chest infection or segmental collapse are recognized complications of cervical sympathectomy.

9.5   Venous Disorders

Varicose veins

The condition   Varicosities are veins in the leg which become dilated and tortuous due to back pressure transmitted from above. Superficial veins are normally protected by valves from the high pressure within the deep venous system. If these valves become incompetent, the deep venous high pressure is transmitted to the superficial veins and their terminal branches become dilated and varicose (Fig. 93).

Common sites for incompetent valves to occur are the following.

1 Where the long saphenous vein joins the femoral vein in the groin.

2 Where the perforator in the lower medial thigh enters the deep system at the adductor canal.

3 Where the short saphenous vein joins the popliteal vein behind the knee.

4 Where several veins perforate the deep fascia of the calf behind the medial border of the tibia (lower leg perforators) (see Fig. 94).

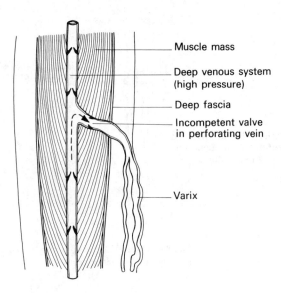

Fig. 93. The mechanism of varicose vein production.

503

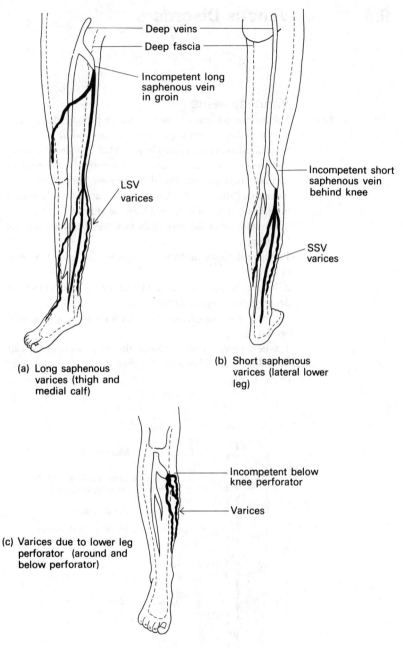

Fig. 94. Three examples of primary varicose veins due to incompetent perforating veins.

Making the diagnosis

The clinician's task is to decide whether the patient's symptoms are due to the varicosities and also to determine where the causative incompetent perforating veins are sited.

The history
Symptoms which may be associated with varicose veins included the following.
1 Disfigurement. The patient is bothered by the appearance of the varices.
2 Pain. Characteristically varicose veins give rise to aching in the calves on standing which is worse at the end of the day and better on elevating the leg. The pain is relieved by elastic stockings.
3 Itching. This often occurs over the varices and may be associated with the presence of varicose 'eczema'.

On examination
The site of the incompetent perforator or perforators is determined.

1 Inspection and palpation
Varices due to long saphenous incompetence are usually in the thigh and on the medial aspect of the calf (Fig. 94a). A dilated sapheno-femoral junction may present as a 'lump in the groin' (a saphena-varix). Short saphenous varices lie below the knee on the posterior and lateral aspects of the calf (Fig. 94b). Above-ankle perforators give rise to bunches of varices on the medial aspect of the calf and there may be palpable 'holes' in the deep fascia due to the enlargement of the incompetent perforating veins.

2 Trendelenburg test
The leg is elevated and the veins emptied. A tourniquet is applied to occlude the superficial veins at three levels:
(a) in the thigh,
(b) below the knee,
(c) lower down the calf.
Observe the highest tourniquet which 'controls' the varices, i.e. prevents them reappearing on standing. The site of incompetence must then be above this. By moving the tourniquet down the leg, the lowest level of incompetence is determined. The varices in Fig. 94c for instance will be controlled by a below-knee, not an above-knee, tourniquet.

Proving the diagnosis

No further tests are usually necessary. However, phlebography may occasionally be useful in selective cases to demonstrate the site of perforators. The procedure carries a morbidity, however, and is not always helpful.

A Doppler ultrasound probe can also be used to detect sites of possible perforators. A tourniquet is placed above and below the suspected site and the ultrasound probe is used to listen over the perforator. The calf is squeezed and retrograde venous flow can be heard if the perforator is incompetent. The findings may be difficult to interpret as to-and-fro flow is also heard over the varices fed by the perforator.

Management

Management

Conservative treatment is advised when the varices are not very severe and when there are no complications such as skin changes, ulceration or haemorrhage. The patient should lose weight and wear supportive stockings. This will usually control symptoms and stop the veins getting worse.

The indications for surgery are severe disfiguring varices, marked and incapacitating aching, and the onset of complications such as ulceration or haemorrhage. Active treatment may then be by injection sclerotherapy or by open operation.

Operation: injection sclerotherapy

This is an outpatient procedure. Sclerosant is injected into the superficial veins immediately over incompetent perforators in the calf. After injection the patient wears compressive bandages for 6 weeks. The technique is not suitable for treating incompetence of the long saphenous vein in the groin or the short saphenous vein due to the danger of causing thrombosis in femoral or popliteal deep veins. Its main use is for treating perforators in the lower leg.

Operation: for varicose veins

Open operation is the method of choice for varicose veins where the primary site of incompetence is in the long or short saphenous veins.

Preoperative management

Varicose veins are not visible during the operation as the patient is recumbent. The veins must therefore be marked with an indelible pencil indicating the exact sites of the major varicosities and perforators. The surgeon will use these markings to expose the superficial varices at operation and will usually do the preoperative marking himself. The patient should be warned that he will have to wear supportive bandages for about 6 weeks after the operation if this is the practice in your unit.

Operation

A variety of terms are used in varicose vein surgery.

1 *High tie of long saphenous veins.* The long saphenous vein is ligated at its origin flush with the femoral vein and all its tributaries are tied off.

2 *Flush ligation.* The ligation of the long or short saphenous veins flush with the deep veins into which they flow.

3 *Multiple avulsions.* Individual varices may be avulsed through multiple small stab incisions over the veins. Accurate preoperative markings are essential for this procedure.

4 *Stripping.* The long saphenous vein may be removed by passing a wire down its lumen attached to a stripping head. As the stripper is pulled up the leg it cuts the branches of the long saphenous vein. This procedure is done in order to disconnect the main vein from its dilated varicose branches and from any remaining incompetent lower-leg perforators.

5 *Subfascial ligation* (Cockett's operation). The lower-leg perforator is approached by incising the skin and deep fascia and ligating the incompetent vein beneath the deep fascia. In this way damaged skin associated with ulceration is subjected to minimal dissection.

Codes

Blood	0 . . . .
GA/LA	GA . . . .
Opn time	1−2 hours . . . .
Stay	2−5 days . . . .
Drains out	0 . . . .
Sutures out	7 days . . . .
Off work	2 weeks . . . .

Postoperative care

The legs are bandaged at the end of the operation and should be kept elevated in the postoperative period. This minimizes bruising from disconnected varices. It also helps to maintain a higher deep venous blood flow and protect against thrombosis. Further protection is provided by applying blue line compression bandages and then encouraging the patient to walk actively from 24 hours postoperatively. The patient is taught to reapply these bandages, which should be continued to be worn for 6 weeks. This helps small remaining dilated superficial veins to regain their tone.

Venous ulceration

The condition

Venous hypertension leads to the development of hyperpermeable capillaries and fibrin leaks into the interstitial tissue, resulting in oedema and induration.

The fibrin sheath around the capillaries is thought to block oxygen diffusion so that, although the skin is often warm due to the high blood flow, it becomes relatively ischaemic and ultimately necroses and ulcerates. Malignant change can occasionally occur in the edge of a chronic ulcer (Marjolin's ulcer).

Venous ulceration typically occurs on the medial side of the lower limb above the ankle. It is most commonly due to venous stasis, either following deep vein thrombosis or secondary to chronic varicose veins.

Recognizing the pattern

The patient
Women are more commonly affected and usually present over the age of 40. They are often overweight.

The history
There is chronic painful reddening or discoloration of the skin which slowly enlarges in the affected area. An ulcer is commonly precipitated by minor trauma. It is frequently painless, but any pain or discomfort that does exist is worse with the leg dependent. There is often a past history suggesting venous thrombosis.

On examination
The typical site for venous ulceration is the lower third of the lower leg, on the medial side. The ulcer is shallow with a ragged shelving edge which is usually dusky blue. The base is covered by granulation tissue. There may be a thin seropurulent discharge.

The surrounding skin is reddened or pigmented (due to haemosiderin) with a thickened or eczematous surface. It is usually warmer than normal skin, and tender. There may be varicose veins and, if present, the site of the incompetent valves must be established (see p. 505).

Proving the diagnosis

In patients where the diagnosis is uncertain, investigations include a full blood count and ESR, culture of the ulcer, WR, Mantoux test and eventually biopsy. The perforators may be demonstrated by ultrasound or phlebography.

Management

There are three aspects to the management of venous ulceration.

1 Treatment of reversible pre-ulceration skin changes
Patients with reddened warm eczematous skin which has not yet ulcerated need elastic, fully supportive knee-length stockings to give a graduated compression of the leg (up to a

pressure of 40−80 mmHg). This helps restore the venous drainage. If there is a surgically remediable cause (see below), this must be corrected. Stanozolol (dose 5 mg 12-hourly) is an anabolic steroid that enhances fibrinolysis and may be given. These measures may be required for up to 6 months before the skin improves.

2 Treatment of an established ulcer

An established ulcer is treated by elevating the leg, bed rest and regular cleaning and dressing. Any pus must be cultured. There are many topical preparations available to clean, soothe and dry the area, e.g. zinc oxide paste (Viscopaste). Skin grafting may be required. Topical antibiotics should be avoided as sensitivity often develops. Systemic antibiotics are only indicated if secondary systemic infection is present. After 1−2 weeks the patient is mobilized with support stockings or Viscopaste bandages.

If ulceration is secondary to varicose veins with a normal deep venous system, then surgical correction (e.g. high saphenous ligation or Cockett's operation for incompetent calf perforators) may result in prolonged cure. However, when the deep venous system is disrupted, there is no effective surgical correction and recurrence of the ulcer is common. Patients should wear supportive stockings for the rest of their life.

3 Prevention

Anyone who develops a deep venous thrombosis should wear 'blue-line' elastic bandages until the tendency to swelling is controlled. They should then be encouraged to wear good supportive stockings until all tendency to oedema formation has disappeared. If the tissues are adequately supported in this way (for 3−6 months) induration can be prevented and ulceration avoided. 'Tubigrip' elastic supports are not adequate (see p. 511).

9.6 Lymphoedema

The condition

Interstitial fluid is normally produced as blood passes through the capillary bed. It is eventually collected up in lymphatic channels and returned to the circulation after being filtered through lymph nodes. Obstruction to the flow of lymph produces a chronic oedema. Causes may be grouped as follows.

1 *Primary*. This is a rare condition affecting 1 in 33 000 of the population. It is due to deficient lymphatic channels. The deficiency may be either due to fibrosis ('acquired') or due to congenital causes such as absent or hypoplastic lymphatics or deficient lymphatic valves.

2 *Secondary*. The lymphatics are blocked due to an external cause such as:
   (a) fibrosis — e.g. following infection or radiotherapy;
   (b) infestation — e.g. filiariasis;
   (c) infiltration — by secondary malignant neoplasm, e.g. malignant melanoma;
   (d) trauma — e.g. following block dissection of the groin or axilla.

Recognizing the pattern

The patient

Primary lymphoedema frequently affects females. The condition may present in the teens or at any time up to middle age. Secondary lymphoedema can occur at any age when the relevant cause is present.

The history

The patient notices painless swelling of one or both limbs. Primary lymphoedema always presents in the legs. The swelling is worse at the end of the day. Occasionally the condition presents with a secondary cellulitis, in which case the leg is acutely painful.

On examination NOW PITTING OEDEMA

The oedema is brawny and typically non-pitting. Measure and record the diameter in centimetres at recorded points from bony landmarks (e.g. medial malleolus, lower border patella, etc.).

Proving the diagnosis

It is necessary to exclude other causes of oedema such as hypoproteinaemia, renal failure or venous insufficiency. A

510

positive diagnosis of lymphoedema can be obtained by a radionucleotide clearance test. Radiolabelled sulphur colloid is injected in a web space of a foot and its uptake is monitored in the groin after 30 minutes. Lymphangiograms may also demonstrate hypoplastic or varicose lymphatics or abnormalities in the proximal lymph nodes.

Management

The management is conservative and operative procedures are only rarely indicated.

Conservative treatment
1 Elevate the foot of the bed 25−30 cm. This makes sure the oedema is minimal by the morning.
2 External elastic compression of the limb. Initially this may be with 'blue-line' bandages but, once the limb diameter becomes stable, a fully supportive fitted elastic stocking should be used. Constant-diameter 'Tubigrip' elastic support is contraindicated as it produces the maximum pressure at the level of the calf muscle, and therefore impairs drainage from the foot and ankle.
3 Early treatment of any infection. Cellulitis is a common complication and this may obliterate further lymphatics. Some clinicians keep patients on long-term low-dose penicillin.
4 Intermittent diuretics. These are occasionally of value.

Operative treatment
There is no truly effective method of restoring lost lymphatic channels and the patient should be told this. Attempts have been made to implant skin or omentum for this purpose with limited success in proximal disease. Occasionally it is necessary to operate to reduce the bulk of swollen subcutaneous tissue in the lower leg.

Two operations will be briefly described. The operations are done under tourniquet control and the limb elevated using a Kirschner wire through the calcaneum.

Homan's operation
An area of skin and a wider area of subcutaneous tissue is excised from the medial aspect of the lower leg, thus reducing its bulk. A similar procedure may be carried out on the lateral aspect.

Charles' operation
All skin and subcutaneous tissue from the knee to the ankle joint is excised, and split skin grafts applied.

10 The Skin

10.1 **Benign lesions of the skin**
Skin lumps

10.2 **Pigmented naevi and malignant skin conditions**
Pigmented naevi
Other malignant skin conditions

10.3 **Skin infections and hyperhidrosis**
Skin infections
Conditions of the nails
Hyperhidrosis

10.1   Benign Lesions of the Skin

Skin lumps

A wide variety of different pathologies present in the skin as lumps. Because of this, 'lumps and bumps' in the skin are popular subjects for examinations. It is important to develop a good routine technique for the examination of skin lumps. This should include the determination of the following.

1 Shape — rounded, irregular, elliptical, etc.
2 Size — in cm, including depth, width and length.
3 Surface — smooth, nodular, irregular, ill-defined.
4 Consistency — hard, soft, fluctuant.
5 Colour.
6 Edge — well-defined, ill-defined.
7 Fixation — to superficial layers of skin or deep to the muscle or fascia.
8 Transillumination.

Make a habit of running through each of these headings each time you encounter a lump in the skin.

Papilloma (skin tag)

The condition   This is a benign tumour due to overgrowth of all elements of the skin. It consists of a core of connective tissue and blood vessels with a lining of skin epithelium.

Recognizing the pattern   *The patient*
The patient can be of any age although it is more common in the elderly.

The history
The papilloma may have been there for years and usually the patient presents asking to have it removed for cosmetic reasons. Occasionally the lump gets in the way and may bleed due to regular trauma (e.g. by clothes). It may become infected.

On examination
Papillomata are usually pedunculated and are smooth, soft and solid. They can occur anywhere and may be of any shape or size. There may be surface ulceration due to trauma.

515

Management

Operation: removal of skin papilloma

The skin is cleaned and an elliptical incision is made around the base of the papilloma. The apices of the ellipse should be in line with Langer's lines. The wound is closed with fine sutures. The papilloma should be sent for routine histology.

Codes

Blood	0	
GA/LA	LA	
Opn time	15 minutes	
Stay	Outpatient	
Drains out	0	
Suture out	3–7 days (depending on site of wound)	
Off work	Less than 24 hours	

Seborrhoeic keratosis (senile wart, basal cell papilloma)

The condition

This is a benign overgrowth of the basal cells of the epidermis, which form swollen, abnormal epithelial cells.

Recognizing the pattern

The patient

The patient is usually elderly. The common complaint is that the lesion is unsightly or gets in the way. It tends to slowly increase in size.

On examination

It is a flattened well-defined plaque raised above the skin and has a rough greasy surface. It may be darker than the surrounding skin due either to pigmentation or to bruising. It occurs on skin that is not usually touched or rubbed regularly, e.g. the back.

Management

A characteristic feature of this condition is that, with gentle traction, the edge can often be peeled off the underlying skin leaving a pink area with a few tiny bleeding points. It can therefore be removed by curetting. This characteristic also confirms the diagnosis. If the lesion does not curette off easily, then it should be excised and sent for histology.

Infective warts

The condition

This is a common lesion due to a papovavirus infection. It is contagious and is often seen in children on the hands. Older people tend to develop immunity to the virus. It may also appear on the feet. On the plantar surface of the foot pressure causes it to grow inwards (verruca).

Recognizing the pattern	*The history* It is a slow-growing nodular lesion of the skin which regresses spontaneously after a number of months. It may bleed on trauma. It also catches on the patient's clothing. *On examination* There is a hard keratinized papillary outgrowth of the skin with a surface made up of short fronds.
Management	Simple reassurance that it will eventually regress is usually sufficient. Regression can be hastened by topical application of silver nitrate or the lesion may be curetted. There are a wide variety of folklore remedies for getting rid of warts.

Keloid

The condition	Keloid is an exuberant overgrowth of fibrous tissue in a scar. It is more common in scars that cross skin creases. The tendency to form keloid scars runs in families.
Recognizing the pattern	*The patient* The patient can be of any age. Keloids are common in people of African or Asian origin. *The history* The lump is slow-growing and there is a history of previous trauma or surgery. The scar may be tender or itch. *On examination* Red-brown or purple firm scar tissue is heaped up above the level of the epidermis and it may even become pedunculated. Keloid can occur anywhere in the skin where there is a scar. The whole scar or part of the scar may be involved.
Management	The condition is difficult to manage and the patient should be reassured that it will eventually settle although the scar will always remain wide. If the scar is still very ugly 15 months to 2 years after the initial injury, it may be worth attempting cosmetic removal. The patient should be warned that recurrence is not uncommon. Sometimes the keloid formation can be decreased by treating the scar with radiotherapy immediately after excision. Local infiltration of the skin around the scar with steroid preparations has a variable affect.

Lipoma

The condition	This is a benign tumour composed of fat cells divided into large lobules by loose fibrous septa. Lipomata are frequently

multiple and the condition tends to run in families. Sometimes these multiple lipomata are painful (Dercum's disease).

Recognizing the pattern

The patient
The patient is usually an adult. The lesion is rare in children.

The history
The lump is often noticed because it gets in the way while washing or because it is unsightly. The lesion is usually slow-growing and there may be a family history of similar lesions.

On examination
Lipomata occur anywhere there is adipose tissue but are commoner on the upper limb and trunk. They may be of any size from a few millimetres to several centimetres in diameter. Occasionally a lipoma arises in the muscle or close to the deep fascia, in which case it appears to be attached to the muscle. The tumour has a smooth, lobulated surface with a well-defined edge. It is usually soft although small lipomas may be quite firm. It often lies in the dermis, and the skin can then be moved over it.

Management

If the lipoma is causing trouble it should be removed.

Operation: removal of lipoma
An incision is made over the lipoma in the direction of the skin crease. The incision is deepened until the capsule of the lipoma is encountered. The capsule is then gently freed from the surrounding skin and quite often it is possible to squeeze the lipoma out by pressure applied to its sides. There should be little bleeding but if a large lipoma has been removed the cavity may be drained.

Codes

Blood	0 . . . .
GA/LA	LA or GA (depending on size) . . . . . .
Opn time	10−30 minutes . . . .
Stay	Outpatient or 24 hours . . . .
Drains out	0−24 hours . . . .
Sutures out	5−7 days . . . .
Off work.	1−2 days . . . .

Sebaceous cyst

The condition

A sebaceous cyst is said to be formed when the duct of a sebaceous gland, responsible for producing the oily sebum protecting the skin, becomes blocked and distended with its own secretion. The cyst lies deep to the skin but is firmly attached to it by the original blocked duct, which is usually visible as a 'punctum'.

Recognizing the pattern

The patient
Sebaceous cysts occur at any age although, because they are slow-growing, they are rare in children.

The history
They may be multiple and the patient usually presents because they are unsightly. They may have been infected or have discharged a creamy material.

On examination
The lump is a spherical, smooth, well-defined swelling of variable size which stretches the normal overlying skin. A punctum is visible. Sebaceous cysts occur where there are sebaceous glands and are commonest in hairy skins, particularly on the scalp. The cyst may discharge and the creamy material dry up in the centre to form a sebaceous horn.

Management

An infected sebaceous cyst must first be drained and then excised later. A non-infected sebaceous cyst should be removed using a local anaesthetic.

Operation: excision of sebaceous cyst
This can be done as an outpatient procedure using a local anaesthetic (1% xylocaine with 1/200 000 adrenaline). Surrounding hairs are removed and the local anaesthetic injected so as to partly separate the skin and the cyst wall. The lump is then incised and the contents emptied. The lining of the cyst is then grasped with artery forceps and enucleated completely. This procedure should be carried out carefully and slowly so that all the wall is removed. Pressure is applied to secure full haemostasis although this is not usually a problem if removal is confined to the wall of the cyst. The skin can usually be closed with one suture.

If the cyst has ruptured previously or been infected, it should be excised intact rather than enucleated as above.

Codes
Blood . . . . 0 . . . .
GA/LA . . . . LA . . . .
Opn time . . . . 15–30 minutes . . . .
Stay . . . . Outpatient . . . .
Drains out . . . . . . 0 . . . .

Sutures out ..... 5−7 days ....

Off work .... 1−2 hours ....

Keratoacanthoma (molluscum sebaceum)

The condition This nodule is formed by a benign overgrowth of a sebaceous gland which subsequently becomes necrotic in its centre and regresses, leaving a deep scar. A lump appears and grows rapidly, reaching 2 cm in diameter within a few weeks. The central core then becomes necrotic and black and hardens.

Recognizing the pattern *The patient*
The patient is usually elderly and complains of a rapidly expanding lesion with a dark central core. The short history differentiates this lesion from a basal cell carcinoma (see p. 531).

On examination
The nodule is rounded with a smooth surface and a dark brown or black necrotic centre. The condition is confined to the skin and does not extend into the subcutaneous tissue.

A keratoacanthoma can occur anywhere where there are sebaceous glands. It is more common on the face and nose (75%).

Management Because of its rapid growth the lesion is often believed to be malignant. It can, however, be differentiated from a squamous cell carcinoma because the latter has a rather longer history and does not develop a necrotic, central plug. Keratoacanthomas can be curetted but are often removed by excision biopsy to be sure of the diagnosis.

Dermoid cyst

The condition This is a developmental abnormality arising at embryological lines of skin fusion when a piece of ectoderm comes to lie beneath the skin's surface. A cyst is formed, lined by stratified squamous epithelium, and there are usually other skin elements within its wall (i.e. sweat and pilosebaceous glands). The cyst contains keratin.

Recognizing the pattern *The patient*
The patient is often a child between the ages of 1 and 2 and the lump has caused the parents concern. However, dermoids can also appear later in life. It takes some time for the lump to grow large enough to be noticed.

On examination
The cyst is often about 1 cm in diameter, spherical and

smooth. It is usually hard but occasionally soft and indentable. It is not attached to the skin. This differentiates it from a sebaceous cyst. Dermoid cysts usually occur on the face and neck. They are common at the outer edge of the eyebrow where the maxillary facial process fuses with the frontal process (see p. 178). They can, however, occur anywhere in the midline.

Management

The cyst needs to be removed but this is not urgent. If the patient is a child, this is usually done under a general anaesthetic.

Operation: excision of dermoid cyst
The skin is incised in Langer's lines and the cyst enucleated.

Codes

Blood	0 . . . .
GA/LA	GA . . . .
Opn time	30 minutes . . . .
Stay	About 24 hours . . . .
Drains out	0 . . . .
Sutures out	3–7 days (depending on site) . . . .
Off work	24 hours . . . .

Implantation dermoid

The condition

This is an acquired condition due to implantation of epidermis into the subcutaneous tissue. The epidermis continues to grow and forms a cyst which is lined with stratified squamous epithelium. There are no other skin elements in the wall and the cyst contains keratin.

Recognizing the pattern

The patient
The patient is usually adult and may be a gardener or manual worker likely to suffer injury to the hand.

The history
The patient may or may not remember the injury which resulted in the implantation. The lump grows very slowly and tends to cause symptoms by 'getting in the way'. It may become infected.

On examination
The cyst is a small, spherical, smooth swelling in the subcutaneous tissues. It is usually quite hard and may be attached to the skin under an old scar. The age of the patient helps differentiate it from a dermoid cyst. Its site, history and absence of a punctum differentiate it from a sebaceous cyst.

| Management | The cyst is excised under a local anaesthetic. |

Ganglion

The condition   This is a myxomatous degeneration of fibrous tissue commonly arising close to a joint capsule or tendon sheath. The cystic lesion contains glairy, sticky, clear fluid.

Recognizing the pattern

The patient
He may be of any age (usually adult) and presents with a lump which may be disfiguring or painful or restrict movement.

On examination
The lump is commonly around the hand or wrist or on the foot, close to joints. Ganglia can, however, occur anywhere. The swelling is lobulated with a smooth surface and a well-defined edge. It may be of any size and consistency. It often becomes more tense when the joint is flexed or extended. It is attached deeply but not to the skin.

Management   A ganglion can sometimes be dispersed by pressure or by aspiration with a needle, but tends to recur. The favoured method of treatment is excision.

Operation: removal of a ganglion
It is usually possible to remove the ganglion under a local anaesthetic but, where it is situated in a difficult site or in a young patient, it may be more advisable to operate under a general anaesthetic. An exsanguinating tourniquet is used where possible. Ganglia are often intimately related to tendons, arteries and nerves and must be dissected out with great care.

Codes

Blood	0 ....
GA/LA	LA or GA ....
Opn time	30 minutes ....
Stay	Outpatient ....
Drains out	0 ....
Sutures out	5–7 days ....
Off work	Depends on occupation: a typist with a ganglion on the wrist may be advised to stay off work for a week, otherwise about 24 hours ....

Neurofibroma

This is a benign tumour arising from the nerve sheath and

consisting of both neural and fibrous elements. As it grows, it either displaces the nerve fibres to one side or else enlarges amongst them. Neurofibromas may be single or multiple.

Multiple neurofibromatosis (von Recklinghausen's disease) is a rare autosomal dominant condition where the neurofibromas are congenital and familial. They are associated with skin tags, 'café au lait' patches, phaeochromocytoma and deeper neuromas (e.g. an acoustic neuroma). The neurofibromas may undergo sarcomatous change.

Recognizing the pattern

The patient
He may present at any age but is usually adult.

The history
A neurofibroma is often asymptomatic. It may be disfiguring or become tender and cause tingling. It may rarely cause motor weakness in the distribution of the nerve involved. If there are multiple neurofibromata, ask if there is a family history.

On examination
A neurofibroma is usually a firm, fusiform swelling in any site. It is usually subcutaneous although it can lie in the skin itself. It is mobile in a direction which is at right angles to the direction of its nerve of origin. Pressure on it may cause tingling in the nerve distribution.

If there are multiple neurofibromata look for 'café au lait' patches, which are brown areas of pigmentation. Take the blood pressure.

Management

A single neurofibroma is usually excised for biopsy to confirm the diagnosis. Multiple neurofibromatosis does not need confirmation by biopsy unless there is clinical evidence of sarcomatous change. This is suggested by increasing pain and increasing size and the development of motor paralysis or peripheral sensory loss.

Preoperative management
Warn the patient of the possibility that there may be temporary or permanent loss of function of the nerve involved.

Operation: excision of a neurofibroma
The neurofibroma can either be enucleated or excised. The nerve ends may be resutured if the function supplied is vital.

Excision should be complete because of the slight danger of sarcomatous change in any remnants left.

Codes

Blood	0 ....
GA/LA	LA or GA ....
Opn time	30 minutes ....
Stay	Inpatient/outpatient ....
Drains out	0 ....
Sutures out	5–7 days ....
Off work	Variable, 24 hours for a small cutaneous lesion ....

Postoperative care
The patient may occasionally need admitting and the limb immobilizing to protect a nerve anastomosis. Patients with multiple neurofibromatosis need regular follow-up to detect sarcomatous change.

10.2   Pigmented Naevi and Malignant Skin Conditions

Pigmented naevi

Introduction and terminology

Pigmented naevi arise from a proliferation of the melanocytes in the skin. Benign overgrowths of melanocytes (hamartomata) are common during childhood and usually stop growing when the skin stops growing. A malignant naevus (malignant melanoma) can arise either spontaneously or in an existing benign naevus.

A number of histological terms are applied to naevi and tend to cause confusion. The melanocytes are situated in the basal layer of the epidermis, i.e. next to the dermis. Proliferations at this site are called junctional naevi (Fig. 95a). These usually become incorporated into the dermis and as the cells mature they form an intradermal naevus (Fig. 95b).

A blue naevus refers to a deep intradermal collection of melanocytes which appear pale blue on the surface.

Some naevi consist of both junctional and intradermal collections and are called compound naevi (Fig. 95c).

The melanocytes in the basal layer of the epidermis may show junctional activity. This is characterized by the following:

(a) pleomorphic cells;

(b) mitoses;

(c) intradermal invasion with loss of maturity of melanocytes;

(d) invasion of single cells or groups of cells into the epidermis;

(e) lymphocytic infiltration.

If this occurs in children before puberty it is, despite its histological appearance, benign, and is called a juvenile melanoma. In adults, such activity is a definite indication of malignant change. The distinction between juvenile melanoma and early malignant change is often very difficult.

Benign naevus

The condition   Benign naevi can occur anywhere, especially in the limbs, on the face and at mucocutaneous junctions. The lesions can be flat or raised and have a rough or smooth surface, with or without the presence of hairs.

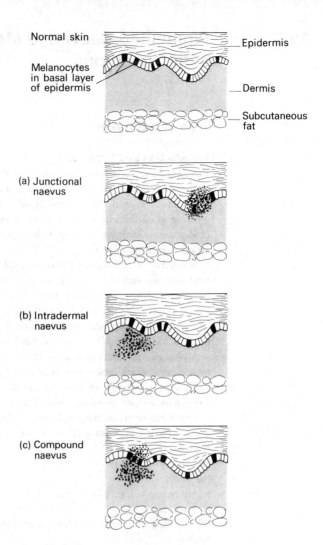

Normal skin

Melanocytes in basal layer of epidermis

Epidermis

Dermis

Subcutaneous fat

(a) Junctional naevus

(b) Intradermal naevus

(c) Compound naevus

Fig. 95. Different types of melanoma.

Management

A benign naevus that is causing no symptoms can be left alone. The lesion is usually excised either because it is cosmetically unattractive, or because it is showing some signs suggestive of malignant change (see Malignant melanoma).

Operation: removal of benign naevus

The lesion is removed under a local anaesthetic using an elliptical incision parallel to Langer's line. The specimen should always be sent for histology. If this does show evidence of malignant activity, then the area is re-excised and skin grafted.

Malignant melanoma

The condition   Malignant melanomas can arise either spontaneously or in an existing benign naevus. They can occasionally be unpigmented although the cells are still able to manufacture melanin and are dopa-positive. An electron microscope will reveal melanosomes.

Malignant melanomas may either spread superficially through the epidermis, with deep invasion to the dermis, occurring late, or become nodular in which case early dermal invasion is usual. The tumour then spreads via the lymphatics and the bloodstream, and secondaries are common in the liver, lungs and brain.

Tumour staging

The stage of a melanoma refers to its extent of spread and gives some indication of prognosis. There are three clinical stages:

Stage 1. Confined to the primary lesion (including satellite lesions within a radius of 5 cm).

Stage 2. Involvement of the first single group of regional lymph nodes and cutaneous secondaries in this course.

Stage 3. Involvement of two or more groups of lymph nodes with visceral metastases.

Malignant melanomas may also be staged histologically.

1 Epidermis only involved.

2 Epidermis plus invasion into the papillary dermis.

3 Epidermis plus deeper invasion into the reticular dermis.

4 Invasion to the base of the reticular dermis.

5 Involvement of the subcutaneous tissues.

The thickness in mm (Breslow) correlates with the incidence of recurrence and metastasis.

Recognizing the   *The patient*
pattern   The patient can be of any age although a malignant melanoma usually occurs in patients over the age of 20. It is commoner in white-skinned people exposed to the sun.

The history

There may be a family history of the condition. The patient usually presents because the lump has changed in some way. Symptoms typical of malignant change are as follows.

1 An enlarging lesion.

2 A change in colour.

3 Itching.

4 Bleeding.

On examination

The malignant lesion can occur anywhere but is more common on the limbs, head and neck. Pigmented lesions in the palms, soles and nailbeds are particularly suspicious as these areas are not normally pigmented.

The typical malignant melanoma is pigmented and may show signs of spread with a halo of pigment in the surrounding skin and/or satellite nodules around the original naevus. The lesion may have an irregular surface, be ulcerated or show evidence of recent bleeding. Occasionally the patient presents with an unnoticed primary lesion and signs of spread of the disease such as enlarged regional lymph nodes, weight loss or systemic symptoms of carcinomatosis.

Management

The patient should be fully investigated to look for evidence of metastatic disease. The naevus should then be removed.

Operation: excision of malignant melanoma

If necessary, a split skin graft is taken from the opposite limb. The lesion is then widely excised with a 1−5 cm margin of skin and the excision carried down to the deep fascia over the muscle. The defect is closed with the split skin graft.

Codes

Blood .... 0 ....

GA/LA .... GA ....

Opn time .... 1−2 hours (depending on site) ......

Stay .... 7−14 days ....

Drains out ...... 0 ....

Sutures out ..... 7−10 days ....

Off work........ 6 weeks......................

Operation: block dissection of the groin

If there is evidence of spread to the regional nodes, a block dissection may be performed. This procedure is carried out both for secondary melanoma and involved lymph nodes from other lesions such as a squamous cell carcinoma.

The enlarged node is first biopsied. If a frozen section report is positive for growth, the main mass of nodes in the groin is then excised. The long saphenous vein is tied lower down the thigh and a block of tissue removed from the front of the femoral vein and artery. The upper end of the saphenous vein is again divided as it enters the femoral vein.

The block may be continued up under the inguinal ligament to remove nodes in the iliac region.

Codes

Blood..........	2 units ....
GA/LA	GA ....
Opn time	2–3 hours ....
Stay	7–10 days ....
Drains out	2–5 days ....
Sutures out	7–14 days ....
Off work........	4–6 weeks ....

Postoperative care
The leg will tend to swell due to lymphoedema. It is important to keep it elevated postoperatively and to apply heavy-duty elastic bandages before the patient is mobilized. The patient should continue to have the foot of the bed raised for 2 or 3 months after the procedure until the tendency to oedema has subsided. If the leg is allowed to become chronically swollen postoperatively, it can be impossible to get rid of the oedema later on.

Block dissection of the neck is described on p. 195

Other methods of treatment
There are a few other methods of treatment which can be tried when the disease is widespread. They all, unfortunately, have limited success.

1 *Radiotherapy*. This is useful for the treatment of bone pain or cerebral metastases.

2 *Immunotherapy*. This is still being evaluated and the results are unpredictable. Malignant melanoma is a tumour which tends to regress for several years at a time and histologically the tumour often shows lymphocytic infiltration. It has been postulated, therefore, that the tumour can be kept under control by an immune reaction mounted by the patient. Attempts have been made to treat melanomas by boosting immunity using BCG or other antigens.

3 *Chemotherapy*. This can occasionally be helpful in advanced disease. The effective agents are the following:

(a) Dacarbazine — which has a short-lived effect on subcutaneous lesions.

(b) Vindesine — which has similar effects.

(c) Nitrosoureas — which have sometimes been found useful in conjunction with radiotherapy for the treatment of cerebral metastases.

Other malignant skin conditions

Squamous cell carcinoma in situ (Bowen's disease)

The condition

This is a thickening of the skin which will eventually develop into a squamous cell carcinoma. Microscopically there may be activity in the prickle cell layer with large clear cells and squamous cells showing early signs of malignancy.

Recognizing the pattern

The patient
The patient is almost always elderly.

The history
The history is of a thickening of the skin, looking like eczema. The patient often regards it as eczema and therefore tends to present late. The lesion gradually spreads.

On examination
There is a brown, crusted, raised lesion with a well-defined edge. Under the crust the lesion is moist and papilliform.
The area must be biopsied and preferably removed. If it is very large, it can be treated with radiotherapy.

Squamous cell carcinoma

The condition

This is a malignant condition of stratified squamous epithelium, characterized by the proliferation of the prickle cell layer (acanthosis) and the formation of keratin. It is locally invasive and also metastasizes via the lymphatics and the bloodstream.

Recognizing the pattern

The patient
He is usually elderly.

The history
There is often a history of exposure to sunlight or chemical carcinogens, particularly the polycyclic aromatic hydrocarbons (e.g. coal, tar and oil). The condition used to be common in people who worked with X-rays and also appeared as cancer of the scrotum in chimney sweeps and mechanics. The lesion enlarges slowly and has usually been present for 1 or 2 months.

On examination
A squamous cell carcinoma is a nodular lesion or a circular ulcer with a raised everted edge. The base of the ulcer is shallow and necrotic and produces an offensive discharge. There may be evidence of local or distant metastases.

Management	The lesion can either be excised or treated with radiotherapy.

Basal cell carcinoma (rodent ulcer)

The condition

This is a locally malignant condition arising in the basal cell layer of the epidermis. Histologically it consists of uniform round cells with no prickle cells or keratin. It grows into surrounding tissues and can cause extensive local destruction but it does not metastasize.

Recognizing the pattern

The patient
The patient is usually elderly. The condition is more common in males, especially white-skinned people who have spent some time in a sunny climate.

The history
This is a very slow-growing lesion which has usually been present for several years before the patient consults his doctor. It may occasionally bleed or itch.

On examination
The lesion is initially nodular but then the centre ulcerates leaving raised, rolled, pearly edges. The long history and characteristic rolled edge distinguish it from squamous cell carcinoma.

Management

The lesion can either be treated with radiotherapy or by excision.

Operation: excision of basal cell carcinoma
The tumour is excised with a 5 mm margin and the defect closed either directly or with a skin graft.

Codes

Blood	0 ....
GA/LA	GA or LA.......................
Opn time	Depends on size and need to skin graft, 30–90 minutes ....
Stay	Day case or 24–48 hours ....
Drains out	0 ....
Sutures out	4–7 days (skin graft 10 days) ....
Off work........	1 day or more depending on size of lesion ....

Skin metastases

Metastases from visceral carcinoma can present as a swelling or ulceration in the skin. The treatment consists of chemotherapy or radiotherapy appropriate to the original primary tumour. The diagnosis is made by biopsying the lesion and by discovering the primary malignancy.

10.3 Skin Infections and Hyperhidrosis

Skin infections

Skin abscess

The condition
A skin abscess is a collection of pus surrounded by granulation tissue lying in the subcutaneous tissues or dermis. The usual organism is *Staphylococcus*. A boil (furuncle) is a small abscess developing in an infected hair follicle.

Recognizing the pattern

The history
There is a painful swelling. The pain is throbbing and characteristically worse at night or if the affected part is dependent. It may have discharged pus.

On examination
There is a localized swelling which is warm, red and tender. It is initially firm but as suppuration occurs it becomes softer, spherical and fluctuant. It may later discharge. The patient is usually pyrexial and the regional lymph nodes become enlarged and tender.

Management
The abscess must be drained unless it ruptures spontaneously. A swab should be sent for culture and sensitivity.

Operation: incision and drainage of abscess
An incision is made over the most fluctuant area. A closed haemostat is inserted into the cavity and then opened. A drain is inserted.

Codes

Blood	0 . . . .
GA/LA	LA . . . .
Opn time	15 minutes . . . .
Stay	Outpatient . . . .
Drains out	48 hours . . . .
Sutures out	0 . . . .
Off work	1–2 days . . . .

Postoperative care
Any predisposing cause should be treated. Antibiotics are only appropriate if there is associated cellulitis or constitutional disturbance.

Hydradenitis suppurativa

This is a troublesome recurrent infection affecting areas where there are sweat glands (e.g. axillae, groins and perineum). Treatment is with antibiotics according to sensitivities, and areas of recurrent sepsis may eventually need to be excised.

Pilonidal sinus

The condition

In this condition broken-off hairs come to lie in a subcutaneous sinus. The lesion characteristically occurs over the sacrum in the gluteal cleft. It can also occur in the hands, axillae or umbilicus.

The lesion in the sacral area probably starts as a preformed congenital pit. Hairs break off the head and back and tend to gravitate towards the cleft. It seems likely that the barbed surface of the hair results in it working its way under the skin once its tip has become lodged in the pit. Several hairs follow down the sinus, which then becomes infected. The patient complains of recurrent abscesses in this area. The abscess usually points to the skin at the side of the midline. Pilonidal sinuses also occur in barbers and in this case the sinus lies between the fingers. The hairs are derived from the customer rather than the sufferer.

Recognizing the pattern

The patient
The patient is typically male with thick black hair. The condition is more common between the ages of 15 and 40.

The history
There are recurrent episodes of pain and sepsis, often with several months between each episode. As the sinus becomes larger, the episodes become more frequent.

On examination
On careful inspection the pit is seen in the midline. There may be several such pits. The abscess is visible and palpable laterally.

Management

A small sinus may settle with antibiotic treatment but once the condition has become recurrent surgery is required. An acutely inflamed abscess will need to be drained.

Three possible operative procedures may be used. The sinus may be incised and laid open, it may be completely excised or it may be curretted and injected with phenol.

Operation: for pilonidal sinus
When the lesion is laid open, a probe is passed along the

track and an incision is made on to it from above. Granulation tissue in the base of the sinus is preserved but the hairs and debris are removed. Any lateral extensions into an abscess cavity are also laid open.

If the sinus is excised, the skin is closed directly over the wound.

Codes

Blood	0 . . . .
GA/LA	GA or LA, depending on size . . . .
Opn time	30−45 minutes . . . .
Stay	3−7 days depending on size . . . .
Drains out	0 . . . .
Sutures out	If present 7−10 days . . . .
Off work	About 3 weeks depending on size of sinus and occupation of patient . . . .

Postoperative care

If the sinus has been excised, and if the wound heals by primary intention, the postoperative care is uncomplicated. Unfortunately, it is not uncommon for the wound to break down as it is usually under some tension and frequently becomes infected. In that case it will have to heal by secondary intention as below.

If the sinus has been laid open, it is dressed daily by inserting a plug of tulle gras or silastic foam. As the wound granulates and the epithelium grows in from the edges, the bulk of the dressing is reduced. It is important to make certain that no 'bridging' of the skin edges occurs as this will lead to renewed pit formation and a recurrent sinus. Similarly, the hairs around the wound must be shaved regularly to prevent them sticking into the granulation tissue and reforming a sinus.

Operation: phenol injection of pilonidal sinus

The surrounding skin is carefully protected using petroleum jelly. Phenol (80%) is injected and left in the sinus for 1 minute. The sinus is then gently curretted and the hairs removed. A small drain may be inserted. This process is repeated three times.

Codes

Blood	0 . . . .
GA/LA	GA . . . .
Opn time	10 minutes . . . .
Stay	24 hours . . . .
Drains out	0 or 24 hours . . . .

| Sutures out ..... | 0 .... |
| Off work .... | 48 hours .... |

Postoperative care
After phenol injection the area remains painless as local nerves are destroyed by the phenol. Occasionally a sterile abscess develops, which requires drainage. The recurrence rate is about 17% if the sinus has fewer than three openings.

Carbuncle

The condition
A carbuncle is a lesion caused by spreading subcutaneous infection and necrosis. It often develops from a furuncle. The infective organism is usually *Staphylococcus*, which produces a coagulase and hence a localized ischaemia.

Recognizing the pattern

The history
The presentation is initially similar to a skin abscess. There is a spreading, very painful lesion of the skin. There are constitutional disturbances. Carbuncles are more common in diabetics.

On examination
The neck is the most common site affected. The lesion is diffuse, hard and reddened with a central area of slough surrounded by multiple sinuses extruding pus.

Proving the diagnosis
The pus should be cultured. The white cell count is usually elevated. The urine must be tested to exclude diabetes.

Management
The initial management is conservative with regular cleaning and dressing and a course of antibiotics (flucloxacillin) to attempt to control the spread of infection. The necrotic central area of skin may need excising and the area covering with a skin graft. Any predisposing cause such as diabetes must also be treated.

Conditions of the nails

'Ingrowing' toenail

The condition
This is usually seen on the big toe where the distal edge of the nail digs into the lateral skin-fold. This causes ulceration which becomes secondarily infected and swollen with granulation tissue.

The term 'ingrowing' is misleading. The trouble is usually due either to trauma or to the patient cutting his nails back in the corners. This leaves a sharp angle to the distal edge of the nail. As the patient walks the skin under the nail rolls over this sharp angle and is traumatized (Fig. 96). It becomes macerated and infected and this infection may damage the nail edge further. The condition is made worse by tight shoes, excessive sweating, and poor hygiene. There is a familial predisposition.

Recognizing the pattern

The patient
The patient may present at any age though the condition is unusual before the age of 5.

The history
The usual complaint is of a painful big toe which is swollen and red and intermittently discharges pus. There may be a past history of ingrowing toenail.

On examination
The nail-folds are affected to a variable extent on one or both sides of the nail.

Management

Conservative management consists of the following.
1 Keeping the feet dry.
2 Avoiding tight shoes or socks.
3 Antibiotics.
4 Cutting the nail across straight and allowing the corners to grow out.
5 Packing the edge of the nail.

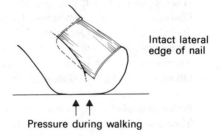

Intact lateral edge of nail

Pressure during walking

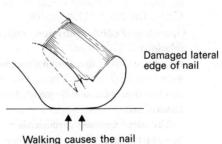

Damaged lateral edge of nail

Walking causes the nail edge to macerate skin

Fig. 96 One mechanism producing an 'ingrowing' toenail.

Packing is carried out using cotton wool pledgets moistened with surgical spirit or tincture of iodine. These are placed under the corner of the nail. They protect the skin from the nail edge and the antiseptic helps to dry up the infection.

If these measures fail, surgical removal of the nail is necessary. This may be either temporary or permanent, and treatment policies vary between surgeons. In the senior author's unit, temporary avulsion is performed for any nail where there is active infection, whether or not permanent excision of the nail is planned. Permanent excision of the nail is done if the condition recurs following avulsion and despite conservative treatment. Excision of the nail-bed is usually performed two months after avulsion of the nail to allow time for any sepsis to settle down. The whole nail-bed may be removed (Zadik's operation) or only on one side of the nail (wedge excision).

Operation: avulsion of the big toenail

The toe is anaesthetized by digital nerve block and a tourniquet applied. A haemostat is passed under one edge of the nail, the nail is grasped and twisted off to the other side. The toe is dressed with paraffin gauze, a gauze pad and then a bandage.

Codes

Blood	0	
GA/LA	LA	
Opn time	15 minutes	
Stay	Outpatient	
Drains out	0	
Sutures out	0	
Off work	1−2 days	

Postoperative care

The patient is advised to keep the foot elevated overnight and the toe is redressed within 48 hours.

Operation: Zadik's operation (radical nail-bed ablation)

This is removal of the germinal matrix to prevent regrowth of the toenail (Fig. 97). The nail is removed as above and then the skin is incised diagonally from each corner of the proximal end of the nail-bed. The proximal skin flap is lifted and separated from the germinal matrix down to the base of the distal phalanx. The germinal matrix is then excised. Care must be taken to excise the matrix laterally enough at the

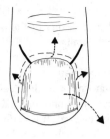

Skin incision
avulsion of nail
reflection of skin folds

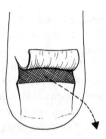

Removal of germinal matrix

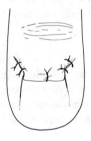

Closure

Fig. 97. Zadik's procedure.

sides of the nail-bed. The skin edges are then stitched loosely together. The dressing is as for nail avulsion.

This procedure is not usually performed in the presence of active infection as there is a risk of osteomyelitis in the distal phalanx.

Codes

Blood	0 . . . .
GA/LA	LA or GA . . . .
Opn time	30 minutes . . . .
Stay	Outpatient/inpatient . . . .
Drains out	0 . . . .
Sutures out	7 days . . . .
Off work	2–5 days . . . .

Postoperative care
The dressing is changed either by the ward staff or by the district nurse after 24 hours.

Operation: wedge excision
This is an operation similar to the Zadik's procedure described above except that only one side of the germinal matrix of the nail is removed. It is performed for recurrent ingrowing toenail where only one side of the nail-fold is involved. It has the effect of narrowing the big toenail.

Topical application of phenol
Phenol can be used to destroy the germinal matrix of the nail. An exsanguinating tourniquet is applied and the nail avulsed as described above. A cotton wool bud soaked in phenol (88% in water) is then placed beneath the proximal skin flap on the germinal matrix. This is left in place for 3–4 minutes. Care must be taken not to get any phenol on the skin and if this occurs it must be washed off with a spirit-based cleansing agent.

The results of this procedure are good and it has the advantage that it can be done at the same time as nail avulsion, requiring the patient to attend hospital on only one occasion.

Paronychia

The condition

This is an infection of the nail-fold, usually seen in the hand. It is commonly due to a *Staphylococcus* or occasionally a *Streptococcus*. These enter following a minor injury. Pus may track from the nail-fold to beneath the nail.

Recognizing the pattern

The patient may be of any age and presents with a painful finger, which on examination shows erythema, swelling and tenderness in the nail-fold. There may be visible pus. If pus has spread under the nail, pressure over the nail will be painful. Advanced infection may spread to the pulp space.

Management

In the first 48 hours the infection may resolve with antibiotic therapy. Splinting the finger and elevation of the limb will help to relieve the pain. Once pus has formed it must be drained.

Operation: incision and drainage of a paronychia
Under digital nerve block and with a tourniquet applied, the skin is incised at one or both proximal corners of the nail-fold and a flap raised to release the pus. All the slough must be excised. If pus is trapped beneath the nail, that part of the

nail must also be removed. The finger is dressed with paraffin gauze. Inadequate primary treatment may result in a chronic paronychia.

Codes

Blood	0 . . . .
GA/LA	LA . . . .
Opn time	10 minutes . . . .
Stay	Outpatient . . . .
Drains out	0 . . . .
Sutures out	0 . . . .
Off work	1−2 days . . . .

Postoperative care
The district nurse is requested to change the dressing daily until the finger heals.

Subungual haematoma

The condition

This is a collection of blood beneath the nail following a crushing injury to the finger tip. It is painful as the tissues are not able to expand.

Recognizing the pattern

The history
There is a history of trauma and the patient presents complaining of a painful finger, the pain often being severe.

On examination
There is a collection of blood beneath the nail and the area is tender to touch.

Management

The digit must be X-rayed to see if the phalanx beneath has been fractured. Then the blood is released by making a hole in the nail over the clot with a red-hot needle. This procedure is painless.

A fracture of the phalanx beneath does not usually require manipulation and the nail provides sufficient splintage. However, a finger splint and elevation of the arm in a sling for 24−48 hours will help to ease the pain.

Hyperhidrosis

The condition

This is excessive sweating. The three most troublesome areas affected are the axillae, hands and feet. The condition causes embarrassment due to the odour produced and also soiling and damage to clothes. Permanently wet hands can be disabling to someone whose job involves fine hand movement.

Management

Medical management is not very effective. Aluminium chloride (Anhydrol forte or Driclor) is an antiperspirant that is applied at night and may be effective in some cases.

When conservative measures fail, hyperhidrosis of the hands or feet can be treated by cervical or lumbar sympathectomy. These operations are described on p. 481 and p. 500 respectively. Hyperhidrosis of the axilla is treated by local excision of the sweat glands. This operation is described below.

Preoperative management
The day before operation the sweat gland area is mapped out. This is done by painting the skin with tincture of iodine, allowing it to dry, and then sprinkling starch powder (e.g. glove powder) over the axilla. The water produced by the sweat glands turns the starch and iodine blue. The area can then be mapped out. An alternative application is quinizarin compound, which is a powder that changes colour when it is moistened.

Operation: excision of axillary sweat glands
The marked area of skin and sweat glands is excised and the wound closed with suction drainage to the subcutaneous space. In the Hurley Shelley operation a smaller area of skin is excised and the sweat glands are removed by an undercutting procedure.

Codes

Blood	0 . . . .
GA/LA	GA . . . .
Opn time	1 hour . . . .
Stay	3—5 days . . . .
Drains out	48 hours . . . .
Sutures out	10 days . . . .
Off work	2 weeks . . . .

Postoperative care
After the wound has healed (usually about 2 weeks after operation), active shoulder exercises with or without physiotherapy may be required to restore full movement to the arm.

11 Conditions of Children

11.1 **Surgical conditions of children**
Congenital hypertrophic pyloric stenosis
Intussusception
Inguinal hernias and hydrocoeles
Umbilical hernias
Umbilical discharge
Rectal bleeding
Rectal prolapse
Necrotizing enterocolitis

11.2 **Congenital obstruction of the gut**
Neonatal intestinal obstruction
Oesophageal atresia
Duodenal atresia
Small bowel obstruction
Malrotation
Meconium ileus
Hirschsprung's disease
Rectal agenesis (imperforate anus)

Congenital hypertrophic pyloric stenosis

The condition

There is obstruction of the pyloric outlet of the stomach by extreme hyperplasia of the circular muscle of the pylorus. The aetiology of this interesting condition is still unclear.

Recognizing the pattern

The patient

The baby is usually between the ages of 3 and 8 weeks, although the condition may rarely occur immediately after birth or up to 5 months of age. Males are more commonly affected than females and the first-born is more commonly affected than later siblings.

The history

There is projectile vomiting of non-bile-stained vomit. The baby fails to gain weight. There may be a family history of the condition.

On examination

The baby may become dehydrated and cachectic if the condition is not recognized early. After a feed with the baby's abdomen relaxed, a rounded tumour may be felt in the right hypochondrium close to the umbilicus. A test feed should be given in order to elicit this physical sign.

Proving the diagnosis

The presence of a palpable tumour and the characteristic history is sufficient. Experience is necessary in order to feel the pyloric mass and this is usually best done by a paediatrician.

Management

Atropine drops (Eumydrin (Winthrop) 1 drop = 200 µg atropine methonitrate: dose: 2−4 drops every 4 hours) have been used in an attempt to relax the pyloric muscle but, generally speaking, surgery is the treatment of choice.

Preoperative management

It is important that any electrolyte disturbances are corrected and the baby is rehydrated before any operation is begun. With prolonged vomiting the baby will be potassium-deficient. Correcting the electrolytes may take as long as 48 hours.

Operation: Ramstedt's operation

It is possible to do this operation under a local anaesthetic, but with a skilled anaesthetist a general anaesthetic is now preferred. A transverse incision is used and the 'tumour' delivered into the wound. The muscle layer is split down to the mucosa and the stomach replaced in the abdomen.

Codes

Blood	0 . . . .
GA/LA	GA . . . .
Opn time	1 hour . . . .
Stay	3−5 days . . . .
Drains out	0 . . . .
Sutures out	5−7 days . . . .

Postoperative care

Clear oral fluids can be started 8 hours postoperatively. If the baby has had a severe gastritis preoperatively, he may continue to vomit a little after the operation. In that case, he should stay on clear fluids until the vomiting ceases. In most cases, however, half-strength and then full-strength milk can be reintroduced by 24−36 hours after the operation.

Intussusception

The condition

An intussusception is a condition in which a segment of proximal bowel is 'swallowed up' by the distal bowel (see Fig. 98). Ninety-five per cent of intussusceptions begin near the ileocaecal valve and are either ileo-ileal or ileo-colic. A causative lesion is found in only 5% of cases. Such lesions include intestinal polyps, Meckel's diverticulum, ectopic pancreas, enterogenous cyst or a swollen lymphoid patch (Peyer's patch). The condition often follows an upper respiratory tract or gastrointestinal infection and in these cases the intussusception may be started by one piece of bowel going into 'spasm' and being propelled within the lumen of the adjoining segment.

Recognizing the pattern

The patient

The patient may be of any age although intussusceptions are commonest in children. The male to female ratio is 3:2. Sixty-five per cent occur in the first year of life, usually between the ages of 5 and 9 months.

The history

There is a classic triad of symptoms.

1 *Pain.* A normally healthy child suddenly screams with pain and draws its legs up and may adopt a squatting

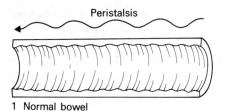

1 Normal bowel

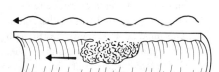

2 Enlarged Peyer's patch or polyp in wall

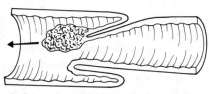

3 Formation of intussusception

Fig. 98. The production of an intussusception.

position. The spasm passes off and the child returns to normality. Recurrent spasms then continue to distress the patient.

2 *Vomiting.*

3 *Bleeding per rectum.* Eighty-five per cent of patients with intussusception pass 'red currant jelly'. The jelly consists of bloodstained mucus produced by the congested intussusceptum. Initially the patient may have his bowels open normally but later he becomes obstructed.

On examination
The presence of a mass is usually diagnostic. It feels like a hard sausage in the right hypochondrium stretching across to the midline. It is tender. The right iliac fossa feels 'empty'. Rectal examination may disclose bloodstained mucus. The apex of the intussusception may be felt.

Proving the diagnosis
A plain X-ray of the abdomen shows signs of intestinal obstruction and an empty right iliac fossa. The diagnosis is

proved on a barium enema which shows the intussusceptum progressing along the colon.

Management The patient may be ill and dehydrated and resuscitation with fluids and blood transfusion may be necessary. A nasogastric tube is passed and the stomach emptied.

Reduction by barium enema
Some intussusceptions can be reduced using the hydrostatic pressure generated during the barium enema examination. This method is certainly worth trying within the first 24 hours of the onset of symptoms. It should be carried out by a skilled radiologist working in co-operation with the surgeon. The head of barium is raised up 110 cm above the baby and no higher. The progress of the intussusception is observed on fluoroscopy. It is important to observe complete reduction of the intussusception, including seeing barium in the ileum.

Operation: reduction of intussusception
A transverse abdominal incision is used and the intussusception reduced manually. If the head of the intussusception has become gangrenous, it is resected. If there is a causative lesion, this will be resected.

Codes

Blood	1−2 units depending on age and size .
GA/LA	GA ....
Opn time	60−90 minutes ....
Stay	5−7 days ....
Drains out	0 (or 6 days if resected) ....
Sutures out	5−7 days ....

Postoperative care
In most cases recovery is quite straightforward. The recurrence rate is about 3% and the intussusception usually recurs at the same place as the previous lesion.

Inguinal hernias and hydrocoeles
The condition An inguinal hernia is the most common paediatric surgical referral. Such hernias are much more common in boys and represent a failure of closure of the processus vaginalis. The latter is a peritoneal pouch which remains attached to the testis as it descends into the scrotum. The upper end of the pouch is in communication with the peritoneum (see Fig. 99).

Hernias and hydrocoeles in infancy are therefore closely related conditions and all require the same management,

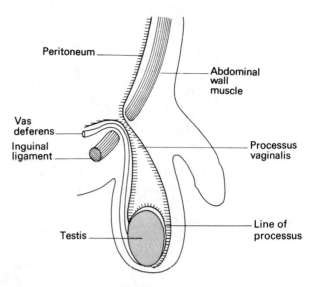

Fig. 99. The processus vaginalis.

which is to close the patent processus. The various types of abnormality are shown in Fig. 100.

Recognizing the pattern

The patient
Most hernias in children appear in the first year of life. The incidence in boys is 1 in 50 and in girls 1 in 500.

The history
The history is of an intermittent swelling in the groin which appears when the child cries or strains. Incarceration is not uncommon and the child may present as an emergency.

On examination
The swelling may or may not be visible. If it is visible, it may be reduced. In girls a sliding hernia of the ovary is not uncommon and the ovary may be felt as a hard 1 cm diameter mass in the inguinal canal.

Proving the diagnosis

The diagnosis is proved by feeling the swelling. If no swelling is present, the characteristic history from the mother is diagnostic. There is really no other lesion which produces intermittent swelling in the groin and which appears on straining.

Management

Hernias and hydrocoeles in infancy should be treated by operation. If there has been an episode of strangulation

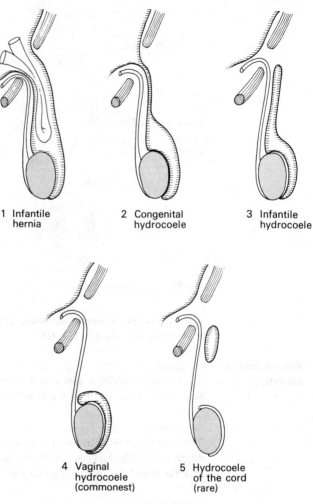

1 Infantile hernia   2 Congenital hydrocoele   3 Infantile hydrocoele

4 Vaginal hydrocoele (commonest)   5 Hydrocoele of the cord (rare)

Fig. 100. Types of inguinal hernias and hydrocoeles.

which has been successfully reduced, the operation should be performed on the next available list.

Preoperative management
Check that both testes are satisfactorily in the scrotum.

Operation: herniotomy in children
The spermatic cord (or round ligament in girls) is exposed in the groin through a transverse incision. The hernial sac is separated from the gonadal vessels and vas and tied off at the internal ring. At the end of the operation make certain the testis has been pulled down to the bottom of the scrotum.

Otherwise it may be caught up in the fibrosis of the hernia repair and become 'undescended'.

Codes

Blood	0 . . . .
GA/LA	GA . . . .
Opn time	15−30 minutes . . . .
Stay	24 hours . . . .
Drains out	0 . . . .
Sutures out	5 days . . . .
Off school	2 weeks . . . .

Postoperative care
Babies and young children recover very rapidly from hernia repairs and no special management is required.

Umbilical hernias

The condition

Umbilical hernias in children are of two types.
1 *Central.* This hernia represents failure of fusion of the various processes of the abdominal wall at the umbilical scar. Such fusion is often delayed beyond the time of birth and may occur as late as two or three years of age. Central hernias therefore usually close spontaneously.
2 *Para-umbilical.* This is a true defect in the linea alba close to the umbilicus and this type of hernia will not resolve.

Recognizing the pattern

The history
The child has a bulge in the region of the umbilicus which has often been present from birth. When this is large, the mother is very concerned about its appearance and the effect on the child.

On examination
The hernial defect is usually quite small compared with the size of the hernia. Central umbilical hernias never strangulate. A para-umbilical hernia can strangulate but this is rare in children and more common in adults.

Management

The mother of a baby with a central umbilical hernia should be strongly reassured that the lesion is likely to settle on its own. Not infrequently she is reluctant to accept this advice. If the hernia persists beyond the age of 3, it is then reasonable to get the child in and repair the defect before he starts school. It must be emphasized, however, that very few hernias will remain until this age.

A para-umbilical hernia is also unlikely to strangulate in childhood and should be repaired by the age of 3 or 4.

Operation: repair of umbilical hernia

A small transverse or semicircular incision is made in the region of the umbilicus and the muscular defect closed.

Codes

Blood	0 . . . .
GA/LA	GA . . . .
Opn time	15–30 minutes . . . .
Stay	24 hours . . . .
Drains out	0 . . . .
Sutures out	5 days . . . .

Umbilical discharge

The condition

Infection of the stump of the umbilical cord can occur in the first few days of life and may persist for a few weeks producing an umbilical granuloma. A swab should be taken and antibiotics given. The granuloma can be cauterized using a silver nitrate stick.

If the discharge is more profuse and persistent then the possibility of a congenital fistula or sinus must be considered. This may be due to a persistent vitello-intestinal duct, a patent urachus or a urachal cyst. The vitello-intestinal duct represents the endodermal connection between the gut and the remnant of the yolk sac, the latter lying outside the embryo close to the placenta. The urachus is an endodermal cavity which develops into the bladder and its proximal end is attached to the umbilicus.

Proving the diagnosis

If there is an obvious opening, a cannula can be inserted and an X-ray contrast study may show the deep connection. A small bowel barium study or a cystogram may also be helpful. An ultrasound examination may demonstrate a urachal cyst.

Management

If a fistula is present, it must be closed.

Operation: Closure of umbilical fistula

Through a transverse incision the umbilical scar is mobilized. A fine probe can usefully be inserted in the fistula. The latter is isolated, ligated and divided. An associated Meckel's diverticulum should be excised. A urachal cyst is removed, repairing the dome of the bladder if necessary.

Codes

Blood	1 unit . . . .
GA/LA	GA . . . .
Opn time	60 minutes . . . .

Stay	2−3 days
Drains out	3−5 days
Sutures out	7 days

Rectal bleeding in children

Common causes are constipation, fissure, worms, Meckel's diverticulum and rectal prolapse.

Constipation and fissure formation are quite common in children and bleeding may be noted. Intestinal worms can give rise to rectal bleeding, in which case the worms may be seen in the stool. Rectal prolapse is not uncommon in children under the age of 2 and is dealt with below.

Investigation
Stool softeners should be given to treat constipation before further investigation is undertaken. Proctoscopy and sigmoidoscopy are performed, under a general anaesthetic if necessary, to look for a fissure or rectal lesion.

If bleeding continues in spite of regulation of bowel habit, fuller investigation is indicated, including a barium enema and a technetium scan for Meckel's diverticulum. If these investigations fail to provide a diagnosis, it may be necessary to undertake a laparotomy to exclude a Meckel's diverticulum or a haemangioma of the bowel. In cases of profuse bleeding, it may be worth while performing an acute angiogram to look for the bleeding point.

Rectal prolapse

The condition
Rectal prolapse in children is associated with a lack of the sacral spinal curvature which develops about the age of 2 as the child begins to walk upright. The condition is usually a mucosal prolapse rather than a complete prolapse (p. 368).

Recognizing the pattern
The child is usually in the first year of life and the mother either notices rectal bleeding or the strawberry-coloured prolapse during defaecation. She is often extremely alarmed by this. Where no prolapse has been seen, there may be a history of excessive straining by the child. The prolapse usually reduces spontaneously.

Proving the diagnosis
If you are lucky enough to see the prolapse, there is no problem. Otherwise the diagnosis can only be made on the mother's history. It is important for the clinician to have this condition in mind.

Management
The management is to reassure the mother and to take no further action apart from making sure the stools are kept

soft. This can be achieved by giving extra roughage in the diet and making sure the child has enough fluid to drink.

The mother should be told that a prolapse is not uncommon in the first year of life and that it should settle as the baby begins to adopt the upright posture. The child is followed up at 3–6-monthly intervals and in most cases the condition resolves spontaneously.

If the prolapse persists, injections may be required.

Operation: injection of rectal prolapse in children

The child is given a general anaesthetic and the anal canal inspected. A nasal speculum can be useful for this. Submucosal injections of phenol in almond oil are inserted.

Codes

Blood	0	
GA/LA	GA	
Opn time	15 minutes	
Stay	24 hours	
Drains out	0	
Sutures out	0	

Necrotizing enterocolitis

The condition

This condition may occur as a complication in any baby requiring postnatal intensive care. It particularly affects babies of low birth weight and those who have suffered from hypoxia or who have had umbilical arterial or venous catheters in place. The aetiology is not clearly understood. There appears to be ischaemic necrosis of the mucosa in various parts of the bowel and this occurs with, or is complicated by, spreading infection along the bowel wall. Multiple areas of perforation can occur.

Making the diagnosis

The baby becomes ill and distended with a clinical picture of intestinal obstruction. The abdominal wall may show a bluish discoloration. An X-ray shows loops of bowel with gas trapped in the bowel wall. If perforation occurs, there may be air seen beneath the anterior abdominal wall on a lateral decubitus view.

Management

This is conservative in the first instance, with adequate fluid replacement and broad-spectrum antibiotic therapy. Where perforation occurs, operation is mandatory and in that case the affected bowel is resected. The proximal bowel can be brought out as an ileostomy and continuity restored later.

Babies who develop necrotizing enterocolitis and who do not actually go on to perforate the bowel may later develop strictures at the site of the disease.

11.2   Congenital Obstruction of the Gut

Neonatal intestinal obstruction

The condition

Obstruction in neonates may be due to defects in the development of the bowel such as an atresia, stenosis or web (Fig. 101). In an atresia a segment of the bowel is missing and the two ends may be connected by a fibrous cord. The proximal end becomes grossly dilated and the distal unused end remains tiny. With a stenosis the bowel is narrowed but there is continuity of the lumen and the obstruction is incomplete. A web is a mucosal barrier across the lumen of the bowel and it may be complete or perforated.

Other causes of obstruction include compression of the bowel from outside by bands, a volvulus, or a malrotation, and obstruction within the lumen from an inspissated meconium in cystic fibrosis. In Hirschsprung's disease there is a defect in the conduction mechanism within the bowel wall. These conditions will be dealt with briefly in the subsequent pages.

Recognizing the pattern

There may be signs that an abnormality in the child is a possibility before birth. Indications include a family history

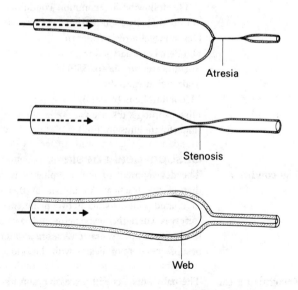

Atresia

Stenosis

Web

Fig. 101. Some different forms of neonatal intestinal obstruction.

of congenital defects, a history of maternal disease or drug-taking during the first trimester of the pregnancy or poly-hydramnios in the mother. The latter is more common with high intestinal obstruction in the foetus.

After delivery the baby will present the classic signs:
1 bile-stained vomiting;
2 abdominal distension;
3 failure to pass meconium. Meconium should be passed within the first 24 hours of life.

Proving the diagnosis

A straight abdominal X-ray taken in the supine and erect positions will show the presence of distended bowel loops and fluid levels.

Management

This is dealt with under the individual presenting conditions. An operation will almost always be required. The baby must be adequately rehydrated and proper electrolyte balance restored before this is undertaken.

Laparotomies in neonates are usually undertaken through transverse muscle-cutting incisions as these give the best exposure of the whole of the neonatal peritoneal cavity.

The pre- and postoperative management of feeding and electrolyte balance in these babies is a paediatric speciality and is beyond the scope of this book.

The baby's nutrition may need to be assisted for several days either intravenously or by a trans-anastomotic tube before normal oral feeding can be instituted.

The following are common conditions causing neonatal intestinal obstruction and are discussed below.
Oesophageal atresia (p. 556).
Duodenal atresia (p. 558).
Small bowel atresia (p. 559).
Malrotation (p. 560).
Meconium ileus (p. 563).
Hirschsprung's disease (p. 564).
Imperforate anus (p. 565).

Oesophageal atresia

The condition

The development of the oesophagus is closely allied with that of the trachea. An atresia at this site is frequently associated with a fistula between the two. The commonest variety is where the oesophagus ends as a blind pouch at the level of the fourth thoracic vertebra and the lower end of the oesophagus communicates with the trachea (Fig. 102).

Recognizing the pattern

The baby presents with excessive salivation and if he is fed there is an attack of choking, coughing and cyanosis.

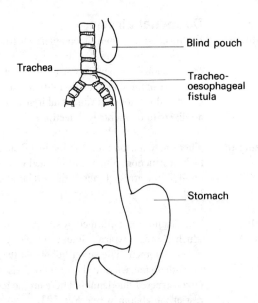

Trachea

Blind pouch

Tracheo-
oesophageal
fistula

Stomach

Fig. 102. The most common form of oesophageal atresia.

**Proving the
diagnosis**
The diagnosis is proved by attempting to pass a nasogastric
tube. If the lower end of the oesophagus opens into the
trachea, a plain X-ray of the abdomen will show normal
bowel gas patterns. If there is no fistula, however, the
abdomen will remain opaque.

Operation: repair of oesophageal atresia
The method of treatment depends on the length of gap
between the two ends of the oesophagus. If this is small,
immediate resection is possible with end-to-end anastomosis
of the oesophagus and closure of the fistula. If the gap is
larger, however, it may be necessary to perform a temporary
gastrostomy together with closure of the fistula. The gap
between the ends of the oesophagus can later be bridged
using a graft of stomach, colon or small bowel.

Codes

Blood	1–2 units . . . .
GA/LA	GA . . . .
Opn time	2–3 hours . . . .
Stay	Very variable – 2 weeks minimum . . .
Drains out	Pleura 24 hours, anastomotic drain 7
	days . . . .
Sutures out	5–7 days . . . .

Duodenal atresia

The condition　In this condition there is complete obstruction of the duodenum around the level of the entry of the bile duct. This is the junction between foregut and midgut. There is a high incidence of this condition in children with Down's syndrome but this does not mean that children with duodenal atresia are likely to be mentally defective.

Recognizing the pattern　There may not be much abdominal distension with such a high obstruction. The vomit is usually bile-stained but may not be if the atresia is above the level of the entry of the bile duct.

Proving the diagnosis　The diagnosis is confirmed by straight X-ray of the abdomen which shows a typical 'double bubble' gas shadow in the upper abdomen. The larger bubble on the left is due to the distended stomach and the distended viscus on the right is the obstructed duodenum. There are no gas shadows in the rest of the abdomen (see Fig. 103).

Operation: for duodenal atresia
The empty distal duodenum is brought up and a side-to-side anastomosis is made between it and the distended first part of the duodenum.

Codes

Blood	1 unit . . . .
GA/LA	GA . . . .
Opn time	60−90 minutes . . . .
Stay	2−3 weeks . . . .
Drains out	5−7 days . . . .
Sutures out	7 days . . . .

Postoperative care
It usually takes 2−3 weeks before the over-distended stomach and duodenum manage to propel gastric contents through the anastomosis into the tiny distal gut. Intravenous feeding or trans-anastomotic enteral feeding is continued during this time.

Small bowel obstruction

The condition　As mentioned above, this may be due to an atresia, a web or stenosis. With an atresia the obstruction is complete and the proximal bowel is grossly distended down to the level of the lesion.

　　In webs and stenoses there may be a small lumen, in which case the obstruction is incomplete.

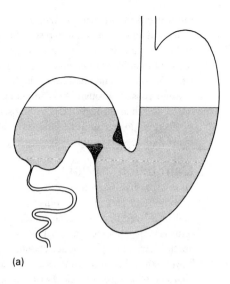

(a)

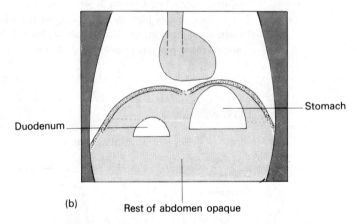

Stomach

Duodenum

(b)   Rest of abdomen opaque

Fig. 103. Duodenal atresia: the 'double bubble' seen on erect X-ray.

Making the diagnosis	In these babies there will be abdominal distension and the lower the atresia, the more the distension. A straight X-ray of the abdomen shows clear evidence of intestinal obstruction. A barium enema will show the typical 'micro-colon'. This simply indicates that the colon has never been used and is therefore small and empty.

Management	**Operation: for intestinal atresia**

At operation it is important to resect the over-distended loop of bowel immediately proximal to the obstruction, as this segment is unlikely to be able to conduct normal peristalsis later. An end-to-end anastomosis is then performed. A tube may be passed through the abdominal wall and into the bowel and then through the anastomosis. This can be used for feeding postoperatively. The residual bowel often takes many days to start to function normally.

Malrotation (Fig. 104)

The condition During normal development the gut is originally a midline structure and part of it lies outside the anterior abdominal wall in a large developmental umbilical hernia. As the gut returns to the abdomen the small bowel enters first and takes up the lower left part of the abdominal cavity. The large bowel returns last and as it does so the caecum rotates three-quarters of a turn anti-clockwise around the axis of the superior mesenteric artery. It thus comes to lie in the right iliac fossa. Abnormalities of this mechanism of rotation can lead to congenital obstruction in one of two ways.

1 The caecum lies high in the right hypochondrium and its peritoneal attachments (Ladd's bands) obstruct the duodenum. These patients present with intermittent intestinal

LATERAL VIEW

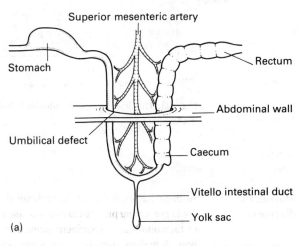

Fig. 104a Normal development of the gut: lateral view. The midgut is originally a midline structure protruding through the umbilical defect.

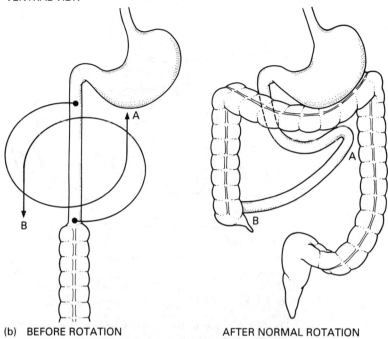

(b) BEFORE ROTATION   AFTER NORMAL ROTATION

Fig. 104b Normal development of the gut: ventral view, before and after normal rotation. Points A and B rotate 300° anticlockwise to achieve the adult position of the gut. The colon comes to lie over the proximal gut.

obstruction. The abdominal X-ray shows the 'double bubble' appearance of duodenal obstruction but there will also be gas in the distal bowel.

2 The second type of obstruction associated with malrotation is a volvulus. The duodeno-jejunal flexure and the caecum are closer together than usual and as a result the base of the small bowel mesentery is shorter, thus making a volvulus more likely.

Recognizing the pattern

Fifty per cent of malrotations present in the first week of life and the rest mostly present in the first year of life. They can, however, present at any time, even in adults. Males are more commonly affected than females in the ratio of 2:1.

   The presenting picture may be of acute complete intestinal obstruction or of intermittent subacute obstruction. The diagnosis may be difficult.

   A volvulus may occur *in utero* or at any time after birth. In the latter case the presentation is with acute intestinal

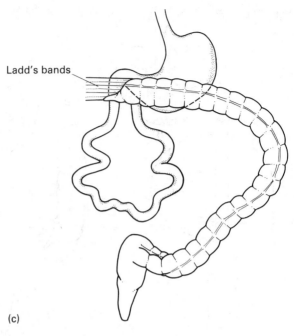

Ladd's bands

(c)

Fig. 104c Malrotation. The caecum lies over the duodenum. The duodeno-jejunal junction is close to the ileo-caecal valve.

obstruction, abdominal pain and distension. With a postnatal volvulus the baby will often have had normal bowel actions previously.

Proving the diagnosis

Where there is duodenal obstruction by Ladd's bands, a straight abdominal X-ray will show the double bubble appearance already described for duodenal atresia. There will be gas in the distal bowel, however, as the obstruction is incomplete.

A volvulus presents the picture of small bowel obstruction. If the bowel has become ischaemic *in utero*, its wall may be calcified and visible on X-ray.

A barium enema confirms the high position of the caecum.

Management

Operation: for malrotation and intestinal obstruction
If there is a volvulus present, this will have to be reduced and any necrotic bowel resected.

If the duodenum is obstructed by Ladd's bands, these are divided. The large bowel is then replaced in the lower left side of the abdomen and the small bowel in the upper right side of the abdomen. No attempt is made to create normal anatomical relationships.

Codes

Blood	1 unit . . . .
GA/LA	GA . . . .
Opn time	90 – 120 minutes . . . .
Stay	2 – 3 weeks . . . .
Drains out	Wound 2 days, deep 5 – 7 days . . . . . .
Sutures out	7 days . . . .

Meconium ileus

The condition

This occurs as part of the syndrome of cystic fibrosis (mucoviscidosis). There is a deficiency of pancreatic enzyme secretion and the meconium in the bowel is hard and sticky. It becomes inspissated in the terminal ileum and complete obstruction results.

Making the diagnosis

The condition usually presents in the neonatal period. The meconium pellets may be visible on plain abdominal X-ray, giving a ground-glass appearance. The sweat test for mucoviscidosis is positive.

Management

The meconium plugs can sometimes be freed by giving the baby a gastrografin enema. If this is unsuccessful, the baby may require operation.

Operation: for intestinal obstruction due to meconium ileus

An ileostomy is made (see Fig. 105). This is done in such a way that the distal bowel can be washed out through it. The proximal bowel is inserted into the side of the ileostomy so that bowel continuity is restored once the distal obstruction has dispersed. While distal obstruction remains, the ileal contents can escape via the stoma. Once normal feeding has been established (including the necessary pancreatic enzymes), the ileostomy can be dropped back and closed. Respiratory complications are common in these babies and they may require oxygen and antibiotics. The long-term prognosis is poor, although improving with modern methods of management.

Hirschsprung's disease

The condition

In these children there is an absence of intramural ganglia in the distal bowel. The rectum is affected in 15% of cases, the rectum and lower sigmoid in 70% of cases, and the upper colon and even small bowel in another 15%. The aganglionic

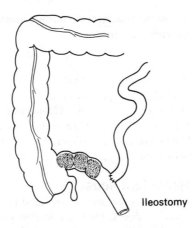

Fig. 105. Ileostomy for meconium ileus.

segment is in spasm and not able to propel faeces in the normal way. The bowel above it becomes grossly dilated and hypertrophied (megacolon). The condition has a familial incidence and often presents as chronic constipation with secondary spurious diarrhoea later in childhood. Presentation in the neonatal period is rare. Left alone, the child may progress to gross malnutrition and eventual death.

Making the diagnosis

The diagnosis can be made on a barium enema which shows the dilated bowel above the tapering 'transition zone' and the narrowed bowel distally. Full-thickness rectal biopsy confirms the absence of ganglia in the bowel wall distally.

Management

In small babies a colostomy early in life may be required. The definitive operation is performed later. This consists of resecting the aganglionic segment and anastomosing the normal bowel to the anal canal. This operation must be carried out without damaging the pelvic splanchnic nerves and a variety of different techniques have been described (Swenson, Duhamel and Soave techniques).

Rectal agenesis (imperforate anus)

The condition

The commonest site for congenital obstruction of the large bowel is the anal canal. There are two varieties of abnormality, the high and low types of imperforate anus. In the high abnormality the rectum ends as a blind pouch above the levator ani and there is no anal canal. In the low abnormality the anal canal is present but the anus itself is closed by a membrane or stenosed (Fig. 106).

Making the diagnosis

The absent anus is usually noted at birth. If, for some reason, the abnormality is missed, the baby will be noted to pass no meconium and to become increasingly distended.

Investigation
The classic investigation is an X-ray with the baby inverted and a ball-bearing placed in the anal dimple. As the colonic gas rises into the lower rectum it can be seen on a lateral X-ray and the distance between the end of the pouch and the ball-bearing can be measured. If the pouch is above a line joining the pubis to the coccyx, the abnormality is a high one.

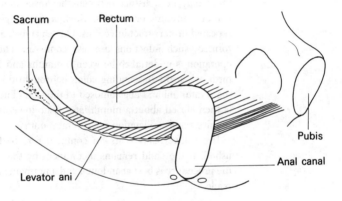

(a)   LOW IMPERFORATE ANUS

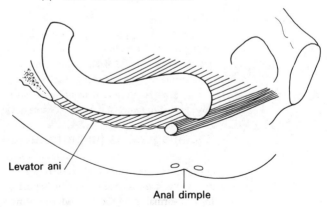

(b)   HIGH IMPERFORATE ANUS

Fig. 106. Two forms of rectal agenesis (imperforate anus).

More recently, ultrasound has provided a useful means of measuring the distance between the anal dimple and the pouch.

Management

Low rectal agenesis

All that is necessary in these babies is to perforate the membrane and dilate up the stenosed anus. Repeated dilatation may then be necessary until the child is old enough to pass a well-formed stool. The prognosis is excellent.

High rectal agenesis

This is a much more serious condition as the baby has been born without the usual muscles and nerves necessary to produce continence. In the immediate postnatal period, a colostomy is required. These babies frequently have other abnormalities associated with the cloacal structures and there may be a fistula between the lower bowel and the bladder, urethra or ureters. Such a fistula gives rise to repeated urinary tract infections. Once a colostomy has been formed, such infections are less common. The definitive operation is undertaken between 6 months and 1 year after birth, when the descending colon is brought down through the levator ani and anastomosed to the skin. The colostomy is then closed about a month later. The lower rectum may require regular dilatation for several months.

It can take many years for continence to be fully established. If the child remains incontinent by the age of 7–8 the procedure is best abandoned and a permanent colostomy made.

12   Trauma

12.1   **Dealing with a major accident**
General principles

12.2   **Head injuries**
Pathology of brain injury
Major head injury
Minor head injury
Intracranial haematoma
Skull fracture

12.3   **Chest and abdominal injury**
Chest trauma
Abdominal trauma

12.4   **Spinal and pelvic injuries**
Fractured spine
Fractured pelvis
Other pelvic injuries

12.5   **Trauma to the skin and limbs**
The management of wounds
Tetanus prophylaxis
Hand injuries
The management of fractures
Fat embolism
Arterial damage
Nerve injuries
Tendon injuries
Burns

12.1 Dealing with a Major Accident

General principles

When a major accident arrives in hospital, there may be many people involved in the initial assessment and resuscitation. There is often great danger for the patient and urgent decisions need to be made. Good organization is imperative, and action, however rapid, has to be methodical and thoughtful. Priorities must be decided and ideally one doctor should assume overall control and assess the progress of resuscitation without being too embroiled in the action.

Accurate notes are important, particularly for victims of assault, road accidents or industrial injuries. Legal action may be taken many months after the injury when the actual details have been forgotten.

How do you cope when the victim of a major accident suddenly comes under your care? The following is a basic plan which may be helpful. There are seven overall steps.

1 *Assess* vital functions and overall injuries.

2 *Resuscitation*.

In practice these two steps are virtually simultaneous.

3 *Review*: a full examination and review of the whole situation.

4 *X-ray*.

5 *Investigate*: relevant blood tests including grouping and cross-matching.

6 *Decide* on priorities for management.

7 *Treat*.

These steps will now be considered in more detail.

1 Assess vital functions

Remember to assess one A, two Bs and one C: airway, blood, brain and chest.

Airway

• Check the airway. Is it clear?

• Is the patient breathing? Is mechanical ventilation effective?

• Is there adequate gaseous exchange, i.e. is the patient cyanosed or adequately oxygenated?

Blood

• Check the blood pressure and pulse.

Brain
- Check the level of consciousness.
- Look at the pupils and limbs for evidence of extradural haemorrhage (see pp. 581 and 582).

Chest
- Check whether there is any injury to the chest which may embarrass respiration.
- Does the patient have a pneumothorax or haemothorax?
- Order an immediate portable chest X-ray to check for these conditions.

2 Resuscitate

Action on:
(a) airway
(b) circulation

Airway

Clear the airway of all potential obstruction, including broken teeth, debris, vomit, etc. The airway may need frequent aspiration. If there is any problem with respiration, give the patient oxygen. If the patient is still not breathing adequately and remains cyanosed, consider intubation and ventilation. Severe maxillary facial injuries are also an indication for intubation.

Treat any life-threatening injury of the chest immediately, e.g. tension pneumothorax or haemothorax (see p. 587).

Circulation

Put up at least one good intravenous infusion. You may use this opportunity to take blood for cross-matching and investigations. Treat any hypovolaemia by plasma expanders such as Haemaccel, plasma or blood. The longer the delay in instituting such therapy, the more collapsed are the veins and therefore the more difficult intravenous cannulation will be.

- Loosen the collar and check that there is unimpeded cerebral perfusion.
- Stop any external bleeding with small clamps or sterile gauze and tight bandages.

By now there should be adequate cerebral perfusion of oxygenated blood, and a fuller assessment of all the injuries can begin.

3 Review

A full history and examination are undertaken together with documentation of the injuries. The exact order in which this is done will be governed by events. However, it must be thorough and, if urgent treatment interrupts it, it must be completed at the earliest opportunity. Patients have, for instance, had a fractured finger left untreated because in the excitement of the initial effort to save life, no one has had time to examine the digits.

The history

Try to determine exactly what happened and how long ago. Obtain a detailed account of the time and nature of the accident including the mechanism and direction of injury. This may be obtained from the patient, from the ambulance man or from the police. A description of the patient's condition when first found is useful and should be recorded.

If the patient is conscious, question him about any areas of particular pain. If his condition deteriorates, this information may be valuable later.

Remember to find out the patient's normal medical condition including any past history (e.g. diabetes, myocardial ischaemia or previous chest injury) and any current medication such as insulin or steroids.

The examination

The examination must be thorough and include all systems. The findings should be accurately recorded, ideally at the time the examination is being carried out.

Examine the patient methodically, starting with the head and neck and trunk and working down both arms and both legs, looking for possible injuries. This is especially important in an unconscious patient.

Use what is known of the mechanism of the accident to predict sites of injury, e.g. a person hit by a car bumper while standing may have ligament injuries to the knee. A passenger in a car hit on the left side may have a ruptured spleen or kidney.

Start with the head, looking for lacerations, bruising, haematoma or deformity. Check the pupil reaction and size.

Next examine the neck, including a careful palpation of the cervical spine for localized tenderness or deformity. Then feel the thoracic and lumbar spine for any possible fracture. If there is any likelihood of an unstable spinal fracture, this must be stabilized before the patient is moved (see p. 600).

Examine the upper limbs next, including the clavicle, joints, bones and soft tissues down to the individual fingers.

Re-examine the chest for rib, lung or mediastinal injury and then feel the abdomen. Palpate methodically around the various organs observing the patient's reaction for any sign of a localized site of tenderness.

Finally examine the pelvis and the lower limbs.

4 X-ray

Send the patient for X-rays.

1 The following are routine in all cases of major trauma:
(a) skull,
(b) cervical spine,
(c) chest,
(d) pelvis.

2 Include the following, depending on injuries observed:
(a) thoracic spine,
(b) lumbar spine,
(c) limbs.

5 Investigations

Send off blood to the laboratory for haemoglobin, cross-matching (the number of units required depends on the injuries observed), urea and electrolytes.

6 Decide

Decide on the priorities for management. This can be done whilst the patient is being X-rayed. It may well be difficult.

The order should be as follows:
(a) conditions threatening life,
(b) conditions which are at present stable but could threaten life if they deteriorate,
(c) major injury, no threat to life,
(d) minor injury.

7. Treat

The management of injuries will be considered under the following headings.

Head injury (pp. 573–584).

Chest trauma (pp. 585–593).

Abdominal trauma (pp. 593–599).

Spinal injury (pp. 600–601).

Injuries to the pelvis (pp. 602–605).

Trauma to the skin and limbs (pp. 606–614).

Burns (pp. 614–619).

12.2　Head Injuries

A head injury may present in isolation or in association with other major injuries.

Brain survival depends on adequate perfusion with oxygenated blood. This is governed by the intracranial pressure (ICP), the mean blood pressure and respiratory function. The brain compartment in the skull is of constant volume, with limited room for expansion either by brain swelling or haematoma. As additional volume is added, cerebro-spinal fluid (CSF) shifts into the spinal compartment, the venous sinuses are compressed and there may be some vaso-constriction. There is thus little initial change in intracranial pressure. Once this leeway is taken up, the intracranial pressure starts to rise, until eventually a small increase in volume causes a dramatic rise.

The brain perfusion pressure (BPP) is the sum of the mean blood pressure minus the intracranial pressure (ICP). A minimum of 40 mmHg is required for adequate brain function. Less than this causes first electrical, and then structural damage. In a major injury with head involvement the intracranial pressure may rise and the mean blood pressure fall, resulting in inadequate brain perfusion.

Pathology of brain injury (Fig. 107)

Brain damage is divided into primary damage sustained at the moment of injury, and secondary damage sustained following the injury.

Primary brain damage occurs by distortion and sudden movement within the dura and skull. Damage may be focal (for example after assault injury), the rest of the brain being relatively normal, or may be a combination of focal and diffuse injury typical of a high-momentum impact. There are three categories of primary injury.

1 *Concussion.* This is a generalized injury resulting in diffuse loss of nerve function. It is an electrical injury which is reversible.

2 *Contusion.* This is more localized and consists of bruising of the cortex.

3 *Laceration* of the cerebral cortex. This is always associated with bleeding into the subdural space. This is structural damage, and thus is irreversible. Diffuse axonal

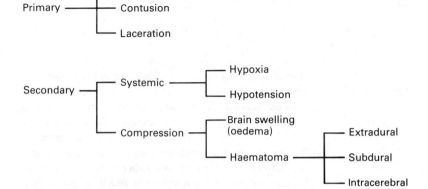

Fig. 107. Pathology of head injury.

injury is included in this category and is seen after high-momentum rotational injuries.

Secondary brain damage is caused by:

1 *Systemic factors*, including:
   (a) hypotension
   (b) hypoxia.

2 *Compression*, either by brain swelling or by haematoma.

If brain compression is asymmetrical, focal shift occurs between the various brain compartments, the most important of which are the medial temporal lobe, herniating beneath the falx and pressing on the third nerve, the temporal lobe, herniating through the tentorial hiatus and compressing the midbrain, and the cerebellar tonsils, herniating through the foramen magnum ('coning').

The assessment and management of head injury is governed by the need to prevent, detect and treat this secondary injury. Systemic and local factors responsible for secondary brain damage are correctable. The prevention of hypoxia and hypotension is crucial to the outcome of brain damage and is most important in the first few hours after head injury.

Head injuries can be divided into major head injuries, where the patient is unconscious on arrival, and minor head injuries, where the patient is conscious.

Major head injury

Assessment

The initial assessment is combined with resuscitation. The following steps are performed.

1 Is the airway patent? If not, an airway must be inserted or the patient intubated.

2 Is the patient breathing effectively? There may be active breathing movements but respiratory effort is wasted due to a flail chest.

3 Is ventilation adequate? Central cyanosis indicates inadequate gaseous exchange, which may be due to pulmonary contusion. Blood gases should be performed as soon as possible. Hypercapnia is a potent cause of cerebral vasodilatation and therefore increased intracranial pressure.

4 Chest X-ray. An early chest X-ray is mandatory to exclude pneumothorax or haemothorax.

5 Pulse and blood pressure. Is there a pulse and is it strong? Is there evidence of any external bleeding? If so, this must be controlled, if necessary with artery clips as a temporary measure.

6 Carotid perfusion. Are there carotid pulses? The collar should be loosened to avoid impeding blood flow to the head.

7 Cervical spine. A patient with a major head injury must be assumed to have a cervical spine injury until this is excluded by X-ray. Until this is done a cervical collar should be put on to protect the neck and to remind the medical staff to perform an X-ray.

Emergency management is performed to achieve cardiorespiratory stability. This may include blood transfusion, insertion of a chest drain for a pneumothorax or haemothorax or even laparotomy for ruptured spleen.

History

Establish full details of the injury especially from the ambulance men. Include the position in which the patient was lying (an unconscious patient lying on his back may have aspirated), the time of the injury, any changes in conscious level, any history of fitting and whether the patient was ever cyanosed or unable to breathe.

Find out about any medical illnesses or drugs the patient was taking.

At the end of this assessment and resuscitation, the mean blood pressure should be restored such that cerebral perfusion is improved even though the intracranial pressure may still be elevated.

Once the blood pressure and ventilation are satisfactory carry out a neurological examination.

Neurological examination

Start a chart of the pulse rate, blood pressure, respiratory rate and body temperature as a basis for future observations. Assess the conscious level. Make a note of the eye signs, motor responses and verbal responses. The Glasgow coma scale is the standard method of recording the level of consciousness and facilitates comparisons later on (Table 26).

Table 26. Glasgow coma scale.

Function	Type of response		Points
Eyes	Open	Spontaneously	4
		To verbal command	3
		To pain	2
	No response		1
Best motor response	To verbal command	Obeys	6
	To painful stimulus*	Localizes pain	5
		Flexion − withdrawal	4
		Flexion − abnormal (decorticate rigidity)	3
		Extension (decerebrate rigidity)	2
	No response		1
Best verbal response[†]		Orientated and converses	5
		Disorientated and converses	4
		Inappropriate words	3
		Incomprehensible sounds	2
	No response		1
Total			3−15

* Apply the thumb to the underside of the supra-orbital ridge and press up, observing the arms.
[†] Arouse patient with painful stimulus if necessary.
(From Jennett B. & Teasdale G. (1977) Aspects of coma after severe head injury. *Lancet*, 23 April, 878−81.)

Examine the head for scalp lacerations or bruising. Localized tenderness and a boggy swelling due to haematoma may be felt over a fracture site. You may feel a depression in the outline of the skull if the fracture is displaced. Look in the nose and ears for blood or CSF leakage, which may indicate that the nasal sinuses, nasal cavity or middle ear are fractured.

Anterior fossa fractures, as well as causing traumatic rhinorrhoea, may extend into the orbit and cause an effusion of blood, leading to unilateral exophthalmos, disturbance of eye movements and subconjunctival haemorrhage. The posterior border of this haemorrhage cannot be seen. The cranial nerves may also be affected. Bruising behind the ear (Battle's sign), with or without facial nerve palsy, indicates a fracture through the petrous temporal bone.

Examine the eyes noting the pupil size, equality and reaction to light. Try to assess eye movement. Examine the limb movements, noting the tone and testing the reflexes.

The continual assessment of conscious level is a dynamic process, the main purpose of which is to detect the trend indicating rising intracranial pressure. This is described further on p. 579.

Management

Early management is governed by the stability or otherwise of the patient's conscious level.

If the unconscious patient is stable, investigations can proceed in an orderly fashion. These should include the following.

1 Repeat blood gases to check respiratory function.
2 Haemoglobin.
3 Urea and electrolytes.
4 Blood sugar.
5 Liver function tests.
6 Skull X-ray. Look for evidence of a skull fracture or a shift of the pineal gland. The radiological features of a skull fracture are described on p. 583. If the pineal gland is calcified, it should be central. A shift of the pineal gland is a significant sign of raised intracranial pressure on one side.
7 CAT scanning. The indications for CAT scanning include the following.

(a) A patient who is deeply unconscious (Glasgow coma score less than 7) after resuscitation.

(b) Any patient with a skull fracture that is (i) depressed or (ii) associated with confusion, neurological signs or a fit.

(c) Continuing unconsciousness for more than 6–8 hours.

(d) Depressed skull fracture or clinical evidence of skull base fracture.

(e) A history of penetrating injury such as stabbing or gun shot.

These patients should be discussed with the regional neurosurgical centre.

General care of the unconscious patient

The priorities are to minimize brain swelling, maintain oxygenation and blood pressure and monitor regularly for evidence of deteriorating conscious level.

Nurse the patient with the head elevated 30°. In some centres intracranial pressure monitoring is performed, as discussed on p. 579.

1 Respiration

If respiration is not adequate, the patient will need to be ventilated. This enables better control of blood gases. The patient may be hyperventilated down to a PCO_2 (partial pressure of carbon dioxide) of 30 mmHg. Any further hyperventilation causes vasoconstriction so that brain ischaemia may result. Sedation and analgesia (using benzodiazepines and opiates) are necessary during this period if the patient is restless or in pain. There is no place for steroids in acute head injury.

If ventilation is required for longer than 7 days, a tracheostomy may be required.

The daily assessment of the chest should include:
(a) examination,
(b) chest X-ray,
(c) blood gases.

Chest physiotherapy should be carried out regularly and if possible coincide with turning the patient. Tracheobronchial suction or bronchoscopy may be required.

2 Cardiovascular system

Ensure cerebral perfusion, avoid hypertension. If the blood pressure increases, exclude raised intracranial pressure, pain, hypoxia or a distended bladder and then treat either with a sedative (e.g. chlorpromazine 5 mg i.v.) or hydralazine (5–10 mg i.v.).

3 Nutrition

This may be given either through a nasogastric tube or by an intravenous route. If the nasogastric route is used, it is important to watch for regurgitation. Also remember that patients with multiple injuries may have an ileus.

4 The bladder

This should be catheterized. Retention of urine is a common cause of restlessness.

5 The bowels

They should be controlled by enemas.

6 Fluid balance

A strict watch should be kept on the patient's fluid balance together with measurements of urea and electrolytes and blood sugar, particularly if mannitol is being given. If anything, the patient should be run with a slight fluid deficit to prevent cerebral oedema.

7 General body care

The pressure points on the skin should be looked after by regular turning and putting the patient on a sheepskin and/ or a ripple mattress. The eyes should be cleaned and kept closed to prevent corneal ulceration. The mouth should be regularly cleansed and kept moist to prevent parotitis or stomatitis. Regular limb physiotherapy is needed to prevent contractures developing.

8 Epilepsy

Fits following head injury are common, particularly after conditions such as depressed skull fracture with dural penetration and brain damage. Epilepsy requires treatment with anticonvulsants, such as phenytoin or carbamazepine. In an emergency i.v. diazepam is a safer drug to use. There is now no indication for prophylactic anticonvulsants.

Deterioration in conscious level

Deterioration may be seen in casualty or after a period of observation in hospital. The faster the deterioration occurs, the faster must be the response if one is to save the patient's brain. Deterioration is due to secondary brain damage, often a developing haematoma.

The signs of deterioration are as follows.

1 A decreasing level of consciousness.

2 Bradycardia.

3 Hypertension.

4 Deep breathing.

Changes in the pupillary reactions and focal neurological signs such as arm or leg weakness indicate the probable site of such a lesion, as discussed on p. 581.

Carry out a CAT scan provided the patient's cardiorespiratory system is stable. This is to differentiate between generalized brain swelling, brain contusions and haematoma.

Contact the neurosurgical centre. Transfer of the patient may be discussed. Transfer of patients is potentially dangerous. Ensure the patient is well intubated, ventilated and stable prior to moving off.

Active measures can be taken to reduce cerebral oedema. Mannitol (20% 250–500 ml i.v. over 20–30 minutes) may be given. Frusemide in small doses is also useful. In some centres direct measurement of the intracranial pressure is made through a burr hole.

Haematoma

An haematoma causing cerebral compression must be

removed. This may be done at the referring hospital, or by a neurosurgeon. Usually transfer is advised, following the resuscitation described above. The management of haematoma is described further on p. 582.

This concludes the final step in successful head injury treatment — namely to reduce the elevated intracranial pressure.

Minor head injury

Assessment
This is defined as a head injury where there has been no loss, or only transient loss, of consciousness, with or without loss of memory. The patient is conscious when seen.

History
A careful enquiry as to the nature of the injuries is undertaken. Establish whether the patient remembers the whole event clearly or if there is any retrograde or post-traumatic amnesia. Are there any disturbances of smell or hearing which may indicate a fracture causing damage to the olfactory or auditory nerves? Are there disturbances of vision, photophobia, nausea, vomiting or headache? Has the patient had a fit?

The examination
The examination is performed as for a major head injury, but in this case with the co-operation of the patient.

The indications for skull X-ray include the following.
1 Loss of consciousness or amnesia at any time.
2 Neurological symptoms and signs.
3 Leakage of CSF from nose or ear.
4 History of penetrating injury or scalp bruising and swelling.

The main decision is whether to admit the patient to hospital or to send him home. The indications for admission to hospital are as follows.
1 A history of transient loss of consciousness, with post-traumatic amnesia of more than 5 minutes.
2 Confusion or other impairment of conscious level at the time of examination.
3 Evidence of a skull fracture.
4 Vomiting or headache, or other neurological symptoms or signs.
5 No witness to the accident or an unreliable history (usually due to drunkenness).
6 Lack of adequate supervision at home.

If the patient can go home, then an instruction sheet may be given, which includes the address and telephone number of the hospital, the date, and advice that the patient should return to hospital immediately if he develops symptoms of nausea, vomiting, headache, drowsiness, photophobia or weakness.

Patients who are admitted should have the following observations quarter- or half-hourly (in order to look for signs of raised intracranial pressure).

1 Conscious level, which should be described as in the Glasgow coma scale (p. 576).

2 Pulse, blood pressure, respiratory rate and body temperature.

3 Pupil size, equality and reaction.

4 Limb tone and movement.

Observations should ideally be continued for 24 hours, after which the stable patient can be discharged. Children generally should stay longer because this age-group can suddenly develop raised intracranial pressure within the first 48 hours despite being stable.

Intracranial haematoma

The condition

Haematomas may be either extradural, subdural or intracerebral.

Extradural haematoma occurs between the bone and the dura and is classically due to rupture of the middle meningeal artery following a fractured overlying temporal bone.

Subdural haematoma occurs between the dura and brain, and is usually associated with severe head injury causing cerebral laceration. It is typically less brisk than an extradural haemorrhage.

Intracerebral haematoma is a collection of blood within the substance of the brain and is associated with major brain damage. Occasionally intracerebral haemorrhage due to aneurysm or hypertension is the primary event which caused the head injury.

Recognizing the pattern

A stable patient develops signs of rising intracranial pressure as described above. The other presentation of intracranial haemorrhage is of a patient who is unconscious and begins to show signs of rising pressure.

On examination

Focal signs may indicate the side of the compression.

1 Pupillary size. There is contraction followed by dilatation of the pupil on the side of the haemorrhage (Hutchinson's pupil). As the pressure further increases, the opposite pupil

shows similar signs. Bilateral fixed and dilated pupils may be a sign of brain-stem death, seen as the terminal evidence of coning. Remember, though, the effects of drugs, including alcohol, and of fits.

2 Hemiplegia. This is usually contralateral to the side of the first dilated pupil.

Proving the diagnosis

The diagnosis is made on a CAT scan. If the patient is deteriorating rapidly, he should if possible still be scanned even if this is one or two slices simply to confirm the diagnosis. Occasionally a patient deteriorates so quickly that even this is not possible.

Management

The management is surgical evacuation provided that the patient's clinical condition warrants it. A patient who is found to have a haematoma but is clinically improving can be managed conservatively. Otherwise a craniotomy or exploratory burr holes need to be performed. In determining which side burr holes should be done, the site of a skull fracture or the side of the first dilated pupil are of more significance than localization by observed limb weakness.

An acute extradural or subdural intracranial haematoma is solid and therefore has to be removed by craniotomy, usually by a neurosurgeon. Skilled anaesthesia is mandatory. Frusemide or mannitol is given while theatre is being prepared.

In the rare event of a patient being taken to theatre on clinical grounds only, exploratory burr holes are performed to decompress the cranium.

Operation: cranial burr holes
The burr hole is situated either next to the fracture or at a point 5 cm up from the mid-point of a line drawn between the external auditory meatus and lateral angle of the eye. A linear incision is made in a direction that can be converted into a scalp flap if a craniotomy is to be performed. The temporalis is divided and a burr hole drilled. If a haematoma is found, it is evacuated. If necessary the burr hole may be enlarged (craniectomy) to find and control the bleeding vessel. This is usually beneath the fracture. It is then acceptable to place a swab in the wound and transfer the patient to the local neurosurgical centre. If the wound is closed, the dura must be stitched up to the pericranium around the craniectomy edge to prevent re-accumulation.

If no haematoma is found, other burr holes may be made as appropriate. If haematoma is excluded on each side, the deterioration must be assumed to be due to brain swelling.

Codes

Blood	2 units . . . .
GA/LA	GA . . . .
Opn time	1 hour . . . .
Stay	Variable, depends on other injuries . .
Drains out	0 . . . .
Sutures out	7 days . . . .
Off work	Variable . . . .

Postoperative care
The long-term management of head injuries is multidisciplinary. Complications such as epilepsy, chronic subdural haematoma, external hydrocephalus and infection may occur.

Skull fracture

The condition

A skull fracture can be closed (simple) or open (compound). An open fracture is one where there is an associated scalp injury, rendering the fracture site open to the atmosphere, with the secondary risk of meningitis or abscess formation. Fractures that run into the nose or middle ear are also regarded as open.

A fracture may also be undisplaced (a linear or fissured fracture) or depressed. A depressed fracture will cause local injury and loss of function depending on its site. The site and the presence of dural penetration determine the treatment required.

Making the diagnosis

This is made on the X-ray and the appearances can be difficult to interpret. A linear fracture is characteristically thinner and darker and has a more angular course than the vascular markings. It is straighter and more defined than the cranial suture lines. In inspecting the skull X-ray, it is important to look for a depression in the fracture, or any evidence of dural penetration (which appears as spicules of bone at right angles to the plane of the vault of the skull). Look carefully at the region at the base of the skull as it is easy to miss fractures there. Also inspect the outlines of the orbit carefully and compare the appearance with that on the opposite side. CAT scanning is indicated in a patient whose fracture is depressed or who has confusion, neurological signs or a fit.

Management

A closed linear fracture requires no additional management, other than that already described for head injuries. The patient is admitted and regular observations are carried out.

An open linear fracture requires surgical treatment. The

wound must be thoroughly cleaned and the fracture inspected. If hair is present, it must be removed, if necessary by craniectomy. Broad-spectrum antibiotics are given (e.g. cefuroxime 1.5 g i.v.). If there is cerebro-spinal fluid leakage, the patient remains in hospital until it stops. If the leak persists more than a week, surgical repair of the defect may be necessary.

A closed depressed fracture is managed conservatively unless there is evidence of dural penetration or the fracture is overlying an important area of function, e.g. the speech or motor cortex. In this case surgery is indicated. The depressed fracture is elevated and any fragments of bone or damaged brain removed.

An open depressed fracture requires urgent operation to clean the area and remove any dirty bone, fragmented dura or damaged brain. The wound can be closed and skull reconstruction may be carried out at a later date. Antibiotics are required as above.

12.3 Chest and Abdominal Injury

Chest trauma

With any chest injury there is a danger that respiration may be compromised. You should also consider whether there has been associated injury to the underlying pleura, lungs or mediastinal structures including the heart.

Injuries to the chest involve one or more of the following.

1 Chest wall.
  (a) Fractured ribs (p. 585).
  (b) Flail chest (p. 586).
  (c) Fractured sternum (p. 587).
2 Pleura.
  (a) Pneumothorax (p. 587).
  (b) Tension pneumothorax (p. 588).
  (c) Traumatic haemothorax (p. 589).
3 Lung.
  (a) Pulmonary contusion (p. 589).
  (b) Pulmonary laceration (p. 589).
4 Mediastinal structures.
  (a) Ruptured thoracic aorta (p. 590).
  (b) Ruptured bronchus (p. 590).
  (c) Ruptured diaphragm (p. 590).
  (d) Blunt injury to the heart (p. 591).
  (e) Haemato-pericardium (p. 592).
5 Penetrating injuries: bullet and stab wounds to the chest (p. 592).

Fractured ribs

The condition

Ribs are usually fractured as a result of a direct blow to the chest or a crushing injury. The fractures may be single or multiple and simple or compound. Pneumothorax may occur either due to a compound fracture with air entering through the wound, or due to perforation of the underlying lung by a fractured rib.

Recognizing the pattern

The history

The patient complains of severe, localized, pleuritic pain and difficulty in breathing. The latter may either be due to inability to take a deep breath because of pain, or secondary to a pneumothorax.

On examination
The characteristic sign is of extreme tenderness at one point along the rib. There may also be bruising or laceration at the site of the injury. Remember to look for signs of an associated pneumothorax.

Proving the diagnosis

The fracture is usually seen on a chest X-ray. Special views are often required.

Management

1 Analgesia
Analgesia must be adequate to allow effective respiration. This is especially important in the elderly and debilitated who are likely to develop an underlying hypostatic pneumonia. Intercostal 'Marcain' nerve blocks are very useful but need to be repeated every 6 hours or so. Non-steroidal anti-inflammatory agents such as diclofenac are particularly useful as they do not cause respiratory depression.

2 Breathing
The patient is given breathing exercises and physiotherapy.

3 Strapping
Opinions differ about the value of strapping. This is effective in relieving the pain but it does also further restrict normal chest expansion.

Flail chest

The condition

A flail chest develops when the chest wall has lost its mechanical rigidity due to multiple fractures. One segment of the rib cage becomes separated from its surroundings and can move paradoxically (i.e. inwards on inspiration, outwards on expiration). This results in inadequate ventilation of the lung and retention of pulmonary secretions. There is associated pulmonary contusion. A dangerous vicious circle ensues in which the lung becomes increasingly oedematous, the patient more and more anoxic and respiratory movements increasingly active. This further exacerbates the paradoxical movement, and progressive anoxia ensues.

Recognizing the pattern

The patient has signs of fractured ribs. Initially respiration may be satisfactory but after 24–48 hours there is increasing dyspnoea and the patient becomes more and more distressed. On inspection the flail segment will be seen to move paradoxically.

Proving the diagnosis	The diagnosis is confirmed on chest X-ray. Blood gas estimations are of value and show a low PO_2 (partial pressure of oxygen) and an elevated PCO_2.

Management	The patient should be sat up and given oxygen. As a temporary measure the flail segment can be supported with strapping. Strong analgesia will be required in all cases and is best given either as intercostal blocks or as a thoracic epidural anaesthetic. The patient is observed carefully and, if the respiratory rate begins to climb, further action may be required. Serial blood gas estimations are also used to monitor progress. In severe cases intermittent positive pressure ventilation is needed. A tracheostomy reduces the dead space and facilitates good tracheobronchial toilet. If the flail segment is depressed (stove-in chest), it will require elevation.

Fractured sternum

The condition	This is a rare injury. It commonly follows road accidents where there is a forceful impact against the steering wheel or dashboard.

Recognizing the pattern	The patient complains of pain over the sternum and is usually breathless. On examination the sternum is very tender and there may be a palpable step or deformity. Pulmonary complications are rare, but there may be associated damage to the trachea, great vessels or heart.

Management	The patient is treated with strong analgesia (e.g. pethidine) to allow chest expansion. If there is severe displacement with a reduction in the anterior/posterior diameter of the chest, the depressed segment is pulled forward at open operation and fixed with wires.

Traumatic pneumothorax

The condition	Air may get into the pleura either through a deep wound or through damage to the lung following a penetrating wound or rib fracture. There is frequently an associated haemothorax. If the air leak is valvular, a tension pneumothorax develops (see below).

Recognizing the pattern	Apart from the pain of the original injury, the patient complains of breathlessness and pleuritic pain. On examination the affected side of the chest is not moving and the percussion note is hyper-resonant. The breath sounds are decreased on that side and there may be tracheal displacement towards the uninjured lung.

Proving the diagnosis

This is confirmed on chest X-ray. The absence of lung markings in the periphery of the pleural space is noted, as is the edge of the lung.

Management

A small pneumothorax can be observed and managed conservatively. With a larger pneumothorax the chest must be drained with a large intercostal drain attached to an underwater seal. The insertion and management of a chest drain is described on pp. 231–234.

If the lung has failed to re-expand, suction should be applied to the drain (75–100 mmHg). When the lung has re-expanded (as shown by lack of bubbling from the chest drain on coughing, and confirmed by chest X-ray), the tube is clamped for 12–24 hours. Once the lung has remained inflated, the tube may be withdrawn. If the tube continues to bubble even after the lung has re-expanded, there is probably a tear in the lung. This usually seals off after a few days but, if the tear is major or involves the bronchus, a thoracotomy may eventually be necessary. A small pneumothorax may go unnoticed and only become apparent when it rapidly develops into a tension pneumothorax when the patient is ventilated.

Tension pneumothorax

The condition

A tension pneumothorax develops when there is a one-way valvular leak of air into the pleural cavity. Air rapidly accumulates, compressing the lung, and urgent treatment is required. Severe respiratory embarrassment develops and death can ensue due to kinking of the great veins secondary to mediastinal displacement.

Recognizing the pattern

A breathless patient with the clinical features of a pneumothorax becomes progressively worse with increasing dyspnoea and evidence of increasing mediastinal shift. The patient is very distressed. There may be associated surgical emphysema of the chest wall, neck and face. It is the steady deterioration in symptoms which suggests the diagnosis. Impaired venous return causes a tachycardia and hypotension. The deterioration can occur very rapidly.

Proving the diagnosis

The presence of a pneumothorax is confirmed by urgent portable chest X-ray. The presence of tension is confirmed by inserting a chest drain as below.

Management

No time should be wasted in wondering whether there is tension pneumothorax or not. If this is a possibility, a chest drain should be inserted urgently. In difficult circumstances, a simple needle straight into the pleural cavity will suffice.

The rush of air under pressure confirms the diagnosis. Once the tension has been released, normal chest drainage connected to an underwater seal can be established.

Traumatic haemothorax

The condition
An accumulation of blood in the pleural cavity can occur from injury to the muscles in the chest wall, lung, heart or great vessels. There may also be a pneumothorax.

Recognizing the pattern
The presence of blood is irritant and causes pleuritic pain and breathlessness. The patient may be shocked. On examination there are signs of a pleural effusion with lack of breath sounds and a dull percussion note at the lung base.

Proving the diagnosis
The blood in the pleural cavity is seen on chest X-ray and confirmed on tapping the chest.

Management
Immediate drainage is required. An underwater seal is used and the level of the water in the bottle is marked so that the blood loss can be measured. Further management is usually conservative until the bleeding stops. However, if more than one litre is removed or if the rate of bleeding is more than 250 ml per hour, a thoracotomy may be required.

Pulmonary contusion or laceration

The condition
This is bruising and oedema of the lung beneath chest wall trauma. There may or may not be an associated rib fracture. The injury to the lung has a severe effect on respiration. There may also be an associated pulmonary laceration with blood or air in the pleural cavity.

Recognizing the pattern
The patient is breathless, apprehensive and cyanosed and coughing produces sputum tinged with blood.

Proving the diagnosis
A chest X-ray shows a progression from a patchy diffuse opacity in the lung fields (12−24 hours after injury) to a complete 'white out'. Blood gases show hypoxia and hypercapnia.

Management
It is important to keep the patient relatively dehydrated and diuretics may be helpful. Intravenous fluid therapy must be carefully regulated to avoid overtransfusion. Oxygen, adequate analgesia and physiotherapy will help, but the patient may eventually need ventilating.

Closed chest injury

Closed chest injuries are often caused by shearing forces generated during extreme deceleration. The following will be considered.

1 Rupture of the thoracic aorta.
2 Rupture of the bronchi.
3 Rupture of the diaphragm.

1 Rupture of the thoracic aorta

Rupture of the ascending thoracic aorta is usually fatal. Rupture of the descending aorta usually involves the intima and media only, resulting in a large peri-aortic haematoma.

Recognizing the pattern

The patient complains of severe central chest pain. The diagnosis is made by noting widening of the mediastinum on a chest X-ray and it is important to be aware of this potentially lethal condition. Where there is doubt a repeat chest X-ray may show progressive widening.

Management

After control of blood pressure, urgent operation is required. Under cardiopulmonary bypass repair or replacement of the aorta by a Dacron graft is undertaken.

2 Rupture of the bronchi

This commonly occurs distal to the carina as the bronchus leaves the support of the mediastinum. There is a large escape of air causing bilateral pneumothoraces and mediastinal emphysema. There may be haemoptysis.

Recognizing the pattern

The patient is acutely dyspnoeic and shocked, and surgical emphysema may be felt in the neck.

Proving the diagnosis

This is confirmed on chest X-ray and on bronchoscopy.

Management

Immediate operative repair is required which will restore lung function. Any significant delay will result in infection around the bronchial wound and later stricture formation.

3 Rupture of the diaphragm

This occurs after a crush injury to the abdomen. The diaphragm usually tears on the dome from front to back adjacent to the pericardium. There may be herniation of the stomach or other organs through the rent. The stomach may distend, collapsing the lung and shifting the mediastinum. Occasionally it becomes strangulated.

Recognizing the pattern	The patient presents with increasing respiratory difficulty following an abdominal injury.
Proving the diagnosis	The chest X-ray may show a raised hemi-diaphragm and, if the left side is involved, a stomach bubble may be visible in the chest. If a nasogastric tube has been passed, it will be seen to lie in the chest. A decubitus film will also show a horizontal fluid level in the chest. A barium swallow is useful.
Management	Following resuscitation and passage of a nasogastric tube, surgical repair is required urgently. If there is no other thoracic injury requiring operation, the diaphragm may be exposed from below through the abdomen. This decreases the incidence of pulmonary complications postoperatively and allows the surgeon to check that the spleen is not damaged.

Blunt injury to the heart

The condition	Blunt injury to the heart may cause contusion of the myocardium with necrosis of muscle fibres. Arrhythmia or heart failure may follow. Occasionally there may be rupture of the papillary muscles or interventricular septum. The thin walls of the atria and right ventricle may burst, causing cardiac tamponade (see below). Cardiac concussion is a condition where there may be arrhythmia in the absence of myocardial necrosis.
Recognizing the pattern	The patient may present with an arrhythmia, heart failure, or cardiac tamponade following a blow on the chest. There may be a pericardial friction rub on examination.
Proving the diagnosis	The ECG may show changes typical of infarction if there is a large area of cardiac contusion. Cardiac-specific enzymes (e.g. the cardiac isoenzyme of creatinine phosphokinase) are elevated.
Management	It is most important to be aware of the possibility of a cardiac injury. The patients most at risk from complications are those with ECG changes, particularly if other major injuries are present.
	The patient must be put on an electrocardiograph monitor. Care must be taken during intravenous infusion not to overload the circulation. Measurement of the central venous pressure or intracardiac pressure may be useful. The patient should be examined frequently with particular care taken to

auscultate the heart. A cardiothoracic surgeon should be warned about the case if it is severe and transfer considered.

Haemato-pericardium

The condition

The pericardial cavity fills with blood following a penetrating injury to the heart (e.g. stab wound) or following blunt trauma with rupture of the walls of the atria or right ventricle. The outer fibrous pericardium limits distension of the pericardial sac, and blood in the cavity therefore prevents ventricular filling, resulting in cardiac tamponade with decreased cardiac output, hypotension, cyanosis and elevated jugular venous pressure.

Proving the diagnosis

This is a life-threatening condition. Aspiration of the pericardial cavity with a needle inserted just under the seventh costal cartilage and to the left of the xiphoid process proves the diagnosis and provides temporary relief.

Management

The pericardial cavity is opened through either an anterolateral thoracotomy or a sternotomy, and the defect repaired.

Bullet and stab wounds to the chest

Any penetrating injury to the chest may cause serious complications but the most dangerous are those that occur within the mid-clavicular lines and between the jaw and xiphisternum. These need careful surgical exploration because of the risk to internal organs. The pleura, subcostal vessels, lung, heart, great vessels and main airways may all be involved. Remember that a low or angulated penetrating wound in the chest may have perforated the diaphragm and injured abdominal viscera, especially the liver, stomach and spleen.

Management

Preoperatively a chest and abdominal X-ray must be taken to look for any missiles. Six to ten units of blood are crossmatched but the laboratory is warned that more may be needed urgently later. If a cardiothoracic surgeon is available, his help should be obtained. Set up at least one good intravenous infusion, a central venous pressure line to prevent overtransfusion, and chest drainage if necessary.

Operation: exploratory thoracotomy for penetrating chest injury

The wound is excised and all dirt, rib fragments and debris are removed either through the same wound or through a separate thoracotomy. The pleural cavity is explored and any pulmonary lacerations repaired. Any other damage is treated as necessary.

Codes

Blood	6 – 10 units . . . .
GA/LA	GA . . . .
Opn time	2 – 3 hours . . . .
Stay	About 7 days but variable . . . .
Drains out	Chest drain 3 – 4 days . . . .
Sutures out	7 – 10 days . . . .
Off work	Variable . . . .

Postoperative care
The postoperative care following thoracotomy is described on p. 235.

Abdominal trauma

Abdominal trauma may be due to penetrating or blunt injuries. Different problems arise in these two categories.

Penetrating injuries to the abdomen
These include the following.

Stab wounds.

Gunshot wounds.

Penetration by other foreign bodies.

The patient complains of abdominal pain and may be shocked with signs of peritonism.

Management

All penetrating injuries of the abdomen should be explored after the patient has been resuscitated. The laparotomy is undertaken to exclude damage to any hollow viscus which may result in fluid leakage and peritonitis, and also to stop any haemorrhage. The entrance wound is excised and a full laparotomy is performed.

Blunt injury to the abdomen
The external visible damage may be minimal but the internal injuries serious. There may also be delay between a causative injury and the appearance of signs of damage. Finally, the internal injury may be at a different site from the site of the original trauma. The internal injuries to be considered are the following.

1 Ruptured liver.

2 Ruptured spleen.

3 Traumatic bowel injury.

4 Pancreatic injury.

5 Renal injury.

Ruptured liver

The condition

In blunt abdominal trauma the liver is usually injured by rapid compression and decompression. This tends to produce a ragged tear in its substance. The condition must be suspected in any case of multiple trauma or abdominal injury. This is especially true if there are external marks on the abdomen or if the patient is shocked with no obvious sign of blood loss.

Recognizing the pattern

The conscious patient may complain of abdominal pain situated in the right upper quadrant. The pain is worse on breathing. On examination he will be shocked (pale, sweaty, anxious, with a tachycardia and sighing respiration). The abdomen may exhibit localized tenderness and rigidity in the right upper quadrant. There may also be more generalized tenderness due to a haemo-peritoneum. The abdomen is distended.

Proving the diagnosis

Peritoneal lavage will show blood in the peritoneal cavity. The urinary bladder is emptied by a catheter. This also allows the urine output to be monitored. A cannula is then introduced into the peritoneal cavity and saline injected. This is moved around by gently rolling the patient and then re-aspirated.

Management

The patient is resuscitated. There is some controversy as to the best course to pursue in this dangerous condition. Some favour initial conservative management in which the patient's condition is very carefully monitored in the hope that, as pressure rises within the abdominal cavity, internal tamponade may occur and the bleeding cease. If such management is pursued and the patient's condition continues to deteriorate, urgent laparotomy is required.

Others proceed more rapidly to laparotomy. Fatalities can occur, however, as the patient is anaesthetized and especially when the abdomen is opened and the tamponading pressure is released.

Operation: laparotomy for ruptured liver

The abdomen is opened and the abdominal viscera inspected. If a hepatic tear is confirmed, one of the following procedures is carried out.

(a) The tear is sutured.

(b) The affected part of the liver is excised (partial hepatectomy) (see p. 308).

(c) The liver is packed to control bleeding. Such packs can

be left in place for a few days and then removed at a second laparotomy.

The danger of wide exploration of hepatic tears is that they may extend into the cava. If such a tear is explored at open laparotomy, death from air embolus is common. Elevation of the legs and positive-pressure ventilation can help direct such air embolism into the lower body.

Codes

Blood	10 units . . . .
GA/LA	GA . . . .
Opn time	Variable, 2−3 hours . . . .
Stay	14 days but depends on other injuries . . . .
Drains out	2−7 days . . . .
Sutures out	7 days . . . .
Off work	2−3 months . . . .

Postoperative care
If the hepatic wound has been successfully sutured or if a partial hepatectomy is performed, the postoperative course should be reasonably straightforward, depending on the other injuries.

If a pack has been inserted, this will need to be removed after about 48 hours. In the interim the urea and electrolytes, platelets and clotting screen must be measured frequently.

If there is a large haematoma within the liver substance, the progress of this haematoma can be monitored using repeat radio-isotope liver scans.

Ruptured spleen

The condition

Splenic rupture may occur as part of an abdominal compression injury or due to a localized blow over the left lower ribs. Rupture may follow trivial injury if the spleen is already enlarged, e.g. due to malaria. Occasionally an injury is sufficient to bruise the spleen but not to rupture the capsule. The haematoma thus formed may rupture after 7−10 days (delayed rupture of the spleen).

Recognizing the pattern

There is pain in the left upper quadrant together with localized tenderness and guarding. The tenderness may be more marked on inspiration. Not infrequently there is an associated fracture of the left lower ribs. The patient also complains of pain in the left shoulder tip (Kehr's sign) and both flanks may be dull to percussion with the right flank exhibiting shifting dullness (Ballance's sign).

| **Proving the** | The diagnosis of intraperitoneal bleeding can be confirmed |
| **diagnosis** | by peritoneal lavage. A straight X-ray of the abdomen may |

Proving the diagnosis The diagnosis of intraperitoneal bleeding can be confirmed by peritoneal lavage. A straight X-ray of the abdomen may show an elevation of the left hemi-diaphragm and a diffuse splenic shadow with displacement of the gastric air bubble. An ultrasound or CAT scan can be very helpful in detecting a splenic haematoma.

Management The patient is resuscitated. Continued pain, shock and abdominal distension will indicate the urgent need for laparotomy.

Operation: laparotomy for splenic injury

The abdomen is opened and blood evacuated. If possible the damaged spleen should be repaired but it is often safer to proceed to splenectomy. The spleen may be repaired by one of the following methods.

(a) Direct suture of a laceration over a haemostatic material such as Surgicel (Johnson and Johnson).

(b) Partial splenectomy. The feeding vessels of the damaged area are ligated, the damaged area excised and the cut organ repaired.

If these procedures are not possible, a splenectomy is performed. The bleeding is controlled by grasping the splenic pedicle between the fingers of one hand. The splenic artery, splenic vein and short gastric arteries are ligated and the spleen is removed. Care is taken not to damage the tail of the pancreas, the fundus of the stomach, or the splenic flexure of the colon. A drain is left in the splenic bed.

Codes

Blood	6 units	. . . .
GA/LA	GA	. . . .
Opn time	60−90 minutes	. . . .
Stay	7−10 days	. . . .
Drains out	3−7 days	. . . .
Sutures out	7 days	. . . .
Off work	About 1 month	. . . .

These figures will be prolonged by associated injury.

Postoperative care
See under splenectomy (p. 326).

Traumatic bowel injury

The condition The bowel may be damaged either by direct injury or indirectly due to damage of its feeding vessels. In the latter case there is risk of rupture some days after the initial injury.

Such injuries occur in road accidents when the bowel is crushed against the spine by a seat belt.

Recognizing the pattern

The patient with a bowel injury may have minimal signs at first and the condition may not be suspected in view of other injuries. If the patient deteriorates with increasing abdominal pain and distension after 2−3 days, think of this possibility.

Proving the diagnosis

The diagnosis is confirmed by an X-ray which shows free peritoneal gas. Aspiration of the abdomen produces bile-stained bowel contents.

Management

Ideally this is by early laparotomy and repair or resection of the damaged area together with careful exploration to exclude other abdominal trauma. In cases of multiple trauma it is permissible to leave the bowel injury for 24 hours or so while life-threatening injuries are dealt with.

Operation: small bowel resection
The damaged bowel is resected and an end-to-end anastomosis performed.

Codes
Blood .... 2 units or more depending on extent of injuries ....
GA/LA .... GA ....
Opn time .... 90−120 minutes ....
Stay .... 7 days ....
Drains out ...... Wound 48 hours, intra-abdominal 2−3 days ....
Sutures out ..... 7 days ....
Off work........ 4−6 weeks ....

Postoperative care
A nasogastric tube is aspirated regularly and the patient is kept on minimal oral fluids until flatus is passed. Anastomotic problems are rare.

Pancreatic injury

The condition

The pancreas may also be damaged by a crushing injury from a seat belt or steering wheel. There is a high amylase content in the peritoneal aspirate and the serum amylase may also be elevated. The diagnosis must be excluded by laparotomy.

Management	The pancreas is explored and sutured or partially resected. The lesser sac and pancreatic bed are drained.

Renal injury

The condition	The kidneys may be damaged by blunt injury to the loins or by compression from the front. The injury may then be extraperitoneal although in children the peritoneum is more likely to be breached as there is little perinephric fat. The renal damage may be anything from a subcapsular haematoma to a complete tear. Occasionally the renal vessels are avulsed.
Recognizing the pattern	The patient is shocked and there is tenderness in the loin. Haematuria occurs but may be delayed. There may also be clot colic. On examination a fullness in the loin may indicate a perinephric haematoma.
Proving the diagnosis	An IVP should be done urgently to demonstrate whether the damaged kidney is functioning or not and whether there is a normal kidney on the other side. Ultrasound scanning or tomography may demonstrate a haematoma. Renal artery angiography is occasionally useful.
Management	Having excluded other abdominal trauma, the initial treatment is conservative, comprising bed rest and analgesia. If there has been extravasation of urine, antibiotics such as ampicillin (500 mg 6-hourly) or co-trimoxazole (2 tablets 12-hourly) may be given. Laparotomy is indicated if there is continued uncontrolled bleeding.

Operation: laparotomy for renal injury

If possible, the damaged kidney is repaired, although a partial or complete nephrectomy is often required. A full laparotomy is undertaken to exclude other intra-abdominal injury.

Codes

Blood	6 units . . . .
GA/LA	GA . . . .
Opn time	1 – 2 hours . . . .
Stay	Depends on other injuries . . . .
Drains out	3 days — kidney bed . . . .
Sutures out	7 – 10 days . . . .
Off work	Depends on other injuries . . . .

Postoperative care
A severe ileus may occur which may need treatment with a nasogastric tube and intravenous fluids. The long-term follow-up should include a repeat IVP after 3 months to check on renal function.

12.4 Spinal and Pelvic Injuries

Fractured spine

The importance of spinal injury lies in the danger of associated trauma to the spinal cord or nerve roots. Injury is more common in the cervical or lumbar region because the vertebrae are relatively unsupported.

A stable spinal fracture will not displace further and there is no continuing danger to the spinal cord. With an unstable fracture the deformity can encroach on the vertebral canal with resulting spinal cord damage.

At the scene of the accident, before the patient is moved, a cervical collar should be applied and any movement of the spine kept to an absolute minimum.

Do not move the patient except 'as a log' until an unstable fracture has been excluded.

Recognizing the pattern

Always consider the possibility of spinal injury when a patient has suffered severe trauma.

The patient complains of severe localized pain at the site of the fracture which may radiate along the distribution of the relevant nerve roots. The patient lies still and the pain is worse on any movement. Ask if there is any numbness, tingling or weakness in the limbs.

On examination there may be visible deformity of the spine. Palpation of the vertebral spines may reveal discontinuity or displacement, and localized tenderness.

Tenderness on one side of the midline suggests muscular injury or damaged transverse processes.

If the cord has been damaged, you may find abnormalities in sensation, movement and reflexes in the limbs. In cervical injuries there may be abnormalities in the pulse, blood pressure and respiration.

Proving the diagnosis

Spinal X-rays must be done in any case of possible spinal injury. Antero-posterior and lateral views are usually taken. There are other specialist views for the odontoid peg or lumbar pedicles. A qualified doctor should be present to supervise the movement of the patient.

When inspecting X-rays check for the following.

1 Symmetry between the two sides.

2 Any incongruities in the width of the vertebral bodies.

3 Any incongruities of the joint spaces.

600

4 On the lateral view look for a step in the posterior or anterior longitudinal ligament disclosing displacement of a vertebra. Loss of this alignment and widening of the gap between the spines are typical of an unstable fracture.

5 Look carefully for evidence of injury to the bones themselves.

CAT scanning now provides an alternative to straight X-rays for radiologically inaccessible parts of the vertebral column (e.g. C7/T1 junction, thoracic vertebrae, etc.).

Management

The patient can be rolled but the head, trunk and pelvis are supported so that there is no relative movement of one vertebra on another. Support the patient between sandbags. In a case of a suspected cervical fracture, the head must be held still in slight extension and kept in a straight line with the body axis.

With muscular bruising or a fractured transverse process, the patient may be allowed home, given analgesics and advised to rest on a firm mattress for 7–10 days. Admission may be required if the pain is severe or movement severely restricted.

If there is a stable vertebral fracture, the patient is admitted, given analgesics and put on a bed with a rigid base. Two or three weeks later the patient is re-X-rayed and then mobilized slowly.

In the case of an unstable fracture consider transferring the patient to a spinal centre. External support such as a cervical collar is needed, and active reduction may be required. Skeletal traction with skull callipers is used for unstable cervical fractures. Alternatively vertebrae may be reduced and fused by open operation.

When there is damage to the spinal cord, attention must be paid to the paralysed limbs to prevent contractures or pressure sores. There may be an ileus for 3 or 4 days. A cervical cord injury may mask symptoms due to other abdominal trauma. Bladder and bowel function may need assistance.

Fractured pelvis

A fractured pelvis must always be considered and excluded after multiple trauma. External evidence of pelvic fracture may be slight but the blood loss can be considerable (e.g. 2 litres) and there is a possibility of associated visceral injury to the urethra, bladder or rectum.

Recognizing the pattern	The patient may complain of back pain, particularly if the sacro-iliac joints are involved. Movements are painful. On examination there is pain on compressing the pelvis and deformity may be visible.
Proving the diagnosis	The fracture is seen on pelvic X-ray. An IVU will exclude damage to the bladder or ureters.
Management	A careful examination should be made of both legs, particularly of the arterial supply and nerve supply. A rectal examination should be performed. Ask about bleeding from the urethra or micturition problems which may indicate associated visceral damage.

The patient may be shocked and require initial transfusion. Four units of blood should be cross-matched and a good intravenous infusion line set up.

If the pelvic ring is intact, a fracture usually occurs through either the superior or inferior pubic ramus, the ileum or the anterior inferior iliac spine. The treatment is conservative with bed rest, analgesia and lower limb exercises. The patient is mobilized as the improvement in pain permits.

A pelvis fractured in more than two places results in disruption of the pelvic ring. The management is designed to encourage closure. The patient can be supported in a pelvic sling or encased in plaster of Paris, which may be tightened by a rubber tourniquet. Upward displacement of part of the pelvis is treated by downward traction through a skeletal pin in the tibia.

Other pelvic injuries

Damage to the urethra

The condition	The urethra may be partially or completely torn. The two sites commonly affected are the membranous urethra at the apex of the prostate (following bilateral fracture of the pubic rami) or the bulbous urethra (following a blow in the perineum).
Recognizing the pattern	There is a history of inability to pass urine, meatal bleeding and a distended bladder. A high-riding, mobile prostate on rectal examination suggests a complete membranous urethral tear. When the bulbous urethra is ruptured, a tense perineal haematoma or a swollen, bruised penis and scrotum are seen.

Proving the diagnosis	If there is a high index of suspicion, the patient should be told not to pass urine. If he has already micturated, a history of painful or bloodstained micturition supports the diagnosis. An intravenous urogram should be carried out on all patients with a pelvic fracture. This should demonstrate any rupture of the membranous urethra or trauma to the bladder. If a bulbous urethral injury is suspected, a cautious attempt can be made to pass a catheter. This should be done in theatre with full aseptic technique. If the catheter passes easily, leave it in the bladder. If it does not pass easily, do not persist, as this may cause further damage and convert a partial tear into a complete one. A urethrogram may also help in suspected bulbous injury.
Management	1 Resuscitation of the patient is the first priority. The urethral repair can wait 12–24 hours if necessary. 2 Antibiotics must be started (e.g. sulphamethizole 500 mg four times a day). 3 If catheterization was not attempted, or was unsuccessful, urine is drained through a suprapubic cystostomy. 4 A ruptured membranous urethra is usually repaired around a catheter which is used as a splint. A ruptured bulbous urethra can be repaired or may be treated conservatively, in which case it should be re-assessed at 10–14 days. If there is associated rectal damage, the definitive repair is delayed until any infection has been treated. Any collection in the retropubic space, such as extravasated blood or urine, is drained. Stricture is a common sequel to any urethral trauma, and a follow-up urethrogram or urethroscopy is required. The treatment of stricture is described on p. 443.

Trauma to the bladder

The condition	There are two mechanisms of bladder injury. A direct blow to the lower abdomen, when the bladder is distended, causes the viscus to burst with leakage of urine into the peritoneum. A fractured or dislocated symphysis pubis may also pierce the bladder causing extraperitoneal leakage. When there is extraperitoneal leakage, the patient may have a strong desire to void urine but is unable to do so. Intraperitoneal leakage causes very few symptoms other than anuria, and the diagnosis may be missed, particularly in a trauma victim, where the anuria may be put down to shock.
Proving the diagnosis	The diagnosis is proved by an intravenous urogram. This should be done if there is any suspicion of bladder injury.

Management	Antibiotics should be commenced. Urgent laparotomy and repair are required. The urethra is catheterized at operation and the peritoneal and extraperitoneal spaces are drained.
	A follow-up urethroscopy must be done. Twenty per cent of patients have accompanying urethral damage and there is a risk of stricture formation.

Injuries to the rectum

These are rare. The damage is usually done by a spike of bone perforating the rectum.

Recognizing the pattern	The patient may have bleeding from the anus and shows signs of a pelvic peritonitis. Rectal examination discloses a fragment of bone in the lumen.
Management	The treatment is laparotomy, repair of the rectal tear and a defunctioning colostomy.

Damage to blood vessels

Management	The internal or external iliac artery can be damaged by a spike of bone.
	The artery is either repaired or ligated. The procedure may involve considerable blood loss and 6−10 pints of blood should be cross-matched.

Nervous injury

The sciatic nerve may be damaged by a traction force or posterior dislocation of the hip. This is usually neuropraxia or axonotmesis (see p. 612) with eventual recovery. Severe disruption of the sacro-iliac joints can cause a nerve root injury where the damage is permanent.

Recognizing the pattern	The hamstrings are paralysed with marked weakness of knee flexion. All the muscles of the lower leg and foot are paralysed and the presenting sign is of foot drop. There is a partial or complete loss of sensation down the leg, apart from the medial surface which is supplied by the long saphenous nerve (a branch of the femoral nerve).
Management	Neuropraxia or axonotmesis should eventually recover. Meanwhile, physiotherapy to the limb maintains the mobility and prevents any contracture deformity. The nerve must be explored if it is thought likely that it is severed, but this is unusual.

Injury to the hip joint

Fractures involving disruption of the acetabulum may later result in osteoarthritis. This risk is lessened if an accurate reduction of the fracture is achieved.

The management of wounds

The management of skin wounds depends on whether they are clean or contaminated and whether the skin edges are intact (incisional wound) or damaged (crushed or torn wound). There may also be skin loss. The aim is to heal the wound as perfectly as possible and prevent secondary infection by pyogenic bacteria or organisms causing gas gangrene and tetanus.

Assessment

Ask the patient how it happened and how long ago. Is it known to be clean or dirty? Could there be any foreign body in the wound? Ask if the patient has been immunized against tetanus, and if so when the last injection of tetanus toxoid was given. (Tetanus prophylaxis is dealt with on p. 608.) Examine the wound edges and look for evidence of contamination or infection. Examine closely for any injury to underlying arteries, nerves or tendons, especially in the hand.

Management

All wounds are carefully cleaned and debrided, removing dead tissue and foreign matter. Haemostasis is secured. Further management depends on the age of the wound and whether it is contaminated or not.

History of less than 8 hours
A *clean or lightly contaminated* wound is then closed in layers by primary suture. If the skin defect cannot be closed, the area may be covered by a split skin graft (see below). Antibiotics (amoxycillin and flucloxacillin) are given if the wound is lightly contaminated rather than clean.
   A *heavily contaminated* wound is then left open and dressed. Antibiotics are given as above. It is then re-examined in 3–5 days and if no infection is present the edges are cleaned and the wound closed by delayed primary suture.

History of more than 8 hours
A *clean* wound cannot be closed as it must be assumed that any potential infection has become established. It should be either treated with delayed primary suture, or closed with drainage, and antibiotic cover given.
   A *heavily contaminated or infected* wound is packed and dressed. It is redressed daily after cleaning with Eusol until

the infection has cleared. Then, usually 10 days later, the wound is opened, the granulation tissue removed, the skin edges cleaned and the wound closed by secondary suture. Skin defects are closed by split skin grafts.

Operation: simple suture of a skin wound

The skin is cleaned with a suitable agent (e.g. chlorhexidine, cetrimide or povidone iodine). The area is draped off and local anaesthetic is injected around the edges of the wound, using a puncture site outside the wound. The skin edges are debrided of all dead and contaminated tissue. The wound edges are then opposed, using interrupted mattress sutures. In the head and neck multiple small sutures are used so as to minimize 'cross-hatching' in the scar later.

Codes

Blood..........	0...............................
GA/LA........	LA............................
Opn time.......	30−60 minutes..................
Stay..........	Variable.......................
Drains out......	3−5 days......................
Sutures out.....	Head and neck 3−4 days, elsewhere 5−7 days, if the wound is under tension 10−14 days.............
Off work........	Variable.......................

Operation: split skin graft

Donor sites are usually the upper arm or thigh and a graft may be taken using a special knife, under a local or general anaesthetic. It is important to learn how to do this and this is best done by observation and assisting an experienced surgeon. The donor site is dressed with tulle gras and left for 10 days. The split skin graft is placed raw face uppermost on tulle gras and then cut to size. Haemostasis in the recipient area is important to prevent blood from lifting the graft. If a mesh graft is used, a larger area can be covered and any haematoma can escape through the holes in the graft. The graft is applied and stitched at the edges with silk, one end of each stitch being left long to tie over a sponge or pad soaked in antiseptic lotion.

Codes

Blood..........	0...............................
GA/LA........	GA or LA.......................
Opn time.......	30 minutes to 2 hours depending on size of graft...................
Stay..........	7−10 days depending on size of graft.

Drains out ...... 0 ....

Sutures out ..... 7–10 days ....

Off work .... Variable ....

Postoperative care

The top ties are divided and the tulle gras and sponge removed at between 5 and 7 days. The graft can then be inspected and if healing is satisfactory the rest of the sutures are removed.

Tetanus prophylaxis

Tetanus is a disease characterized by muscle spasm caused by the toxin of *Clostridium tetani*, a Gram-positive, anaerobic, sporing bacillus. The spores appear in animal faeces and therefore contaminate earth. Extensive wounds with heavy contamination are typically affected, although tetanus can follow small penetrating injuries. Active immunization with toxoid is now a routine part of the triple vaccine given to children. A booster dose should be given every 10 years. The organism is sensitive to penicillin, metronidazole or tetracycline.

A high-risk wound is one that is heavily contaminated, deep and more than 8 hours old, and contains dead tissue.

Management

Surgical debridement and toilet must be performed for all wounds.

The type of tetanus prophylaxis given depends on the nature and age of the wound and the immune category of the patient. The measures available include the following:

(a) a booster dose of tetanus toxoid;

(b) a complete course of tetanus toxoid;

(c) penicillin;

(d) antitetanus globulin.

1 Patients with active immunity who have received a dose of toxoid within the last 5 years need no further prophylaxis.

2 Patients who last had toxoid more than 5 years ago require a tetanus toxoid booster and, if the wound is old or deep, or contamination is present, a course of penicillin.

3 Non-immune patients should be given a tetanus toxoid course and a course of penicillin for all but the most minor wounds.

4 Human antitetanus globulin has been produced for passive immunity but it is rarely used now because it is expensive, not readily available and not without risks.

Hand injuries

These are commonly seen in casualty. The importance of

careful assessment, particularly of associated injury to artery, tendon or nerve, has been mentioned. The hand should be cleaned, cooled and elevated and interference kept to a minimum. Severe hand injuries should be referred for a consultant plastic surgeon's opinion. Amputated finger tips are commonly seen. If the bone is exposed it is best trimmed back and the tip covered with a split skin graft. If the wound is less than 1 cm in diameter and particularly in children, re-epithelialization will be satisfactory. If a whole finger has been amputated, re-implantation is possible. The finger should be cooled and the patient referred to a microsurgery unit.

The management of fractures

This section covers the general principles of fracture management as far as these may be required by the general surgical houseman treating a patient with multiple trauma. For the management of specific fractures the reader is referred to a textbook of orthopaedics.

Individual fractures may be either simple (closed) when the skin is intact, or compound (open) when the skin surface over the fracture has been broken. Other terms which may be applied to fractures describe the type of break as either transverse, spiral, oblique or comminuted (see Fig. 108).

Recognizing the pattern

The history
The patient complains of localized pain at the fracture site and is unable to use the affected limb. The mechanism of

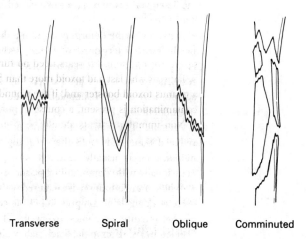

Transverse   Spiral   Oblique   Comminuted

Fig. 108 Types of fracture.

injury should be ascertained as this will give a clue to the type of fracture expected.

On examination
There is swelling, bony deformity and loss of function of the affected limb. Abnormal mobility and crepitus at the fracture site may provide incontrovertible evidence of a fracture.

Note whether there is a skin wound. If there is, the fracture must be regarded as compound whether or not the bone is visible.

Management

The precise management depends on the site of the fracture and other associated injuries. In general, however, the steps in management of any fracture are as follows.

1 *Resuscitation and temporary splinting.* Fractures of long bones are associated with a significant blood loss which may require replacement. The pain resulting from a fracture is extreme and analgesic therapy is important. A temporary splint gives relief and protects against further damage whilst the patient is transferred to hospital and to the X-ray department.

2 *X-ray.* Having detected the sites of fractures by clinical methods, an X-ray is essential to define exactly what injury has been sustained.

3 *Repair of skin wounds.* Any skin wound must be carefully cleaned and all dirt and devitalized tissue must be removed. Associated arterial, nerve and tendon injuries will need to be repaired (see pp. 612–614). The method of wound closure will depend on the time after the injury and the extent of contamination. Clean, recent wounds may be closed immediately, others may have to be closed by delayed primary suture.

4 *Reduction.* If the deformity is putting the overlying skin or neighbouring artery or nerve under pressure, then reduction is urgent. Otherwise it can be delayed whilst more general resuscitative measures are carried out. Reduction may be achieved by closed manipulation under anaesthesia or by open operation.

5 *Fixation.* The aim is to maintain the position of the reduced bone ends until they heal together. External immobilization is usually achieved with plaster of Paris or occasionally with aluminium or plastic splints.

When immobilization is achieved with plaster of Paris, there is a danger of compression of the contents of the limb as the fracture continues to swell. This danger can be avoided by using an initial 'back slab' which can if necessary be completed later. If a complete plaster has to be applied, it must not be too tight and should contain plenty of padding to allow the fracture to swell. A routine 'plaster check' must be carried out after 24 hours and the circulation in the distal limb assessed. If there is any evidence of occlusion, then the plaster must be removed.

Another form of immobilization is the application of traction on each side of the fracture. This may be applied either to the skin or to a pin passed through the skeleton (e.g. a tibial pin for reduction of a fractured femur).

Internal fixation is used when the fracture is reduced by open operation. The bone ends are fixed either by a device placed within the cortex (intramedullary nail, screws or wires) or by a pin and plate placed on the outer cortex.

6 *Rehabilitation.* Any prolonged immobilization of the limb will lead to muscle wasting and joint stiffness. Regular physiotherapy is important, therefore, both during the period of immobilization and once the fracture has healed.

Fat embolism

The condition

Fat embolism is more common than generally supposed and occurs when droplets of fat get into the bloodstream. The fat may be derived from bone marrow or adipose tissue but may also be of metabolic origin, perhaps by aggregation of chylomicrons. The emboli may lodge in the pulmonary circulation or pass through the lungs and lodge in parts of the systemic circulation such as the brain, skin and kidney.

Recognizing the pattern

The patient
The patient is often a young adult with a lower limb fracture, but the condition can also occur in those with severe burns or extensive soft tissue trauma.

The history
There is sudden onset of respiratory distress, drowsiness, restlessness or disorientation 24 to 48 hours following injury.

On examination
Mild pyrexia and tachycardia are early signs. Petechial haemorrhage due to skin emboli is a helpful sign but may not be present. Cyanosis and right heart failure may occur in severe cases.

Proving the diagnosis

Fat droplets may be found in the sputum and urine. The platelet count is invariably low. An arterial blood gas sample will show hypoxaemia, which is the major cause of death. A chest radiograph shows a 'snow-storm' appearance.

Management	Oxygen should be given. Other measures which have been advocated include heparinization and intravenous low-molecular-weight dextran. Severe respiratory distress may require sedation and assisted ventilation.

Arterial damage

The condition	Arteries may be damaged by direct trauma transecting the vessel, by external compression (e.g. from a nearby fracture) or by traction which disrupts the intima. This latter injury is often followed by thrombosis and occlusion of the vessel, even though the outer wall of the artery is intact.
Recognizing the pattern	Penetrating arterial injury is unmistakable. Bright red pulsatile blood escapes from the wound. With an acute arterial occlusion the patient complains of pain in the muscles distal to the damaged vessel. The affected tissues are pale and cold and there are paraesthesiae and paralysis. Distal pulses are absent.
Proving the diagnosis	An emergency arteriogram may be indicated.
Management	An occlusion of a main limb artery needs urgent exploration and repair.

Operation: exploration of traumatic arterial occlusion
The artery is exposed and the site of damage identified. If the artery has been transected, the damaged ends are resected and a vein graft used to bridge the gap created. Attention must also be paid to any venous damage.

If the artery is intact, then an occlusion is due either to external compression or to an intimal tear. If any external compression has been relieved and the distal pulses do not return, an arteriotomy is performed and the damaged segment either excised or bypassed.

Codes
Blood . . . .   2–4 units . . . .
GA/LA . . . .   GA . . . .
Opn time . . . .   1–2 hours . . . .
Stay . . . .   Depends on other injuries . . . .
Drains out . . . . . .   Suction drain 48 hours . . . .
Sutures out . . . . .   7 days . . . .
Off work . . . .   Depends on other injuries . . . .

Nerve injuries

The condition	There are three types of nerve injury.

1 *Neuropraxia.* This is caused by a blunt injury resulting in concussion of the nerve.
2 *Axonotmesis.* This is caused by a stretching injury which ruptures the axons but not the nerve sheath. The axons degenerate distal to the injury.
3 *Neurotmesis.* This is complete severance of the nerve and its sheath.

Recognizing the pattern

The clinical signs of nerve injury are loss of sensation and flaccid paralysis with loss of reflexes. The precise clinical picture depends on the particular nerve which is damaged.

Management

1 Neuropraxia and axonotmesis
If the injury is a neuropraxia, the treatment is conservative and the nerve usually recovers in 7–10 days. Axonotmesis takes longer because the axons have to grow back down the intact nerve sheath. Physiotherapy is required to prevent contractures and maintenance of normal posture until renervation occurs. The patient needs adequate reassurance and should be told that the nerves grow at the rate of about 1 mm/day (or 1 inch/month). Several weeks may therefore be needed for recovery of an axonotmesis in a limb.
2 Neurotmesis
When a nerve has been divided, the wound must be carefully explored to identify the nerve ends. These should be freshened and the nerve sheath resutured accurately to restore continuity. If this is done with care, there is a good chance that the axons will regrow down the distal nerve sheath. They regrow at the rate above.

Digital nerves
A divided digital nerve can be repaired using a microsurgical technique. Digital nerve injuries in the dominant hand involving the thumb, index or middle finger cause serious disabilities and an attempt should be made to repair these.

Tendon injuries

The condition

Tendons may be partially or completely severed in a laceration injury. Such tendon injuries are commonly seen after cuts over the dorsum of the fingers, back of the hand or the wrist. Careful repair is essential.

Making the diagnosis

Complete division of a tendon is made obvious by the loss of function of the affected muscle. Where there is a laceration over the anatomical site of a tendon, careful examination of the function of the extensors and flexors should be carried out.

Management   The treatment of partial or complete tendon rupture is surgical repair. The wound should be explored under a general anaesthetic. If necessary the patient can wait 6−8 hours until the next morning's operating list, providing there is no associated arterial injury. A partial division of a tendon can be repaired by a continuous suture of fine prolene or other similar material. A complete division needs end-to-end anastomosis.

Postoperative care

The limb is splinted so as to relax the affected tendon and minimize any tension across the suture line. Active physiotherapy is commenced at 10−14 days.

Burns

The condition   Major burns are a threat to life. Deterioration can be rapid and the management in the acute stage is critical.

There are five types of burns.

1 Dry thermal − flame.
2 Wet thermal − scald.
3 Chemical.
4 Electrical.
5 Friction.

The damage is caused by coagulation of proteins with cell death. Burns can be of varying depth and any one burn is rarely uniform.

A mild burn causes vasodilatation and diffuse erythema. Kinins are released which cause pain.

Moderate burns cause some cell death with increased capillary permeability and blister and oedema formation. Sensation remains intact and as these burns are of partial thickness the skin will regrow.

Severe burns cause death of cells involving the dermis and deeper tissues, and appear as white insensitive areas. The full thickness of the skin is damaged and the skin will not regrow as the germinal layers have been destroyed. Such a burn heals by fibrosis with resulting contractures.

The main early danger from major burns is the development of 'burn shock'. Burn shock is due to exudation of protein-rich fluid from the surface of the burn and oedema into the tissues beneath the burn. Both these follow increased capillary permeability. The loss of fluid results in hypovolaemia which can develop rapidly, the extent depending on the size of the burn. A patient with 50% burns, for instance, can lose half his plasma volume within 3−4 hours. This fluid loss must be replaced rapidly.

Anaemia can develop due to blood loss, red cell destruction and bone marrow suppression.

Later on the damaged and necrotic tissue, lying in a protein-rich exudate, is an ideal site for infection, which can result in septicaemia.

Assessment

The precise history of the time and cause of the burn must be obtained, including the length of time that the causative agent was active. A rapid initial examination is performed to assess the following.

1 Signs of shock — apprehension, restlessness, thirst, pallor, sweating, tachycardia, hypotension and air hunger.

2 Whether or not the airway is affected by an inhalation burn — stridor, hoarseness, soot in nostrils, pharnygeal erythema.

3 The size of the burn (see Fig. 109). The area of the burn is expressed as a percentage of the total body surface area. It is calculated using 'Wallace's rule of nines' as in the figure. It may be useful to remember that the hand represents 1% of the adult body surface area.

This initial assessment allows burns to be divided into minor or major categories.

Minor burns

These are burns involving less than 10−15% of the adult body surface area (less than 10% in children), with little evidence of systemic upset or disturbance of the airway.

On examination
Draw the size of the burn and map out the areas of definite full thickness, probable full thickness and partial thickness. These are judged by the appearance (erythema, blistering or white areas), and the presence or absence of sensation to pin-prick.

Management

Different centres have different regimes. Below is one possible scheme of management.

1 Local management
(a) Superficial burns of the face and superficial scalds are left exposed to the air. They heal in 10−14 days.
(b) Partial-thickness burns cause erythema and superficial blistering with no break in the skin. They are cleaned with an antiseptic agent and dressed with tulle gras. They are then re-examined in 3−5 days. Check that no areas have become full-thickness. The wounds are then redressed and the burns usually heal with little scarring.

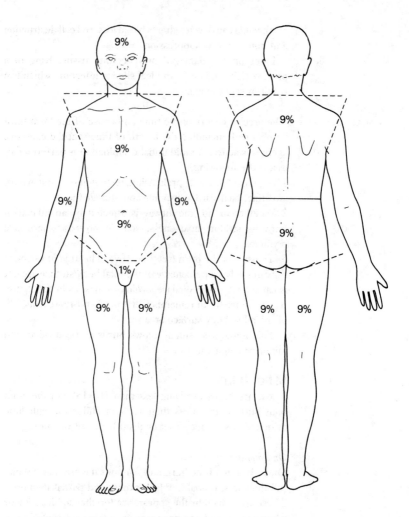

'Wallace's Rule of Nines' (eleven areas of the body, each equal to about 9% of the total surface area).

Fig. 109 A method for measuring the extent of burns on the body surface area.

(c) Deeper burns. Burns with skin loss or those which are dirty must be cleaned with an antiseptic solution and all dirt, large blisters and dead tissue removed. The burn may then be coated liberally with Flamazine cream. This cream contains sulphadiazine and is useful in preventing infection, especially by Gram-negative organisms. It is also useful in treating infected burns. The Flamazine-coated burn is dressed with gauze and ideally is redressed daily. This cream also has a soothing effect. The cream must not be used when a second assessment is required as it is difficult to examine the burn once it has been applied.

(d) Full-thickness burns. These heal by fibrosis, causing contractures and scarring, and are best treated by skin grafting. This is done either at 3–5 days or after 3 weeks when the burnt skin is sloughing.

2 Oral fluids

Those containing sodium are sufficient to counteract any mild hypovolaemia.

Major burns

A burn is described as major when the area involved is more than 15% of the body surface area (10% in children). The Regional Burns Centre should be contacted regarding all major burns.

Management

The main priority is maintenance of the airway and prevention of circulatory collapse. While this is undertaken, the burn is covered with sterile towels.

1 Airway

If the airway is obstructed or the patient has inhaled soot, pass an airway or endotracheal tube. If severe respiratory damage has occurred, an early tracheostomy may be indicated.

2 Analgesia

Burns are very painful and adequate analgesia must be given. Intravenous morphine (0.1 mg/kg) gives instant pain relief. Intravenous chlorpromazine (0.5 mg/kg) sedates the patient and acts as an anti-emetic.

3 Fluid replacement

Delay in replacing the fluid lost can lead to rapid deterioration, renal failure and death.

Set up at least one intravenous infusion with a wide-gauge cannula. Avoid using a CVP line if possible, due to the risk of infection. Catheterize the patient to monitor the urine output.

During cannulation take blood for haemoglobin, haematocrit, urea and electrolytes and serum for grouping and crossmatching blood.

Calculation of fluid deficit

There are many formulae to help you do this. The one below (the Mount Vernon formula) is commonly used and estimates the volume of plasma (colloid) required to replace the predicted plasma loss. Different formulae are required if crystalloid is used, as more fluid will then be needed.

The first 36 hours after the burn are divided up into six 'time units', as shown in Fig. 110. A similar volume of fluid is given for each 'time unit'. This volume of fluid is calculated from the patient's weight and the area of the burn, as follows:

Plasma volume required for each time unit

$$= \frac{\% \text{ Area} \times \text{weight (kg)}}{2} \text{ cm}^3.$$

For example a 50% burn in a 70 kg man needs 1.75 litres of plasma in each time unit.

You will note that the time units immediately after the burn are much shorter than those later on. The first 12 hours is the critical period. If therapy is not started until 4 hours after a burn, then the fluid deficit must also be replaced. Therefore the calculated volume required for the first 12 hours must be given in the remaining 8 hours.

One of the problems with a formula that predicts the rate of plasma loss is that, if fluid replacement is not started early, the patient will become hypovolaemic and this in itself will reduce the rate of fluid loss. The above formula will then over-estimate the plasma requirements. In this situation the actual (static) plasma deficit may be calculated using the haematocrit, as follows:

Static plasma deficit =

$$\text{blood volume} - \frac{\text{blood volume} \times \text{normal haematocrit}}{\text{measured haematocrit}}$$

For example, knowing the normal blood volume (5 litres) and haematocrit (44) for a 70 kg man, if the above patient's haematocrit was 60, four hours after the burn, then the *actual* plasma deficit is 1334 ml. The *predicted* loss was 1750 ml.

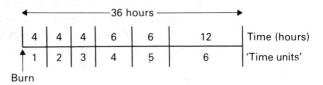

←			36 hours			→	
4	4	4	6	6	12		Time (hours)
↑ 1	2	3	4	5	6		'Time units'

Burn

Fig. 110.

This method gives a prediction of the patient's fluid requirement, and frequent clinical observations must be made to check on the patient's fluid status and urine output. Serial haematocrit estimations are invaluable. As a result of this reassessment, the amount of fluid required in each time unit can be modified accordingly.

Blood requirements
Blood replacement will be required if the burn is deep and more than 10% of the body area. Then, for each 1% burn, give 1% of the patient's total blood volume. The above patient would need 2.5 litres of blood. The blood is usually given in the sixth time unit instead of the equivalent amount of plasma. If the burn is 25% or more, it may be given in the second and sixth time units.

An extensive burn causes an ileus and the patient is not, therefore, able to take oral fluids. In this case the standard body requirements for water and electrolytes must be added to the burn formula regime.

4 Infection
Systemic antibiotics are usually given in extensive burns prophylactically. Penicillin and flucloxacillin are suitable.

The local management of the burn itself has been described on p. 615.

Management of burns in special sites
In deep circumferential burns of the limb or chest, the tight burnt skin may occlude the blood supply to the extremities or affect respiration. The burnt skin must be divided along the length of the limb or in a criss-cross pattern on the chest wall, to release this constricting pressure.

Burns around the eye rapidly result in extensive periorbital oedema. It is therefore essential to examine the eye early before the palpable fissure closes. If the eyelids have been destroyed, the eye must be bathed with artificial tears and the eyelids restored by plastic surgery at the earliest opportunity to prevent corneal scarring.

Burns of the head and neck with severe facial oedema or evidence of inhalation of soot or hot gases require urgent tracheostomy.

Severe burns to the hands must be cleaned, dressed with tulle gras, and elevated to minimize oedema. The patient should be referred to a plastic surgeon.

List of Surgical Procedures

Adrenal glands
  bilateral adrenalectomy for breast cancer
    220
  tumours
    adrenalectomy for Conn's syndrome
      332–3
    adrenalectomy for Cushing's syndrome
      331–2
    excision of a phaeochromocytoma 329–30
Appendicectomy 335–6
Arteries see vascular operations

Bladder
  catherization
    suprapubic 432–3
    via the urethra 431–2
  diverticula resection 424
  stones
    cystostomy 422–3
    litholapaxy 422
  tumours
    cystoscopy and examination under
      anaesthesia 426–7
    Helmstein's procedure 428
    partial cystectomy 428–9
    total cystectomy 429
    trans-urethral resection of tumours
      (TURT) 427–8
  urethro-cystoscopy 430
Bowel
  colon
    colostomy closure 358, 359
    Hartmann's procedure 357, 363
    laparotomy for acute diverticulitis 366
    left hemicolectomy 356
    Paul–Mickulicz procedure 356–7
    right hemicolectomy 354–5
    transverse colectomy 359
    transverse loop colostomy 357–8
  external intestinal fistulae excision 77
  laparotomy for ischaemic 341–2
  malrotation and intestinal obstruction 562
  obstruction 339
  rectum
    abdomino-perineal resection 362–3
    anterior resection 357, 362
    Delorme's procedure for prolapse 370
    injection in children for prolapse 554
    Ivalon sponge repair for prolapse 370–1
    local resection for carcinoma 361
    Thiersch wire for prolapse 369–70
  small intestine
    duodenal atresia 558
    ileostomy for meconium ileus 563–4
    intestinal atresia 560
    intussusception reduction 548
    Meckel's diverticulum 340
    resection 597
    resection for Crohn's disease 344

Breasts
  cancer
    radical mastectomy 216–17
    simple mastectomy 215–16
    wide local excision 215
  drainage of abscesses 225
  lump biopsy 204
  mammodochectomy 223–4
  microdochectomy 223
  subareolar mastectomy for gynaecomastia
    227–8

Carotid body tumours, removal 146–7
Cervical ribs, removal 150
Charles' operation 511
Chest
  exploratory thoracotomy for penetrating
    injuries 592
  insertion of drains 231–4
  median sternotomy 235
  thoracotomy 235
Colon
  loop ileostomy 349
  panproctocolectomy and terminal ileostomy
    348–9
  total colectomy and ileo-rectal
    anastomosis 349
Commando operation 195

Delorme's procedure for prolapse 370
Diaphragm, drainage of subphrenic abscesses
  73–4

Fogarty catheter embolectomy 495

Gall bladder
  cholecystectomy and exploration of common
    bile duct 289–91
  laparoscopic cholecystectomy 291
Genitalia, male
  epididymal cyst excision 458
  herniotomy in children 550–1
  hydrocele removal 456–7
  operation for varicocoele 467
  penis
    circumcision 448–9
    complete amputation 451
    partial amputation 450–1
  testes
    correction of torsion 466
    exploration – ?orchidectomy 460–1
    orchidopexy (dartos pouch procedure)
      453–4
    subcapsular orchidectomy 441–2
Groin
  block dissection 528–9
  see also hernia repair

Hartmann's procedure 357, 363

Head, cranial burr holes   582–3
Heller's operation   247–8
Helmstein's procedure   428
Hernia repair
  epigastric   401
  femoral   394–5
  herniotomy in children   550–1
  incisional   398–400
  inguinal   391–2
  obturator   402–3
  para-umbilical   400
  Spigelian   401–2
  strangulated   397
  umbilical   552
Highly selective vagotomy   270, 272–3
Homan's operation   511

Isulinoma excision   313–14

Jaundice, obstructive   296

Kidneys
  laparotomy for renal injury   598–9
  nephrectomy   415–16
  nephro-ureterectomy   413–14
  stone removal   411–12
  transplantation   419–20
  ureteral stones
    endoscopic removal   410
    uretero-lithotomy   410–11

Laparoscopic cholecystectomy   291
Limbs
  amputations
    above knee   486
    below knee   486
    ray   487
    Syme's   487
    toe   488
    transmetatarsal   487
  vascular operations see under vascular operations
Litholapaxy   422
Liver
  abscess drainage   74–5
  laparotomy for ruptured   594–5
  resection   308–9
  transplantation   310–11
Lord's stretch   381–2, 385
Lymph nodes, cervical, biopsy   153
Lymphoedema, Charles' operation and Homan's
  operation   511

Meckel's diverticulum   340
Mouth
  excision of dermoid cysts   181
  removal of mucous retention cysts   179–80
  wedge excision of lip carcinoma   185–6

Nails
  avulsion of the big toenails   538
  incision and drainage of a paronychia   540–1
  radical nail bed ablation   538–40
  wedge excision   540
Neck
  block dissection   194–5
  excision of cystic hygroma   156
  laryngotomy   236

pharyngeal pouch excision   148–9
removal of branchial cysts   145–6
removal of branchial fistulae/sinuses   144
tracheostomy   236–7

Oesophagus
  atresia repair   557–8
  dilatation of strictures   246
  fibroscopy   239–40
  Heller's operation for achalasia   247–8
  intubation of carcinoma of   255–7
  perforation repair   243
  rigid oesophagoscopy   240–1
  surgical bypass   258
  surgical resection
    oesophago-gastrectomy   252, 253–4
    pharyngo-laryngo-oesophagectomy   252–3
    total oesophagectomy   252, 253
    transection   306
  varices
    oversewing   305
    sclerotherapy   299
Ovaries, bilateral oophorectomy   219–20

Pancreas
  bypass operation for carcinoma   317, 318
  distal pancreatectomy   316, 317
  insulinoma excision   313–14
  pancreatic duct stricture   324–5
  pseudocyst drainage   323
  Whipple's operation   316–18
Parathyroid adenoma, neck exploration for
  176–7
Parotidectomy, superficial   139–40
Paul–Mickulicz procedure   356–7
Perianal region
  anal stretch (Lord's stretch)   381–2, 385
  banding of piles   385
  drainage of abscesses   377–8
  haemorrhoidectomy   385–6
  high perianal fistulae   380
  injection of piles   384–5
  laying open of fistulae   380
  sphincterotomy   382
Phenol injection   535–6
Portacaval shunts
  distal spleno-renal shunt (Warren shunt)   300,
    301
  mesenterico-caval shunt   301–3
  portacaval anastomosis   299–301
  spleno-renal anastomosis   300, 301
Prostate gland
  radical prostatectomy   442–3
  retropubic prostatectomy (Millin's)   438–9
  subcapsular orchidectomy   441–2
  transurethral resection   437
  transvesical prostatectomy   437–8
  trans-urethral resection of tumours (TURT)
    427–8

Ramstedt's operation   546

Skin
  axillary sweat glands excision   542
  basal cell carcinoma excision   531
  benign naevus removal   526–7
  dermoid cyst excision   521

ganglion removal   522
incision and drainage of abscesses   533
lipoma removal   518
malignant melanoma excision   528
neurofibroma excision   523−4
operation for pilonidal sinuses   534−5
papilloma removal   516
phenol injection of pilonidal sinuses   535−6
resuture of abdominal wounds   *70*, 71
sebaceous cyst excision   519−20
simple suture of a wound   607
split skin grafts   607−8
Spleen
    laparotomy for injury to   596
    splenectomy   326−7
Stomach
    highly selective vagotomy   *271*, 273
    partial gastrectomy
        for stomach cancer   282
        for ulcers   266−8, *270*
    pyloric stenosis, Ramstedt's operation   546
    thoraco-abdominal gastrectomy   283
    total gastrectomy   283
    transection   306
    truncal vagotomy and antrectomy   *270*, 271−2
    truncal vagotomy and drainage   271, *272*
Submandibular duct, stone removal   142
Submandibular gland, removal   142−3
Sweat glands, excision of axillary   542

Thiersch wire for prolapse   369−70
Thyroid gland
    excision of thyroglossal cysts   172
    thyroidectomy
        hemi-thyroidectomy   165−6
        subtotal   163−4
        total   166
Toes, amputation   488
Tongue
    block dissection of the neck   194−5
    commando operation   195
    hemi-glossectomy   194
    partial glossectomy for carcinoma   194
Transplantation   310−11

Trans-urethral resection of tumours
    (TURT)   427−8

Umbilicus
    exploration   403
    operation for umbilical discharge   552
    repair of umbilical hernia   551−2
Urethra
    catheterization   431−2
    dilatation   444−5
    internal urethrotomy   444
    open urethroplasty   445
    urethro-cystoscopy   430

Vascular operations
    aortic aneurysm replacement   491−2
    for arterio-venous fistulae   497
    artero-iliac endarterectomy or bypass   481−2
    axillo-femoral bypass   484, *485*
    cardiopulmonary bypass   62
    carotid artery endarterectomy   500
    cervical sympathectomy   502
    Charles's operation and Homan's operation
        for lymphoedema   511
    exploration of traumatic arterial occulusion
        612
    femoro-femoral bypass   484, *485*
    femoro-popliteal bypass   482−*3*
    Fogarty catheter embolectomy   495
    inflow stasis pulmonary embolectomy   61−2
    injection sclerotherapy   506
    injection sympathectomy   481
    lumbar sympathectomy   481
    profundaplasty   483−4
    repair of ruptured aortic aneurysms   493
    for varicose veins   506−7
Veins *see* vascular operations

Warren shunt   *300*, 301
Whipple's operation   316−18
Wounds
    resuture of abdominal   *70*, 71
    simple suture of   607

Index

Abdomen 8
  postoperative sepsis *69*
  resuture of wounds 71
  trauma 539−9
Abdominal pain *261*
  central 334−45
  referred skeletal pain 371−2
  upper 261−2
Abscesses
  alveolar 182−3
  breast 224−5
  hepatic 74−5
  pelvic 75
  perianal 375−8
  skin 533
  subphrenic 72−4
Accidents, major 569−72
Achalasia, oesophageal 238, 239, 246−8
Acid phosphatase, prostatic carcinoma 440−1
Adamantinomas 184−5
Adenocarcinomas
  bladder 424, 428−9
  thyroid 168−9
Adenolymphomas 138
Adenomas
  accessory pleomorphic 183−4
  adrenal 330, 332
  multiple endocrine 177
  parathyroid 173, 174, 175
Adhesions, intestinal 339
Admissions, patient 4−9
Adrenal tumours 328−33
Adrenalectomy 220, 331−3
AIDS patients 30−2
Airways obstruction 235−7, 570
Alimentary system, history 5
Allergies, preoperative assessment 6
Aminoglutethamide 219
Amputation
  limb 485−7
  prophylactic antibiotics *108*
  toes 488
Anaesthesia, respiratory diseases 16−17
Anaesthetists 11, 13
Anal canal, anatomy 375
Anal fissures 381−2
Anal stretch 381−2, 385
Analgesics 101−4
Anaphylactic shock 53
Aneurysms, arterial 489−94
Angina 21
Angiography, digital subtraction 475
Angioplasty, balloon 480
Ankle-brachial pressure index *476*
Antibiotics *106*−7
  bowel preparation 111
  for a fever 10
  prophylactic 22−3, 107, *108*

Anticoagulants 11, 28−9, 107−10
  for deep vein thrombosis 57
  for pulmonary emboli 60−1
Antithyroid drugs 162
Anuria 43, *65*, 429−30
Anus
  imperforate *565*−6
  pain around *375*−87
Appendicectomy *335*−6
Appendicitis, acute 334−6
Arrhythmias 22
Arteries
  acute embolisms 494−5
  aneurysms 489−94
  arterio-venous fistulae 496−7
  carotid artery disease 498−500
  damage 612
  exploration of traumatic occlusion 612
  investigation of disease 475−*7*
  replacement 480
  thoracic aorta rupture 590
Arteriography 475
Aspirin 103
Asthma 19−20
Atresia
  intestinal 555, 558−9, 560
  oesophageal 556−8
Audit, surgical 131−2
Axonotmesis 613

Balanoposthitis (balanitis) 446−7
Ballance's sign 595
Barium enemas 351, 548
Barium swallow 250
Barrett's oesophagus 249
Bassini repair 391
Bed sores 77
Beta blockade 162−3
Bile *292*
  vomiting 284−5
Bile duct surgery 289−91
Bladder
  cystoscopy and examination 426−7
  diverticula 423−4
  stones 421−3, 430
  traumatic damage 603−4
  tumours 424−9, 430
Blood
  culture for septicaemia 78
  preoperative requirements 14−*15*
  requirements, burns 619
  sugar estimation 24
  transfusion reactions 52−3
Blood vessels, traumatic damage 604
Boils 533
Bougies *255*
Bowel
  change in habit 350−2

ischaemic 340−2
obstruction 337−9, 340
congenital 555−6
preparation for surgery 110−11
traumatic injury 596−7
Bowen's disease 530
Brain, pathology of injury 570, 573−4
Branchial sinuses/fistulae 143−4
Breasts 199−200
abscesses 224−5
carcinoma 212−13
in male patients 226
management of advanced 218−21
management of early 214−18
metastatic spread 202, 213
diffuse lumpiness 207
lumps 206−11
assessment 200−5
management 205
lymphatic drainage 202
male, conditions of 226−8
nipple discharge 201, 209, 222−4
pain in 206, 209, 224−5
reconstruction 217−18
Breathlessness, postoperative 40−1
'Brompton's cocktail' 104
Bronchi, rupture 590
Bronchopneumonia 47−8
Buerger's test 472
Buprenorphine 104
Burns 93, 614−19
Bypass 479
aorto-iliac 481−2
axillo-femoral 484, 485
cardiopulmonary 62
femoro-femoral 484, 485
femoro-popliteal 482−3
pancreatic carcinoma 317, 318

Calcium 175
Carbuncles 536
Carcinoid syndrome 345
Carcinoid tumours 344−5
Carcinoma
adenoid cystic 138
adrenal 333
anaplastic 169
bladder 424−9
breast 212−21
male 226
colon 350, 353−9
lip 185
maxillary antrum 187
oesophagus 238−9, 249−58
pancreas 314−18
papillary 168−9
penis 449−51
prostatic 439−43
rectal 359−63
skin 530−2
stomach 281−3
thyroid 167−70
tongue 192−5
Cardiopulmonary bypass 62
Cardiovascular disorders 5, 7, 20−3
postoperative 51−62
Carotid artery disease 498−500

Carotid body tumours 146−7
CAT scans 577, 579
Catheterization, urinary 35, 63, 64, 431−3
Caustic stricture, acute 243−5
Central venous pressure (CVP) 94−6
Cerebral cortex, injury 573−4
Cervical auricle 136
Cervical joint disease 5
Cervical ribs 149−50
Charles' operation 511
Chemotherapy, for breast cancer 220−1
Chest 5
burns 619
drains 231−4
examination 7
flail 586−7
infection 106
postoperative pain 38−9
stove-in 587
thoracotomy 234−5
trauma 585−93
bullet and stab wounds 592−3
closed chest injury 590−1
X-rays 9, 17, 20
Children
intravenous fluids 92−3
surgical conditions 545−66
Chlormethiazole edisylate 105
Cholecystectomy 289−91
Cholecystitis, acute 288, 289
Christmas disease 29
Chvostek's sign 177
Circumcision 448−9
Claudication 471, 478
Cleft lip and palate 178−9
Clotting disorders 29−30
Cockett's operation 507
Codeine 103
Colectomy 349, 359
Colitis, ulcerative 346−9, 350, 351
Collapse, postoperative 42−3, 51
Colon
carcinoma 350, 353−9
Crohn's disease 342−4
diverticular disease 350, 351, 363−6
polyps 350, 352−3
sigmoid volvulus 351, 367−8
ulcerative colitis 346−9, 350, 351
Colostomy 357−9
Coma scale, Glasgow 576
Commando operation 195
Concussion 573
cardiac 591
Confusion, postoperative 41−2
Conn's syndrome 332−3
Consent, patient 12
Constipation, postoperative 40
Contraceptives, oral 6
Contusions
cerebral 573
pulmonary 589
Coroner, informing 128−30
Countryman's lip 185
Cranial burr holes 582−3
Cremation forms 130
Crohn's disease 342−4
Cryptorchidism 451−4

Cullen's sign 320
Cushing's syndrome 330−2
Cylindromas 138
Cystectomy, bladder 428−9
Cystic fibrosis 563
Cystic hygroma 155−6
Cystic medial necrosis 489
Cystoscopy 426−7, 430
Cystostomy 422−3
Cysts
  branchial 144−6
  breast 207−8
  dermoid 181, 520−1
  epididymal 457−8
  lymph, solitary 156
  in the mouth 179−82
  mucous retention 179−80
  renal 416−17
  sebaceous 518−20
  thyroglossal 170−2
  thyroid 166−7
Cytotoxic agents 220−1

Dartos pouch procedure 453−4
De Quervain's thyroiditis 160
Death 125−6
  documentation 127−30
  informing patients and relatives 123−5
Delorme's procedure 370
Dexon 113−14
Dextran 88
Dextrose 86−7
Diabetes 23−7, 322
Diagnoses, pitfalls 9−10
Diamorphine 104
Diaphragm, rupture 590−1
Diarrhoea 287
Diazepam 105
Dichloralphenazone 105
Dihydrocodeine 103
Discharge, patient 99−100, 123
Distalgesic 103−4
Diverticular disease 350, 351, 364−6
Documentation 127−32
Doppler ultrasound probe 506
Drains 34, 35, 117−21
  insertion in chest 231−4
Drip site, infected intravenous 71−2
Drugs
  controlled 99
  on discharge 99−100, 123
  history 6, 10
  postoperative 34, 35
Dukes' classification of rectal carcinoma
    359−60
Dumping 286
Dysphagia 238−58
  post-vagotomy 273

Elderly, intravenous fluids 92−3
Electrocardiograms (ECGs), preoperative 9
Electrolytes 8, 21
Electromagnetic flow meter 476
Embolectomy 61−2, 495
Embolisms
  acute arterial 494−5
  fat 611

pulmonary 58−62
Encephalopathy, signs of 298
Endarterectomy 479
  aorto-iliac 481−2
  carotid artery 500
Enemas, barium 351, 548
Enterocolitis, necrotizing 554
Epididymal cysts 457−8
Epididymis, chronic infections 463−4
Epididymo-orchitis 463
Epilepsy 579
Epispadias 449
Epulis 183
Examination 7−8
  major accident 571−2
  postoperative 35
Exercise, and arterial obstruction 477
Eyes, burns 619

Factors, coagulation 29, 30
Fat necrosis 209−10
Feeding 96−7
Fibroadenomas, breast 210−11
Fibroscopy, oesophageal 240
Finney pyloroplasty 272
Fistulae
  arterio-venous 496−7
  biliary 290−1
  branchial 143−4
  Cimino 496
  external intestinal 39, 75−7
  mammillary 225
  perianal 378−80
  urinary 66−7
Fluids
  ingestion of caustic 243−4
  intravenous see intravenous fluids
  replacement after burns 614, 617−19
  when unconscious 578
Flurazepam 105
Follicular carcinoma 169
Foreskin conditions 446−9
Fractures 609−11
  pelvic 602
  ribs 585−6
  skull 583−4
  spine 600−1
  sternum 587

Galactocoeles 208
Gallbladder, gall-stones 288−91
Ganglia 522
Gangrene 472
Gas bloat syndrome 264
Gastrectomy
  oesophago-gastrectomy 252, 253−4
  partial 266−8, 270, 282
  post-gastrectomy syndromes 283−7
  thoraco-abdominal 283
  total 283
Gastrinomas 311−12
Gastritis 280−1, 284
Gastrointestinal tract 560−1
  haemorrhage 277−81
  obstruction 337−9
  congenital 555−66
  postoperative complications 45−7

Gastro-jejunostomy 272
Genitalia, male, congenital lesions 449
Glossectomy 194
Glossitis, chronic superficial 189−90
Goitres 158−64
Goodsall's rule 379
Graves' disease 160−4
Grey Turner's sign 320
Groin 388−9
   block dissection 528−9
   lumps 389, 390 see also hernias
Gynaecomastia 226−8

Haemaccel 88−9, 93
Haematemesis 277−9, 297
Haematomas
   intracranial 579−80, 581−3
   perianal 386−7
   subungal 541
Haemato-pericardium 592
Haematuria 417−19
Haemoglobin 8
Haemophilia 29−30
Haemorrhage 93
   gastrointestinal 277−81
   intracranial 581
   postoperative 51−2
Haemorrhoidectomy 385−6
Haemorrhoids 382−7
Haemothorax, traumatic 589
Hands
   burns 619
   injuries 608−9
Hartmann's procedure 357, 363
Hartmann's solution 87, 88
Hashimoto's disease 159
Head
   injuries 573−84
   lumps in 135−43, 151−6
Heart
   blunt injury to 591
   haemato-pericardium 592
   murmurs 22
Heartburn 5, 262
Heineke−Mikulicz pyloroplasty 272
Heller's operation 247−8
Helmstein's procedure 428
Hemicolectomy 354−5, 356
Hemi-glossectomy 194
Heparin 57, 107
Hepatitis B 32
Hernias
   epigastric 400−1
   femoral 389, 392−5
   hiatus 239, 262−4, 281
   incisional 397−400
   inguinal 389−92, 548−51
   irreducible 395
   obstructed 395
   obturator 389, 402−3
   reduction en masse 395, 396
   Richter's 395, 396
   Spigelian 401−2
   strangulated 339, 395, 395−7
   umbilical 400, 552
Herniorrhaphy 391
Herniotomy 550−1

Hirschprung's disease 563
History, patient 4−7, 34−5
Hodgkin's disease 153−5
Homan's operation 511
Hormone therapy, for breast cancer 217, 219
Hurley−Shelley operation 542
Hydradenitis suppurativa 534
Hydrocoeles 455−7, 548−51
Hydrocortisone 28
   suppression test 175
Hydrothorax 95
Hygroma, cystic 155−6
Hypercalcaemia 174, 175
Hyperhidrosis 541−2
Hypernephromas 414−16
Hyperparathyroidism 173−7
Hypertension 21
   portal 296−303
Hypnotic drugs 105
Hypocalcaemia 177
Hypoglycaemia 24
Hypoglycaemics, oral 25
Hypophysectomy 220
Hypospadias 449

Ileo-rectal anastomosis 349
Ileostomy 348−9
   for meconium ileus 563−4
Ileus
   gall-stone 288
   meconium 563−4
   paralytic 39, 45−6, 337
Immunotherapy 221
Infarction, myocardial 20−1, 53−4
Infections
   antibiotics for acute 106, 107
   intravenous drip site 71−2
   septicaemia 77−9
   wound 68, 69
'Ingrowing' toenails 536−40
Insulin 26−7
   test 269, 312
Insulinomas 311, 312−14
Intensive care unit 80−2
Intestinal bleeding 340
Intestinal obstruction 337−9, 340
   congenital 555−6, 559−60
Intravenous fluids 86−9
   central venous pressure (CVP) 94−6
   feeding 96−7
   indications 85
   normal daily requirements 85
   regimes 89−93
   monitoring the effect 93−4
Intussusception 342, 546−8
Ischaemia
   of the bowel 340−2
   of the leg 471−7
   amputation for 485−8
   management 478−9
   types of procedure 481−5
   vascular operations 479−81
   myocardial 20−1, 39
   transient attack 499−500
Ivalon sponge repair 370−1
Ivor Lewis operation 253

Jaundice 289, 291–6
Jaws, tumours 187

Kehr's sign 595
Keloids 517
Keratoacanthomas 520
Ketoacidosis 24
Kidney disorders 407–20
  injury 598–9
  renal cysts 416–17
  renal failure 44, 65–6, 93
  renal tract stones 407–9
  kidney 411–12
  ureteral 409–11
  renal transplantation 419–20
  renal tumours 413–16
Koilonychia 248

Laparotomy
  for acute diverticulitis 366
  for ischaemic bowel 341–2
  for renal injury 598–9
  for ruptured liver 594–5
  for spleen injury 596
Laryngotomy *236*
Laxatives 110
Leriche's syndrome 473
Levorphanol 104
Limbs
  burns 619
  fractures *609*–11
  legs
    arterial supply *473*
    ischaemia see under ischaemia
    lymphoedema 510–11
    tendon injuries 613–14
Lipomas 517–18
Lips
  carcinoma 185
  cleft lip and palate *178*–9
  mucous retention cysts *179*–*80*
Litholapaxy 422
Liver
  abscesses 74–5
  function tests 8–9
  jaundice 289, 291–6
  portal hypertension 296–303
  ruptured by trauma 594–5
  transplantation 309–11
  tumours 306–9
Lockwood's operation 394
Lord's stretch 381–2, 385
Lotheissen's operation 395
Lymph nodes, cervical 151–6
Lymphadenitis, tuberculous 153
Lymphadenopathy, cervical 151–6
Lymphoedema 510–11
Lymphoma
  malignant 153–5, 170
  non-Hodgkin's 155, 459

McEvedy's operation 394
Mallory–Weiss tears 280
Malrotation, bowel 339, 560–3
Mammary duct ectasia 209
Mammillary fistulae 225
Mammodochectomy 223–4

Management, patient
  postoperative 10, 34–5
  preoperative conditions 9–10, 11–12,
    16–32
  see also terminally ill patients
Mastectomy 215–17, 227–8
Mastitis, plasma cell 209
Meckel's diverticulum 339–40
Medullary carcinoma 169–70
Melaena 277–9, 297
Melanoma, malignant 186, 449, 527–9
Mendelson's syndrome 49
Mesenteric adenitis 336–7
Mesenterico-caval shunt 301–3
Microdochectomy 223
Micturation 5
  disorders 44, 63–6, 429–33
Mikulicz's disease 137
Millim's prostatectomy 438–9
Molluscum sebaceum 520
Morphine 102, 104
Mouth, conditions of 178–88
  submandibular lumps 140–3
Mumps 136–7, 463
Murphy's sign 289
Myxoedema 157–8

Naevi, pigmented 525–7
Nails, conditions 536–41
Nasogastric feeding 97
Nausea, postoperative *37*, 39–40
Neck
  block dissection 195
  lumps in 136, 143–56
  thyroid lumps 157–72
  tracheostomy 235–7
Needles *117*
Nephrectomy 415–16
Nephro-ureterectomy 413–14
Nephrolithotomy 411
Nerves, injuries 604–5, 612–13
Neurofibromas 522–4
Neuropraxia 613
Neurotmesis 613
Nissen's fundoplication 264, *265*
Nitrazepam 105

Oesophago-gastrectomy *252*, 253–4
Oesophagoscopy 239–41, 247
Oesophagus
  achalasia 238, 239, 246–8
  atresia 556–8
  carcinoma 238–9, 249–51
  palliation 255–58
  radiotherapy 254–5
  surgical resection 251–4
  dysphagia 238–58
  impacted foreign bodies 238, 241–2
  oesophagitis 262, 281
  perforation 242–3
  strictures 238, 239, 243–6
  varices 299, 303–6
Oliguria 43, 63–4, *65*, 429–30
Oophorectomy, bilateral 219–20
Operating lists 12–*15*
Operations, assisting at 33–4
Opiates 102, 104

Orchidectomy 441−2, 460−1
Orchidopexy 453−4
Oxycodone 104

Paget's disease 213−14
Pain
  abdominal see abdominal pain
  breast 206, 209, 224−5
  limb at rest 471, 478−9
  perianal 375−81
  postoperative 37, 38−9
  referred skeletal 371−2
  relief 101−4
Pancreas 317
  benign tumours 311−14
  carcinomas 314−18
  duct stricture 324−5
  inflammation 318−25
  pseudocysts 323
  traumatic injury 597−8
Pancreatectomy, distal 316, 317
Pancreatico-jejunostomy 324−5
Panproctocolectomy 348−9
Papaveretum 102
Papillomas, skin 515−16
Paracetamol 103
Paraphimosis 447−8
Parathormone 173, 175
Parathyroids, lumps in 173−7
Paronychia 540−1
Parotid, region, lumps in 136−40
Parotidectomy, superficial 139−40
Parotitis 136−7
Patey's operation 216
Patients see management, patient
Paul−Mickulicz procedure 356−7
Pelvi-ureteric tumours 413−14
Pelvis
  abscesses 75
  injured 601, 605
  injuries to organs within 602−5
Penis
  amputation 450−1
  carcinoma 449−51
  foreskin conditions 446−9
Pentagastrin test 269
Pentazocine 103
Perianal pain 375−87
Pethidine 102
Phaeochromocytomas, excision 329−30
Pharyngeal pouches 147−9, 238
Pharyngo-laryngo-oesophagectomy 252
Phenol injection of pilonidal sinuses 535−6
Phenoxybenzamine 436
Phimosis 447
Phlebography 505
Phlebothrombosis 95
Phosphate 175
Pilonidal sinuses 534−6
Plasma protein fraction 88, 93
Plethysmography 476
Plummer−Vinson syndrome 248−9
Pneumonitis, aspiration 49
Pneumothorax 49−50, 587−9
Polyposis coli, familial 352, 353
Polyps, colonic 350, 352−3
Portacaval anastomoses 299−300

Post-mortem 126
Postoperative period 34−5
  complications 36−44
  Potassium, extra 92
Prerenal failure 44, 65−6
Prescriptions 34, 98−100
Proctoscopy 350, 351, 384
Profundaplasty 480, 483−4
Prostate gland
  conditions of 63, 433−43
  size 8
Prostatectomy 437−9, 442−3
Prostatitis 433−4
Pseudocysts, pancreatic 323
Puestow's operation 324
Pulmonary collapse 47−8
Pulmonary contusions or lacerations 589
Pyelolithotomy 411
Pyelonephritis 412−13
Pyloric stenosis 275−7
  congenital 545−6
Pyloroplasty 272
Pyrexia, postoperative 10, 36−8

Radiotherapy
  carcinoma of breast 218−19
  oesophageal carcinoma 254−5
Ramstedt's operation 546
Randall's plaques 407
Ranula 180
Raynaud's phenomenon 500−2
Rectum
  agenesis 564−6
  bleeding 349−50, 547
    in children 553
  carcinoma 359−63
  proctoscopy 350, 351
  prolapse 368−71, 553−4
  resections 357, 361−3
  traumatic damage 604
Relatives, dealing with 122−3, 124
Renal disorders see kidney disorders
Respiratory complications, postoperative 47−50
Respiratory diseases 16−19
Resuscitation 570
Ribs, fractured 585−6
Richter's hernias 395, 396
Riedel's thyroiditis 160
Roux-en-Y conversion 284−5

Saline solutions 86−7, 92
Salivary tumours, mixed 183−4
Salt, extra 92
Sclerotherapy
  injection 506
  of oesophageal varices 299
Scrotal conditions 451−67
Sebaceous cysts 518−20
Seborrhoeic keratosis 516
Sedative drugs 105
Seminomas, testicular 458, 459, 461
Sengstaken tubes 304−5
Septicaemia 77−9, 615
Shunt procedures, portal hypertension 299
Sialectasis 138
Sigmoid volvulus 351, 367−8
Sigmoidoscopy 350, 351

Silk sutures 114
Skeletal pain, referred 371–2
Skin
  bed sores 77
  benign lesions 515–24
  burns 614–19
  grafts 607–8
  hyperhidrosis 541–2
  infections 533–6
  malignant conditions 527–32
  pigmented naevi 525–9
  tags 515–16, 523
  see also wounds
Skull fractures 577, 583–4
Smokers, and surgery 7, 17, 18
Sphincterotomy 382
Spigelian hernias 401–2
Spine, fractured 600–1
Spleen 325–7
  ruptured by trauma 595–6
Spleno-renal shunts 300, 301
Splenoportography 298
Squamous cell carcinomas 186, 530–1
Sternotomy, median 235
Sternum, fractured 587
Steroid drugs 27–8
Stomach 261–81
  acidity reduction 266–7, 270, 271–3
  acute postoperative dilatation 46–7
  carcinoma 281–3
  transection 306
  see also gastrectomy
Streptokinase 60–1, 110
Stricture
  oesophageal 243–6
  pancreatic duct 324–5
  urethral 443–5
Strokes, postoperative 55
Submandibular gland, removal 142–3
Submandibular region, lumps 140–3
'Succussion splash' 276
Surgeons, preoperative requirements 12–13
Sutures 33
  figure-of-eight 70, 71
  removal 116–17
  sizes 116
  skin wound 607
  'surgeon's knot' 115
  types 112–16
Sweat glands, excision of axillary 542
Sympathectomy 480–1
  cervical 502
  lumbar 481
Syphilis 464, 489

Tamoxifen 219
Tanner slide 391
Teeth
  cysts 182
  examination 8
Temazepam 105
Tendon injuries 613–14
Tenesmus 360
Teratomas, testicular 458, 459, 461
Terminally ill patients
  with breast cancer 221
  informing 123–5

pain relief 104
Testes
  absent 451–4
  neoplasms 458–62
  painful 462–7
  torsion 464–6
Tetanus prophylaxis 608
Tetany 177
Theatre 13–14, 33–4
Thiersch wire, for rectal prolapse 369–70
Thoracic aorta rupture 590
Thoracotomy 234–5, 235, 592
  exploratory 592
Thrombolytic agents 60–1
Thrombosis, deep vein 5, 55–7
Thyroid gland
  descent 170, 171
  lumps
    carcinoma 167–70
    cysts and adenomas 166–7
    general assessment 157–8
    goitres 158–64
    solitary nodules 164–6
    thyroglossal cysts 170–2
    thyroiditis 159–60, 170
    thyrotoxicosis 157, 160–4
  scan 158
  thyroid crisis 164
Thyroid stimulating hormone (TSH) 158
Thyroidectomy 163–6
Thyrotrophin releasing hormone test 158
Toes, amputation 488
Tongue
  carcinoma 192–5
  chronic superficial glossitis 189–90
  neoplasms 191–2
  ulceration 190–1
Tonsils, malignant disease 187–8
Tracheostomy 235–7, 619
Trans-urethral resection of tumours (TURT) 427–8
Transplantation
  kidney 419–20
  liver 310–11
Trauma 569–72
Trendelenburg test 505
Troisier's sign 281
Trousseau's sign 177
Tuberculosis 464
Tubes 35, 255–7, 304–5

Ulcers
  peptic 264–5
    duodenal 268–73
    gastric 265–8
    perforated 273–5
    pyloric stenosis from 275
  rodent 531
  tongue 190–1
  venous 507–9
Umbilicus
  discharge 403, 552
  hernias 400, 552
Unconscious patients 576–80
Urea 8
Ureter 408, 409–11
Uretero-lithotomy 410–11

Urethra
  epispadias and hypospadias   449
  stricture   443−5
  traumatic damage   602−3
Urethrocytoscopy   430, 441
Urethroplasty, open   445
Urethrotomy, internal   444
Urinalysis   23
Urinary complications, postoperative   44, 63−7
Urine, retention   44, 63−4, 429−33
Urodynamic studies   430

Vagotomy   *270−3*
Varicocoeles   466−7
Veins
  ulceration   507−9
  varicose   503−7
Ventilation perfusion scans   60
Ventricular failure, left   21−2, 54−5
Verrucae   516
Virchow's triad   55−6
Vitalography   *17−18*
Volvulus   339, 561
Vomiting
  bilious, post-gastrectomy   284−*5*
  causing a Mallory−Weiss tear   280
  haematemesis   277−9, 297

postoperative   *37*, 39−40
  inhalation   49

Wallace's rule of nines   615, *616*
Warfarin   107−10
Warren shunt   *300*, 301
Warthin's tumour   138
Warts   516−17
Whipple's operation   316−18
Whipple's triad   312
Wounds   606−8
  dehiscence   39, 69−71
  discharging   39
  drains   118−*20*
  infections   68, *69*
  pain   38
  tetanus prophylaxis   608

X-rays
  chest   9, 17, 20
  major trauma   572, 575
  skull   577
  spinal   600−1

Zadik's operation   538−40
Zollinger−Ellison syndrome   311, 314